Forensic Toxicology

Forensic Toxicology
Principles and Concepts

Nicholas T. Lappas

Courtney M. Lappas

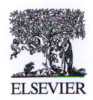

AMSTERDAM • BOSTON • HEIDELBERG • LONDON
NEW YORK • OXFORD • PARIS • SAN DIEGO
SAN FRANCISCO • SINGAPORE • SYDNEY • TOKYO

Academic Press is an imprint of Elsevier

Academic Press is an imprint of Elsevier
125 London Wall, London EC2Y 5AS, UK
525 B Street, Suite 1800, San Diego, CA 92101-4495, USA
225 Wyman Street, Waltham, MA 02451, USA
The Boulevard, Langford Lane, Kidlington, Oxford OX5 1GB, UK

Notices

Knowledge and best practice in this field are constantly changing. As new research and experience broaden our understanding, changes in research methods, professional practices, or medical treatment may become necessary.

Practitioners and researchers must always rely on their own experience and knowledge in evaluating and using any information, methods, compounds, or experiments described herein. In using such information or methods they should be mindful of their own safety and the safety of others, including parties for whom they have a professional responsibility.

To the fullest extent of the law, neither the Publisher nor the authors, contributors, or editors, assume any liability for any injury and/or damage to persons or property as a matter of products liability, negligence or otherwise, or from any use or operation of any methods, products, instructions, or ideas contained in the material herein.

ISBN: 978-0-12-799967-8

British Library Cataloguing-in-Publication Data
A catalogue record for this book is available from the British Library

Library of Congress Cataloging-in-Publication Data
A catalog record for this book is available from the Library of Congress

For information on all Academic Press publications
visit our website at http://store.elsevier.com/

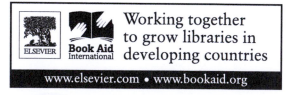

Working together
to grow libraries in
developing countries

www.elsevier.com • www.bookaid.org

Publisher: Shirley Decker-Lucke
Acquisition Editor: Elizabeth Brown
Editorial Project Manager: Joslyn Paguio-Chaiprasert
Production Project Manager: Lisa Jones
Designer: Matthew Limbert

Typeset by TNQ Books and Journals
www.tnq.co.in

For Marcia,
wife and mother extraordinaire,
with gratitude

Contents

Preface

In the preface to their 1981 book *Introduction to Forensic Toxicology*, editors Robert H. Cravey and Randall C. Baselt stated that it was their opinion that up until 1975 "… the only presentations of modern forensic toxicology that could be used for teaching purposes were an 18-page chapter by C.P. Stewart and A. Stolman entitled *The toxicologist and his work* in their book *Toxicology: Mechanisms and Analytical Methods* (1960) and the first two chapters from A.S. Curry's *Poison Detection in Human Organs* (1963)." For one of us who began teaching forensic toxicology at the graduate level in 1975, this lack of textual material suitable for beginning students in forensic toxicology was readily apparent. A great deal of the original literature consisted of case reports, which, although important for practitioners, did not provide students with the principles and concepts that they required.

In the last quarter of the twentieth century and the first years of the twenty-first century, there has been a dramatic increase (an explosion) in the literature of forensic toxicology—journals and books have proliferated. There are several reasons for this upsurge, including rapid advances in methods of analyses, an improved understanding of the interpretation of postmortem and antemortem analytical results, and a better understanding of problems specific to forensic toxicologists, such as postmortem redistribution and factors influencing drug stability.

As significant and important as the advances in the literature of forensic toxicology have been, there has been relatively little literature, other than review articles and portions of a few books, suitable for students and professionals beginning their study of forensic toxicology. Many books on the subject attempt to cover the entire topic in a single volume, incorporating the theory of instrumental methods and immunological analysis, drug disposition, mechanisms of drug action, therapeutic and adverse drug effects (including pathological findings), postmortem analysis, and interpretation as well as chapters on individual drugs of abuse. We are of the opinion that a text suitable for the beginner should introduce the fundamental principles and concepts of forensic toxicology, which introductory texts in forensic toxicology often do not cover adequately. The details of instrumental theory and practice and the toxicology of abused drugs often are included at the expense of the foundational principles of toxicology.

The content in *Forensic Toxicology: Principles and Concepts* is based upon two graduate courses in forensic toxicology that one of us has taught for 40 years to hundreds of master's degree candidates in forensic sciences at The George Washington University. The text is not meant to be encyclopedic in nature, but rather to provide an overview of the largely unchanging core tenets of the discipline: analysis, interpretation, and reporting.

We hope that *Forensic Toxicology: Principles and Concepts* will serve as a core resource not only for upper-level undergraduate students and beginning graduate students studying forensic toxicology and/or forensic chemistry, but also for scientists who are beginning their careers in forensic toxicology laboratories.

We have chosen to focus on topics that beginning toxicology students generally will not have been exposed to previously. As such, our text does not include theories of instrumental methods of analysis, the knowledge of which, although of paramount importance, is common to most beginning students in forensic toxicology who are, or were, undergraduate chemistry majors. These topics are excluded not only because a familiarity with these topics has often been obtained previously by students, but also because they are dealt with in great detail in numerous other excellent sources. However, since these students generally do not have experience with certain foundational subjects important to forensic toxicologists, including pharmacokinetics, pharmacodynamics, immunology, and toxicogenomics, appendices introducing these topics have been included. In addition, an appendix containing a review of selected cases in which the core principles of toxicology were applied is included.

The text contains the following chapters:

Chapter 1, The Development of Forensic Toxicology is an introduction to the discipline with an emphasis on the founding scientists and historical landmarks demonstrating that roughly 200 years ago, the creators of this discipline not only identified problems unique to the field, but also established many of the principles that continue to be employed in modern forensic toxicology.

Chapter 2, The Duties and Responsibilities of Forensic Toxicologists is a summary of the core professional activities of forensic toxicologists—analysis, interpretation, and reporting—each of which is the topic of an entire unit in the book and will be presented in greater detail in the chapters of those units.

Chapter 3, Forensic Toxicology Resources identifies a number of the books, journals, online resources, and organizations from which information of direct or peripheral importance to forensic toxicology may be found.

Chapter 4, The Laboratory examines the administration and functions of a modern forensic toxicology laboratory.

Chapter 5, Analytical Strategy describes the various protocols employed by forensic toxicology laboratories for the detection of drugs in biological samples.

Chapter 6, Sample Handling focuses on the principles underlying the selection, collection, preservation, and transmittal of samples to the laboratory prior to their analysis.

Chapter 7, Storage Stability of Analytes describes the factors that may influence analyte stability in stored samples and provides an overview of the strategies commonly utilized to maximize analyte stability.

Chapter 8, Analytical Samples considers the common and uncommon samples analyzed by forensic toxicologists, including the merits and disadvantages of each.

Chapter 9, Sample Preparation provides an overview of the methods of sample preparation that are most commonly utilized in forensic toxicology laboratories.

Chapter 10, Methods of Detection, Identification, and Quantitation provides an overview of the criteria that should be utilized for selecting a method of analysis, with a focus on the benefits and disadvantages, as well as the sources of error, of several of the methods that are widely employed in forensic toxicology laboratories.

Chapter 11, Quality Assurance and Quality Control describes the components of a quality assurance/quality control program in a forensic toxicology laboratory.

Chapter 12, Types of Interpretations assesses the opinions that can and cannot be made based on analytical results and identifies those factors that may affect the conclusions drawn by forensic toxicologists.

Chapter 13, Reports is a description of the information that should be included in official reports of analytical toxicology results and an overview of the manner by which written reports should be prepared.

Chapter 14, Testifying is a description of the process of giving sworn testimony at deposition or in court. The role of the expert at trial, the preparation for and manner of providing expert testimony, including a presentation of the "shoulds" and "should nots" of testifying, are presented.

Appendix A, Principles of Pharmacokinetics is a presentation of the theories of drug absorption, distribution, metabolism, and excretion, emphasizing those that are of particular importance to forensic toxicologists.

Appendix B, Principles of Pharmacodynamics considers the mechanisms of drug action that are important to interpretations made in forensic toxicology.

Appendix C, Immunoassays explains those aspects of immunology that are of importance to forensic toxicologists, including an overview of the immune system and the theory of immunoassays.

Appendix D, Toxicogenomics examines the effects of genetic differences on pharmacokinetics and pharmacodynamics and describes how genetic polymorphisms may affect the interpretation of analytical results.

Appendix E, Famous Cases in Forensic Toxicology is a presentation of specific cases in which forensic toxicology played an important role.

In reviewing the literature for the preparation of this book, we have been impressed by the intelligence, insights, and intellectual power that so many forensic toxicologists, past and present, have brought to their work and as a result, to the development of forensic toxicology. We are appreciative of their efforts and we hope that we have represented their work accurately.

We are grateful also to our students. As is common for teachers, we have learned far more from our students than they have learned from us. As it is true that the dose makes the poison, it is also true that the students make the teacher: for this we are thankful to our many students.

Nicholas T. Lappas
Courtney M. Lappas

The Development of Forensic Toxicology

Of all of the branches of Medicine, the study of Toxicology is without contradiction that which excites the most general interest.
Mathieu Joseph Bonaventure Orfila

1.1 DEFINITIONS

1.1.1 TOXICOLOGY

The word "toxicology" stems from the Indo-European root word *tekw*, meaning to flee or run from which are derived the Greek *toxon*, bow, and *the* Latin, *toxicum*, poison (McKean, 2005).

Many definitions of toxicology have been proposed, but generally all emphasize that toxicology is the study of adverse effects produced by drugs and chemicals.

- "Toxicology is the study of the harmful actions of chemicals on biologic tissue" (Loomis and Hayes, 1996).
- "Toxicology is the study of the adverse effects of chemical or physical agents on biological systems: it is the science of poisons" (Hayes, 2001).
- "Toxicology is concerned with the deleterious effects of these chemical agents on all living systems" (Plaa, 2007).
- "Toxicology is the study of the adverse effects of chemicals on living organisms" (Eaton and Klaassen, 2001).
- "Toxicology is the study of the adverse effects of chemical, physical or biological agents on living organisms and the ecosystem, including the prevention and amelioration of such adverse effects" (Society of Toxicology, 2005).
- "Toxicology is the science of poisons including their sources, chemical composition, actions, tests and antidotes their nature effects and antibodies" (Stedman's medical dictionary, 2006).

1.1.2 POISON

The word "poison" is the same as the Old French word for magic potion, which stems from the Latin, *potare*, to drink (McKean, 2005). The use of the word "poison" to describe chemicals that cause adverse effects is problematic since it implies that there exist substances that produce *only* adverse effects regardless of the conditions

Forensic Toxicology. http://dx.doi.org/10.1016/B978-0-12-799967-8.00001-3

of exposure—a concept discarded by Paracelsus almost 500 years ago (see below). Unfortunately, the word poisons is used in the title of the standard one-volume toxicology text, *Toxicology: the Basic Science of Poisons*. We will attempt to refrain from the use of the word "poison" in this text as it is now known that all chemicals can produce serious adverse effects if administered in sufficiently large doses by specific routes of administration. In place of the word poison, we will use the words "drug(s)" or "chemical(s)."

1.1.3 DRUG

The word "drug" derived from the Old French *drogue* by way of the Middle Dutch *drogue vate,* which referred to the dried goods contained in vats generally, is taken to mean a chemical that is used for a **beneficial medical purpose**.

Code of Federal Regulations (21CFR210.3, 2015) makes the following definitions under Rules for the Food and Drug Administration (with emphasis added):

- "Drug product means a finished dosage form, for example, tablet, capsule, solution, etc., that contains an *active drug ingredient* generally, but not necessarily, in association with inactive ingredients. The term also includes a finished dosage form that does not contain an active ingredient but is intended to be used as a placebo."
- Active ingredient means *any component that is intended* to furnish pharmacological activity or other direct effect in the diagnosis, cure, mitigation, treatment, or prevention of disease, or *to affect the structure or any function of the body of man* or other animals. The term includes those components that may undergo chemical change in the manufacture of the drug product and be present in the drug product in a modified form intended to furnish the specified activity or effect.
- Inactive ingredient means any component other than an *active ingredient.*

Based on these definitions, we will attempt to adhere to the use of the word(s) "drug(s)" to refer to substances that are intended to furnish pharmacological activity or to affect the structure or any function of the body of man or other animals and are used intentionally or unintentionally for appropriate or inappropriate purposes. We will use the word(s) "chemical(s)" for those substances, e.g., volatile organic compounds, pesticide, carbon monoxide, that are not intended either for medical purposes or to affect the structure or any function of the body of man or other animals, but that are intentionally or unintentionally used or misused for the effects that they produce.

1.1.4 FORENSIC TOXICOLOGY

Forensic toxicology "… has no future as it is now organized and will not have until an adequate definition of forensic toxicology is reached" (Kemp, 1974). This statement demonstrates the confusion among forensic toxicologists that existed in the not-too-distant past as to a definition of their profession. Initially, forensic toxicology was referred to as "postmortem chemistry" and forensic toxicologists were referred to as "coroner's chemists" as the roles and functions that fell within the purview of the science and its practitioners were the detection and/or quantitation of drugs present in postmortem samples and the interpretation of the results obtained. Under these circumstances, forensic toxicology could be defined as the science concerned with determining whether the death of an individual was caused by, or related to, the use of a drug. This "classical" definition is consistent with the role of forensic toxicologists in a coroner's or medical examiner's office in which they are part of the team that investigates the possible role of drugs in fatalities. As a result of the additional demands placed on forensic toxicologists by society, forensic toxicology has become a much broader discipline in that it presently encompasses additional aspects of toxicology, principally as they relate to the living.

Currently, there are considered to be three different types of forensic toxicology: postmortem toxicology, human-performance testing, and forensic urine drug testing. These have been defined as follows (SOFT/AAFS), 2006).

- "Post-Mortem Forensic Toxicology, which determines the absence or presence of drugs and their metabolites, chemicals such as ethanol and other volatile substances, carbon monoxide and other gases, metals, and other toxic chemicals in human fluids and tissues, and evaluates their role as a determinant or contributory factor in the cause and manner of death.
- Human-Performance Forensic Toxicology, which determines the absence or presence of ethanol and other drugs and chemicals in blood, breath or other appropriate specimen(s), and evaluates their role in modifying human performance or behavior.
- Forensic Urine Drug Testing,[1] which determines the absence or presence of drugs and their metabolites in urine to demonstrate prior use or abuse."

The classical definition of forensic toxicology describes the discipline as retrospective, in that its aim is to determine whether there is a correlation between an event of interest and any drugs detected after the occurrence of such an event. The more recent description of the field includes a prospective aspect of forensic toxicology, such as preemployment drug screening, in which an attempt is made to identify the potential hazards of drug use by a person before the drug use causes any adverse effects.

1.2 LANDMARKS IN FORENSIC TOXICOLOGY
1.2.1 EARLY ACTIVITY IN TOXICOLOGY

It seems reasonable to assume that throughout history humans have been concerned with the adverse effects produced by the numerous substances they have

---

[1]This category should be expanded to include the detection of drugs in hair and oral fluid as these samples are being used for the same purposes as urine drug testing.

encountered in their environment. The written expression of this concern dates back at least as far as the *Ebers Papyrus* (Sigerist, 1951, p. 311), which is a record of medical knowledge and practices in Egypt from approximately 1550 BC and which describes naturally occurring toxic substances such as hemlock, opium, and lead as well as their antidotes—including those that are not only ineffective and/or harmful, but also repugnant. In the fourth-century BC, several dangerous plants were described in the *De Historia Plantarum* written by the Greek botanist and philosopher Theophrastus (Gallo, 2001). In the first-century AD, the Greek physician Pedanius Dioscorides, who served with the Roman army of the emperor Nero, wrote the *Materia Medica*—Dioscorides is credited with the first classification of poisons into separate classes such as plants, animals, and minerals (Haas, 1996).

The *Hsi Yuan Lu*, translated variously as or "Translations to Coroners" or "The Washing Away of Wrongs" (Kiel, 1970; McKnight, 1981), a multivolume series of books of legal medicine from the thirteenth-century AD China, is thought to be the oldest extant book on forensic medicine (Agren, 1984). This work includes a list of the duties and responsibilities of the district magistrate, the chief governing official for a governmental administrative area. Among the several duties of the magistrate was the investigation of suspected homicides, including poisonings. In this duty, the magistrate was aided by his assistant, the coroner, in performing the investigation and postmortem examinations as directed by the *Hsi Yuan Lu*. Although the *Hsi Yuan Lu* predates by centuries the scientific era of toxicology, it contains several methods that exemplify early attempts at "scientific" toxicology. One method called for the insertion of a silver needle into the mouth or body cavity of the deceased (McKnight, 1981, p. 135); blackening of the needle was taken as a sign of a poisoning. Although there is a scientific explanation for the blackening of the needle since silver can react with sulfur-containing compounds to form black precipitates, this method is obviously inadequate and falls short of modern requirements of proof, since most likely the black precipitates produced would be due to the reaction of the silver with hydrogen sulfide, a product of putrefaction and not the detection of a poison (Kiel, 1970). A second procedure relied on biological rather than chemical detection (Giles, 1924). Boiled rice was placed in the mouth of the deceased where it was kept for several hours after which it was fed to a chicken. The effect, if any, on the chicken was noted. Although this procedure has not caught on with forensic toxicologists, the use of animals in forensic toxicology persisted for many years (Of Interest 1.1). As primitive as they were, the developers of these early attempts at "scientific toxicology" should be applauded for their ingenious application of observations in an attempt to solve theretofore insoluble problems.

In the sixteenth century, Philippus Theophrastus Aureolus Bombastus von Hohenheim, more commonly and better known as Paracelsus, formulated his famous maxim: "In all things there is a poison, and there is nothing without a poison. It depends only upon the dose whether a poison is poison or not" (Ball, 2006, p. 229). Paracelsus, an alchemist, theologian, physician, and "protoscientist," rejected

---

OF INTEREST 1.1 THE ANALYTICAL FROG

Although the development of the Marsh test and subsequent other tests for the detection of arsenic in biological samples had been developed prior to the middle of the nineteenth century, adequate chemical methods were not available for the detection of many homicidal substances. For this reason, biological tests, somewhat more sophisticated than those described in the *Hsi Yuan Lu*, which were conducted using animals for the detection of these substances, persisted well into the late nineteenth century.

Reese, a leading toxicologist of the time, suggested a number of animals that would be suitable for use in toxicological testing—cats, rabbits, guinea pigs, or mice were recommended, but not birds which were deemed to be unsatisfactory for this purpose (Reese, 1889). One such method, for the detection of strychnine, a convulsive drug, reported by Reese relied on the use of frogs, which were reported to be sensitive to the effects of strychnine. This method was recommended since other substances, such as morphine, were known to interfere with other, nonanimal-based tests for the detection of strychnine in biological samples. The method described by Reese consisted of the subcutaneous injection into a frog of an extract of stomach and stomach contents obtained from the body of a person suspected of having been poisoned by strychnine. A positive result for strychnine by this method was the production of spasms in the animal. Since this test was also nonspecific for strychnine, it was suggested that it should be used in conjunction with smell, taste (the early forensic toxicologists were fearless), and color tests of the extract prepared from the stomach and stomach contents.

---

the works of Galen[2] that had prevailed for centuries and instead promulgated, among several other and generally less accurate theories, a far from modern chemical theory of diseases in his *Opus paramirum* (Ball, 2006, p. 260) in which he considered the cause of disease to be a bodily imbalance of three substances—salt, mercury, and sulfur. During his life, Paracelsus who was at times "looked upon as a magician and quack and sometimes as a physician of genius" by his contemporaries (Sigerist, 1951, pp. 12–14), was drunk for a good portion of his life, was castigated as a disciple of the devil (Ball, 2006), and failed to cooperate with his contemporaries—many of whom he treated with outright contempt and scorn (Davis, 1993). Nonetheless, regardless of his personal and professional shortcomings, this antisocial polymath is remembered today as perhaps the first to recognize the significance of dose and of the harmful potential of all substances. Considering the scientifically barren times in which he lived, we must excuse his failure to recognize that other factors, such as the route of administration, gender, age, and genetics may account for the differentiation among beneficial, innocuous, and harmful effects.

Although alchemists and protoscientists continued their attempts throughout subsequent centuries to understand the effects of chemicals on the human body, it was not until the development of the basic disciplines of chemistry and biology that modern, or truly scientific, toxicology developed. In the early nineteenth century, Mathieu Joseph Bonaventure Orfila (Figure 1.1), generally referred to as "The Father

---

[2]Galen, who lived in the second-century AD, is considered to be the greatest physician and medical researcher of antiquity. Many of his theories of physiology, anatomy, and pathology, although containing several errors and mistaken concepts, persisted in to the sixteenth and seventeenth centuries.

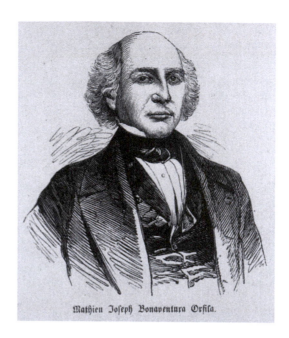

FIGURE 1.1

Mathieu Joseph Bonaventure Orfila.

of Toxicology," was at the forefront of the establishment of the scientific foundation of modern toxicology.[3] He studied the biological and chemical characteristics of several toxic substances and developed and applied methods of chemical analysis of postmortem materials to determine whether death was caused by a toxic substance. One of his most important findings was that drugs were absorbed into the blood and distributed to the tissues of the body and therefore could be detected in tissues other than those of the gastrointestinal tract (Coley, 1991). In 1813—1814, Orfila published his classic two-volume reference, *Traité de Toxicologie: Traité des poisons tires des regnes* minéral, *végétal at animal ou toxicologie générale considerèe sous les rapports de la physiologie, de la pathologie et la mèdicine legale*, which is considered to be the first book of modern toxicology (Borzelleca, 2001). In this work, he classified substances into six categories: corrosives, astringents, acrids, stupefying and narcotics, narcotic-acrids, and septics or putrefiants. This presentation of toxicological principles and concepts was an immediate scientific sensation and translations soon appeared in several countries including an 1817 abridged translation, *A General System of Toxicology, or, a Treatise on Poisons Found in the Mineral, Vegetable and Animal Kingdoms, Considered in their Relations with Physiology, Pathology and Medical Jurisprudence*, in the United States by Joseph Nancrede.

---

[3]Orfila was also active in other areas of forensic science. For example, he published papers on the chemical identification of bloodstains following their aqueous extraction (Gaensslen, 1983, p. 74).

The Industrial Revolution and the continuing development of chemistry and biology in the nineteenth century and the subsequent development of analytical chemistry, biochemistry, physiology, pharmacology, anatomy, pathology, and statistics fostered the inception and growth of diverse toxicological disciplines including analytical toxicology, clinical toxicology, environmental toxicology, veterinary toxicology, genetic toxicology, regulatory toxicology, and forensic toxicology. The interdisciplinary nature of toxicology is demonstrated by the number of scientific disciplines to which it has been applied. It is unlikely that toxicologists will have expertise in all of the foundational disciplines of toxicology, but they must have at least a working knowledge of many and an extensive knowledge of one or more of these disciplines depending upon their areas of specialization.

Orfila and many of the first scientists to refer to themselves as toxicologists were concerned with the detection of homicidal poisonings. These early forensic toxicologists, who generally came from careers in medicine, were crucial to the development and establishment of the three basic roles of their maturing science: analysis, interpretation, and reporting. These forbearers of the discipline developed chemical methods of analysis that could be applied to postmortem samples, applied their knowledge of the basic sciences to the interpretation of the analytical results, and presented their findings in a manner acceptable to and understood by judges and juries. In short, they identified and established the roles and functions of present-day forensic toxicologists.

Presented below is a discussion of a selected group of events and scientists, which when taken together serve to illustrate the early development of forensic toxicology.

1.2.2 ARSENIC

The late eighteenth and early nineteenth centuries saw the continuing development of the biomedical sciences including the "new" science of toxicology, which was heavily dependent upon advances in chemistry and physiology. Prior to the development of chemistry, the absence of reliable chemical and toxicological methods of analysis made the detection of drugs and chemicals, especially in biological samples, difficult and generally unreliable. As a result, suicidal, homicidal accidental poisonings, by means of naturally occurring materials such as minerals and plant-derived substances, were widespread.

Arsenic is one of the naturally occurring chemicals that has been used widely throughout history as a favored instrument of suicide and homicide, perhaps even having had an influence on history.[4] In addition to its homicidal use, it was also

---

[4]Livia, the wife of the Roman emperor Augustus, was rumored to have been one of the most notorious arsenic murderers. She was said to have been responsible for several murders committed with arsenic, including that of Augustus, so that her son could ascend to the throne. Her exploits served as the focus in the historical fiction, *I, Claudius*, by Robert Graves.

widely available during the nineteenth century as a means of rodent control, as the active agent in sheep dip used to prevent infestations of farm animals, in foods, household remedies, and in the form of copper arsenite ($CuHAso_3$), it was the pigment in Scheele's Green, popularly used for imparting a green color to several products including in paints and wallpaper. Because of its pervasiveness in society, arsenic played a central role in the development of legal medicine and because of this was instrumental in the development of forensic toxicology in the nineteenth century.

The popularity of arsenic, usually in the form of the trivalent As_2O_3 or "white arsenic" as a homicidal agent, is illustrated by reports that it was the leading cause of known homicidal poisonings in the early nineteenth century (Watson, 2006a) and that it was the cause of 185 of the 541 recorded cases of fatal poisonings in England in 1837—1838 (Coley, 1991). There were several reasons for the popularity of As_2O_3 as a homicidal agent: it was inexpensive, readily available, had a sugar-like appearance, and had little smell or taste, which enabled the poisoner to mask easily its presence in food or drink. Additionally, the signs and symptoms (Ellenhorn, 1997, p. 1540) produced by arsenic ingestion, including severe abdominal pain, diarrhea and vomiting, and inflammation of the gastrointestinal tract, were similar to other causes such as cholera, the occurrence of which into the nineteenth century was not rare. For these reasons, and, probably most importantly, because of the lack of a reliable method for the detection of arsenic in human remains, the use of arsenic as a homicidal agent flourished in the early nineteenth century.

Physicians recognized that in order to establish that arsenic poisoning was the cause of death in suspected homicides, a reliable method was required by which arsenic could be detected in human samples. This need to identify homicidal poisonings by the reliable detection of arsenic, and by extension of other agents, was an important stimulus to, and paralleled the development of forensic toxicology.

The identification of arsenic in the eighteenth and early nineteenth centuries commonly relied on methods that are now considered primitive, such as the production of a garlic-like (alliaceous) odor when arsenic-containing substances were heated; reduction by which arsenic present in samples was reduced to its elemental form by heating; and prominently, "the liquid tests" that consisted of the use of various reagents that would produce characteristically colored precipitates consistent with the presence of arsenic (Of Interest 1.2).

The liquid tests included the reaction of samples with reagents such as ammoniacal sulfate of copper (copper sulfate in ammonia), ammoniacal nitrate of silver (silver nitrate in ammonia), lime water, or sulfuretted hydrogen (hydrogen sulfate) (Burney, 2002), which were expected to react in the presence of arsenic to produce colored precipitates. These tests were not easily adaptable to the detection of arsenic in biological samples since they were difficult to perform, had relatively high detection limits, were subject to errors of specificity, and were not easily adaptable to colored biological samples (Burney, 2002). Importantly, the end points of the analyses, the formation of precipitates of specific colors, required extensive training to recognize, were by their nature subjective due to interpersonal variation in color

---

OF INTEREST 1.2 *ON THE ROAD TO MARSH* (CAMPBELL, 1965; CAUDILL, 2009; FARRELL, 1994; GOLDSMITH, 1997)

The need for a reliable method for the detection of arsenic produced a number of methods, many of which were in common use prior to Marsh's landmark discovery; all were supplanted by the Marsh test.

Carl Wilhelm Scheele, 1775: Developed a method for the production of arsine (AsH_3) in nonbiological samples.

$$As_2O_3 + 6Zn + 12HNO_3 \rightarrow 2AsH_3 + 6Zn\,(NO_3)_2 + 3H_2O$$

Samuel Hahnemann, 1785: Developed a test in which the passage of sulfureted hydrogen gas through an acidified arsenic solution to produce a bright yellow precipitate of arsenius sulfide.

$$H_2S + HCl \rightarrow As_2S_3$$

Johann Daniel Metzger, 1787: Determined that heating arsenic trioxide with charcoal would reduce it to its elemental form, a method known as the reduction test.

$$2As_2O_3 + 3C \rightarrow 3CO_2 + 4As$$

Benjamin Rush, 1805: Identified the reaction of arsenites and arsenates with alkaline copper sulfate to produce a green precipitate.

$$3Cu_{2+} + 2(AsO_4)^{-3} \rightarrow Cu_3(AsO_4)_2\,(s)$$

Valentine Rose, 1806: Applied the Metzger's method to the detection of arsenic in gastric tissue.

Joseph Hume, 1809: Described the reaction between silver nitrate with arsenites to form a yellow precipitate.

$$3AgNO_3 + AsO_3^{-3} \rightarrow Ag_3AsO_3$$

---

recognition, and were described in specific terms that had unclear meanings, e.g., "the bloom of an Orleans peach," "lively" grass green, and "brilliant" lemon yellow (Burney, 2006).

Although these methods of detection were nonspecific, subject to errors of interpretation and generally not applicable to biological samples, they were accepted as scientific evidence in trials of the time (Of Interest 1.3).

The problems in the application of the "liquid tests" to complex samples served to spur interest in the development of analytical and forensic toxicology. In 1813, Orfila attempted to demonstrate to his students in Paris that the liquid tests could be used to detect arsenic in complex samples (Nieto-Galan and Bertomeu-Sanchez, 2006). To his dismay, the precipitates that formed when the reagents were added to a sample of coffee to which he had added arsenic were not of the anticipated colors. As a result of these unexpected results, Orfila is said to have exclaimed—"Toxicology does not exist." His extensive ground-breaking scientific efforts following this episode were instrumental in the writing of his classic work, *Traité de Toxicologie*. Publication of *Traité de Toxicologie*. This book and Orfila's research, which included the development of analytical methods for the detection of poisons and the demonstration that chemicals were absorbed into the general circulation, were momentous events in the development of toxicology as a scientific discipline and led to Orfila being celebrated deservedly today as the "Father of Toxicology."

OF INTEREST 1.3 WHAT A "GRUEL" DEED (ANONYMOUS, 1752; EMSLEY, 2005, PP. 145–147)

I forgive thee my Dear and I hope God will forgive thee; but thee shouldst have considered better, before thee attemptist any Thing against thy Father; thee shouldst have considered I was thy own Father.

This statement was made shortly before his death by Francis Blandy, who was convinced that his sickness had been caused by his daughter Mary. Mary Blandy, a 26-year-old "spinster" living in Henley-on-Thames fell in love with Lieutenant William Henry Cranstoun, a married man who hid his marital status from Mary. However, Cranstoun did not hide his desire to marry her, in spite of the objections of her father. Cranstoun's ardor no doubt was spurred on by the 10,000 pound dowry that Mary's future husband would acquire. Cranstoun convinced Mary that the "powders to clean Scotch pebbles" that he gave her, if administered to her father would change her father's resistance to their marriage. Mary, apparently extremely gullible, believed him and periodically added the powder to her father's food over a period of months, until a final dose of the powder added to his gruel in August of 1751 proved fatal. Mary was brought to trial in February of 1752 for the fatal poisoning of her father with arsenic trioxide.

Dr Anthony Aldington, who had cared for Mr Blandy, provided medical and scientific testimony for the prosecution. His medical opinions were based both on the classic signs and symptoms of arsenic poisoning—severe pain of the gastrointestinal tract accompanied with severe vomiting and diarrhea—that Mr Blandy exhibited after eating the gruel as well as on postmortem findings that were consistent with arsenic poisoning. Aldington's identification of arsenic was based on the detection of "… the Stench of Garlick" upon heating of samples and the results of several of the chemical color tests commonly used for the identification of arsenic. He summarized his results of these tests by testifying that a known sample of arsenic and the powder found in Mr Blandy's gruel.

… corresponded so nicely in each Trial that I declare I never saw any two Things in Nature more alike than the Decoction made with the Powder found in Mr. Blandy's Gruel and that made with white Arsenic."

Mary Blandy was convicted and subsequently hanged on April 6, 1752.

Additional criticisms of the liquid test were levied by Sir Robert Christison (Figure 1.2), the preeminent forensic toxicologist of the nineteenth century in Great Britain:

If what has been said of the modifications which the liquid tests for arsenic undergo in their action when they are applied to vegetable and animal fluids be reconsidered it will at once be seen that they are quite useless in relation to such fluids. If the solution indeed contains a large proportion of arsenic and is not deeply coloured all the three will act in the usual manner. But in actual practice the solutions are always diluted and in them the liquid tests with the exception of sulphuretted hydrogen gas either do not act at all or throw down precipitates so materially altered in tint from those which alone are characteristic of their action that their employment would lead to frequent mistakes.

Christison (1829)

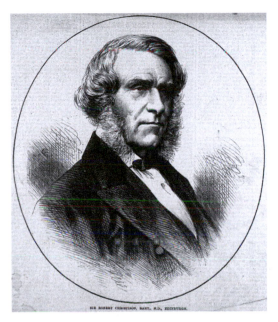

FIGURE 1.2

Robert Christison.

Christison's characterization of the problems of the liquid tests was accurate and carried great weight since Robert Christison was the preeminent toxicologist in Great Britain in the first half of the nineteenth century. His text, *A Treatise on Poisons in Relation to Medical Jurisprudence, Physiology and the Practice of Physic*, which was published in 1829 when he was professor of medical jurisprudence and police at the University of Edinburgh in Scotland, was the first work devoted to forensic toxicology in Great Britain (Anonymous, 1830) and the first book on toxicology written in English and published in the 19th century (Christison, 1829, p. i). This publication, his development of analytical methods, his success as an expert witness in forensic toxicology, and his position as medical adviser to the Crown in Scotland for 37 years (Coley, 1991), brought him such acceptance and fame that he felt "… his reputation in Scottish courts became so overpowering that his evidence was rarely questioned" (Crowther, 2006).

The problems of arsenic detection in human remains raised by Orfila, Christison, and others was successfully addressed first by James Marsh, a low-salaried chemist employed by the English government, whose work in this field was stimulated by the 1832 trial of John Bodle who had been charged with the murder of his tyrannical grandfather (Thorwald, 1964). Marsh had participated in this case as an expert for the prosecution and had conducted the prevailing standard color tests for the detection of arsenic. He reported the presence of arsenic in the coffee prepared by the defendant for his grandfather and he was confident of the defendant's guilt.

However, Bodle was found innocent. Marsh was convinced that his inability to present demonstrable evidence to the jury was instrumental in the acquittal.[5] As a result of his failure to convince the jury of his analytical findings in this case, Marsh worked to develop a method of analysis for the detection of arsenic in human tissues that would solve the courtroom and scientific problems associated with the existing methods. Based on the prior work of Carl Wilhelm Scheele[6] in 1775 and others (Watson, 2006a), Marsh developed a method, which now bears his name, that could be employed for the detection of arsenic in biological samples and would produce demonstrable positive results that a jury could see (Marsh, 1836). The basis of the Marsh test is the reaction of arsenic-containing samples including biological fluids or tissues with hydrogen gas generated by the reaction of zinc with an acid, such as sulfuric acid. When heated, arsine gas (As_2H_3)—the product of this reaction—is reduced to metallic arsenic that may be collected on a solid surface such as a glass or porcelain plate. The presence of the shiny deposit, known as an arsenic mirror, is a positive result. In the paper reporting the development of his method, Marsh stated that

> *Notwithstanding the improved methods that have of late been invented of detecting the presence of small quantities of arsenic in the food, in the contents of the stomach, and mixed with various other animal and vegetable matters[7] a process was still wanting for separating it expeditiously and commodiously, and presenting it in a pure unequivocal form for examination by the appropriate tests.*

The Marsh test was an analytical sensation because it presented forensic toxicologists with a method for the detection of arsenic in biological samples. Although the test was not specific for arsenic, it could be used for the detection of very small amounts of arsenic, was reliable in the hands of an experienced chemist, and produced demonstrable results that could be shown easily and explained to a lay jury comprised of individuals unfamiliar with analytical assays. However, in spite of its analytical merits, the Marsh test initially was met with mixed reviews. Alfred Swaine Taylor (Figure 1.3) (Coley, 1991; Rosenfeld, 1985), who had been appointed lecturer in medical jurisprudence at Guy's Hospital in London in 1831 and subsequently developed a widespread reputation and fame as a forensic toxicologist due to his textbooks in medical jurisprudence as well as his effectiveness as an expert witness, was an early advocate of the Marsh test, although in certain cases he deemed it to be unnecessary and relied on more traditional methods of detection.

---

[5]The ability to convince jurors of the validity of scientific evidence is perhaps the most important role of the expert at trial, but it is also one of the most difficult.

[6]Scheele has been credited with the discovery of oxygen years prior to the claims of Priestley, who is generally credited with the discovery, or Lavoisier, who claimed the priority of discovery (Severinghaus, 2003).

[7]Unfortunately, neither the work of Sheele nor any of the others who developed the methods to which he referred and who laid the foundation for his breakthrough was mentioned by Marsh in the paper describing his method.

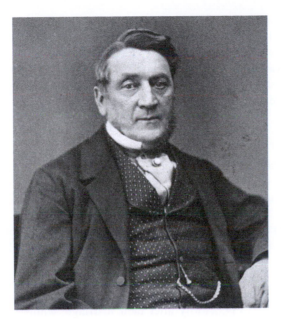

FIGURE 1.3

Alfred Swaine Taylor.

Less enthusiasm for the Marsh test was expressed by Fresenius, the renowned German chemist who created the first journal dedicated exclusively to analytical chemistry. Fresenius opined that the Marsh test was not suitable for the detection of arsenic in organic matter and that there was a possibility that zinc and sulfuric acid used in the test could be contaminated with arsenic (Coley, 1991). However, because Marsh had been aware of the "ambiguity" (false-positive results) that might result if his reagents or apparatus were contaminated with arsenic, he had recommended that the procedure should be performed in the absence of a sample to ensure that any arsenic that was detected did not originate from either of those sources. He described the analysis of a blank (although he did not use that term) consisting of the zinc and sulfuric acid reagents in the absence of a sample as follows:

> *It is, therefore, necessary for the operator to be certain of the purity of the zinc which he employs, and this is easily done by putting a bit of it into the apparatus, with only some dilute sulfuric acid; the gas thus obtained is to be set fire as it issues for the jet; and if no metallic film is deposited on the bit of that glass, and no white sublimate within the open tube, the zinc may be regarded as in a fit state for use.*
>
> **Marsh (1836)**

Marsh's method not only greatly improved existing methods, but it also stimulated the development of other methods for arsenic detection by Berzelius and Reinsch, who developed a method by which arsenic and other metals were detected by their plating onto a copper coil in a boiling HCL solution (Reinsch, 1842). Additionally, Gutzeit developed a semiquantitative method for arsenic detection in which arsine gas is reacted with nitric acid to produce a precipitate, which, with numerous modifications, was used into the twentieth century.

The Marsh test had ushered in the era of scientific analytical toxicology and with it the modern age of forensic toxicology.

1.2.3 THE LAFARGE AFFAIR (SAUNDERS, 1952; THORWALD, 1964)

The Marsh test played a prominent role in a case of homicidal poisoning that came to be known as the LaFarge affair. This case provoked the same type of widespread public attention in the nineteenth century as the O.J. Simpson case did in the twentieth century.

The principal characters in the LaFarge affair were Marie Cappell and her husband, Charles LaFarge. Before they were married, Charles LaFarge had represented himself to Marie as the owner of a thriving foundry and a fine country estate, neither of which was true, and which caused a great distress to Marie when she first saw the "estate" after her marriage to this man who she hardly knew. In December 1839, shortly after their marriage, while Monsieur LaFarge was in Paris on a business trip, he received a cake prepared for him by his wife. Charles became ill after eating the cake and returned home where he was cared for by Marie. In spite of or, as later was charged, because of Marie's care, Charles died on January 13, 1840. Some of the servants on the LaFarge estate were suspicious of Madame LaFarge's behavior (she would not allow anyone other than herself to care for her husband) and suspected foul play. As a result of their investigation, which, among other findings, revealed that Madame LaFarge had purchased arsenic in December 1839—prior to Monsieur LaFarge's trip to Paris, the authorities concluded that Madame LaFarge had poisoned her husband and she was charged with homicide.

In addition to the nonscientific evidence that they uncovered, the authorities made several attempts to determine whether the remains of Charles LaFarge contained arsenic. A panel of "experts" comprised of physicians from Brives was called upon to conduct analyses of the exhumed remains of Charles. They reported that they had detected arsenic in LaFarge's stomach and stomach contents. However, Orfila, who was consulted by the defense, concluded that these physicians, who were unaware of the Marsh test, had used an outdated and nonspecific method of detection and their results were therefore not reliable. The court then appointed a second panel of "experts" consisting of two apothecaries and a chemist from Limoges. Responding to the criticism of the results produced by the physicians from Brives, they applied the Marsh test, a method they had never used before; they reported that they did not detect arsenic in LaFarge's stomach or stomach contents. In order to resolve the several discrepancies among the analytical results, the court then ordered a "tie-breaker" in which the "experts" form Brives and Limoges would work together to analyze samples from LaFarge's exhumed body to determine whether arsenic was detectable in any of the organs. The combined experts reported that arsenic was not detected in the organs obtained from the exhumed body. However, arsenic was detected in eggnog prepared for Charles by Marie and also in Marie's malachite box, which contained a white powder she had been seen putting in the eggnog.

In the midst of this scientific chaos, Orfila was called upon to examine LaFarge's remains. Employing what was then the state-of-the-art Marsh method for his determination of arsenic, Orfila analyzed the samples obtained from LaFarge's body and testified that he had detected arsenic in them.[8] Based on Orfila's scientific testimony and the investigative findings, Madame LaFarge was convicted and sentenced to life in prison, although her sentence was commuted after she had served a few years. Marie LaFarge's case was a *cause célèbre* and generated extensive scientific and popular tumult since she had many supporters who defended her innocence. She even wrote a memoir that was a popular success.

Orfila's work in the LaFarge case was received enthusiastically by many who welcomed it as the dawn of modern toxicology, which held the promise of detecting poisons as widely used as arsenic in the tissues of a victim by means of state-of-the-art chemical methods. Orfila's role in this case contributed to his eminence as "… one of the first international stars of science" (Crowther, 2006). However, the analytical results and the verdict were also greeted with controversy by those who argued that the Marsh test was subject to numerous errors of procedure and interpretation (Of Interest 1.4). Among the criticisms of the results obtained by Orfila by means of the Marsh test were (1) that the results did not agree with those produced by original experts and (2) the method was so sensitive that contamination of the postmortem samples by arsenic in the reagents or in the cemetery soil could have produced false-positive results. However, Orfila had conducted analyses and obtained data that anticipated and blunted these, as well as other criticisms. He explained that the inconsistency between his results and those of the local "experts" was due to their lack of expertise in the performance of the test, e.g., they used samples that were too small, they used a flame that was too large, and they did not wait long enough for the formation of the arsenic deposit. The second criticism was discounted since he had demonstrated that neither the reagents he used nor the soil from the cemetery contained arsenic, as determined by the Marsh test (Of Interest 1.5). In addition, Orfila explained that the arsenic he had detected in the samples taken from LaFarge's body was present in a quantity that was much greater than the amount of arsenic found naturally in the human body.

The LaFarge affair demonstrated that newer methods of chemical analysis employed in the detection of chemicals from postmortem samples were reliable only if precautions were taken to avoid contamination of samples and if they

---

[8] Orfila was eminently qualified for these analyses since he was the first to extract arsenic from nongastrointestinal organs (Eckert, 1980).

OF INTEREST 1.4 HE SHOULD HAVE TAKEN THE TRAIN (WEINER, 1959)

One of Orfila's leading critics was François Vincent Raspail, a distinguished scientist in his own right who has been called the "founder of microchemistry" and who formulated an early version of the cell theory.

Orfila and Raspail disagreed not only about scientific matters, but they also held differing political views, which may have exacerbated their scientific disagreements—Raspail was an antimonarchist republican who was jailed and exiled for his political views, whereas Orfila supported the monarchy. One of the longest boulevards in Paris is named for Raspail.

Raspail was to testify for the defense in the LaFarge case, but did not arrive at the court in time to do so because he fell from his horse in his haste to reach the court in Tulle (Thomas, 1974).

OF INTEREST 1.5 THE SOIL DID IT

Although the criticism in the LaFarge affair that arsenic in the soil had contaminated the remains of Charles LaFarge was answered by Orfila, the "soil did it" defense persisted into the twentieth century in the case of Marie Besnard (Thorwald, 1964) who was accused of the fatal arsenic poisoning of her husband and several relatives and neighbors. The exhumed bodies of several of her alleged victims were found to contain elevated concentrations of arsenic. After 3 trials, over a period of 9 years, Marie was acquitted of all charges, in part as a result of the defense position that the presence of arsenic in the exhumed bodies of the alleged victims may have resulted from the action of soil microbes that caused the diffusion of arsenic from the soil into the buried bodies.

---

were performed by scientists who were well trained, experienced, and expert in their use. These caveats remain to this day.

1.2.4 THE BOCARME CASE (ANONYMOUS, 1882; THORWALD, 1964; WENNING, 2009; WHARTON AND STILLÉ, 1855)

A second "crime of the century," the Bocarme case, was significant not only for its sensationalism, but also for its impact on the development of analytical and forensic toxicology. In 1843, Alfred Juliet Gabriel Hippolyte Visart, the Count de Bocarmé, married Lydia Fougnies, the daughter of a prosperous grocer, in the anticipation that financial gifts from her father would enable him to maintain his lifestyle—one that included a large mansion staffed with many servants, elaborate parties, and hunting expeditions. The Count soon realized that his wife's yearly income from her father's estate coupled with his own income was insufficient for the maintenance of his preferred lifestyle and he generated huge debts of several thousand francs. Gustav Fougnies, the Countess' brother, who had inherited the major portion of their father's estate was unmarried and had been in poor health since the loss of his leg. Bocarmé became impatient waiting for Gustav to die a natural death and therefore planned to murder him since Lydia, her brother's only heir, would inherit his sizable estate. His plans had to be accelerated when Gustav surprisingly announced his plans to marry. Of course, Bocarmé, who wished to spend his anticipated largess, desired to commit the murder in a manner that could not be identified as a homicide. He determined that poisoning would be the best way of achieving his goal.

Using an assumed name, Bocarmé approached Professor Löppens, a chemist, in Ghent for information concerning the preparation of nicotine from tobacco leaves.[9] Löppens described him the method to be used, and Bocarmé had the equipment necessary for the procedure manufactured. His first attempts were not successful, but ultimately, after almost a year of effort, Bocarmé obtained a sample of nicotine that was lethal to the animals on which he had tested it. After Bocarmé had prepared two vials of nicotine, an amount he judged to be sufficient for his purpose, he and his wife invited his brother-in-law to dinner at which time they attacked him and attempted to pour the nicotine down his throat. The brother-in-law resisted (some people just will not cooperate) and in the ensuing struggle, nicotine was splashed on his clothing and body as well as the floor. However, a sufficient amount was forced into the Gustav's mouth and he died. The Countess told the servants that her brother had died of apoplexy. After Gustav's death, Lydia directed the servants to wash or burn her brother's clothing and crutches and to wash the floor with vinegar. Vinegar was forced into Gustav's mouth and his body was washed with vinegar. The servants thought that the events of that evening and the behavior of the Bocarmés were unusual and suspicious and, therefore, reported their concerns to the authorities who initiated an investigation. Due to the suspicious behavior of the Count and Countess, the presence of chemical burns on the side of Gustav's mouth and a human bite mark on his hand, the authorities suspected that the cause of death was not apoplexy. Therefore, they had the body examined by physicians who concluded that there was no sign of natural death and that poisoning was indicated.[10]

Jean Servais Stas, a 37-year old, brilliant chemist at the École Royale Militaire was asked to determine whether any poisons could be detected in the tissues of Gustav Fougnies. It was widely accepted at this time that "vegetable alkaloids," i.e., nitrogenous bases found in plants, could not be detected in human tissue because of the complexity of the tissue matrix with its many potentially interfering substances that made it difficult to purify the alkaloids sufficiently to apply available methods of detection. Even the great Orfila, whom Stas had assisted in Paris, was of this opinion and had stated only a few years earlier that there was no accepted method for the extraction of vegetable alkaloids, such as nicotine, from human remains, and that the detection of these materials from human remains might never be possible (Wenning, 2009)!

---

[9]Bocarmé developed his methods under the ruse that he was preparing a unique *eau-de-cologne* or pesticide (Wenning, 2009)!

[10]The physicians erroneously surmised that the chemical burns were due to sulfuric acid; it was later concluded by Stas that they were due to the vinegar used by the Bocarmés.

However, Stas developed a method, now known as liquid—liquid extraction, by which the nicotine was extractable from samples into organic solvents. The method involved the separation of the nicotine from "animal matter" through a series of extractions of an alkalinized aqueous portion of the sample with ether. The residue that remained after the evaporation of ether was tested not only with the standard tests of the day for the identification of pure nicotine, but also by the odor of nicotine and that of mouse urine, an odor associated with nicotine—a unique *eau-de-cologne* indeed (Wenning, 2009)! On the basis of his analysis, Stas concluded that the body of the brother-in-law contained nicotine.

Based on the evidence presented by Stas as well as additional evidence developed by the investigators, the Count de Bocarme was convicted and guillotined. However, the Countess de Bocarme who said that she knew of her husband's activities and goals, but did nothing to stop him because her husband had threatened her and she feared for her life, was acquitted. Lydia indeed led a charmed life; shortly after her acquittal she received a bequest of several hundred thousand francs from the estate of an Englishman whose prior proposal of marriage she had refused (Anonymous, 1885).

The method of Stas was modified in 1851 by Otto for the removal of fats. The so-called Stas—Otto liquid—liquid extraction, although modified several times in the ensuing years, remains the basis for the liquid—liquid and solid-phase exactions used in forensic toxicology laboratories to this day.

Apart from its significance in the development of analytical toxicology, it is also of interest to note that the method developed by Stas, which was largely responsible for the conviction of Count de Bocarme, had been developed specifically for this case and had not been evaluated previously by other forensic toxicologists prior to the time at which the results obtained from its use were presented and accepted as trial evidence. The use and acceptance of a novel, untested analytical method in a criminal investigation was also significant in a case—the murder trial of Carl Coppolino—that would occur almost 100 years later.

In the nineteenth century, the work of Orfila, Christison, and Marsh spearheaded the development of forensic toxicology. The authors of several texts of medical jurisprudence attempted to incorporate forensic toxicology as an integral component of medical education and practice. However, by the late nineteenth and early twentieth centuries, the complexity of forensic toxicology had become "… too delicate for the medical profession" (Crowther, 2006), and it was entrusted to those scientists whose training and education had prepared them for this specialized profession. Forensic toxicology had become a science unto itself.

1.3 FORENSIC TOXICOLOGY IN THE UNITED STATES

The development of forensic toxicology which was taking place in Europe in the nineteenth century was slow in crossing the Atlantic. The publication of books in the United States in the mid-eighteenth century on the topic of medical jurisprudence (Niyogi, 1980) such as Dean's *A Manual of Medical Jurisprudence* in 1845 and *A Treatise on Medical Jurisprudence* in 1855 coauthored by Wharton, an attorney, and Stillé, a physician, devoted significant space to forensic toxicology issues, including general concepts of forensic toxicology and the diagnosis of poisoning by elements, organic and mineral acids, and various natural products. However, the book considered to be the first American book devoted to toxicology, *Microchemistry of Poisons*, by T.G. Wormley, was not published until 1867—more than 50 years after Orfila's classic work (Borzelleca, 2001). Wormley's text included a thorough presentation of the chemistry and toxicology of a number of poisons, as well as an overview of detection methods including, as appropriate, drawings of the crystals produced by the reaction of various substances with specific reagents. The success of the first edition led to the publication of a second edition in 1885 that was praised as meriting "… a separate place in medical literature occupying the middle ground between legal medicine and medical chemistry. To each of these branches it is an invaluable, and, we may say indispensable adjunct" (Anonymous, 1885). Subsequently, in the early twentieth century, several texts and research papers dealing with the symptoms and detection of poisons were published.

The landmark event in the development of forensic toxicology in the United States was the establishment of a forensic toxicology laboratory in the New York City Medical Examiner's Office in 1918, which followed the establishment of a medical examiner's system in that city (Freimuth, 1983). Alexander Gettler, the first director of this laboratory, took on this duty in addition to his duties as a pathological chemist at Bellevue Hospital and an instructor at the Bellevue Medical School (Freireich, 1969). Gettler and his laboratory staff developed or adapted methods for the detection for a number of substances including ethanol, methanol, carbon monoxide, cyanide, and chloroform and provided interpretations of analytical results. The thoroughness of Gettler's work is exemplified by his report that he evaluated 58 methods for the identification of methanol in approximately 250 liquors and more than 700 samples of human organs (Gettler, 1920)! In later life, he recounted the circumstances of several cases in which the presence or absence of substances such as fluoride, chloroform, and carbon monoxide led to the resolution of the cases (Gallo, 2001; Gettler, 1956). Not only was Gettler's direct influence on analytical and forensic toxicology extensive, but his influence ultimately spread far beyond New York as several of the forensic toxicologists whom he had trained disseminated their knowledge and skills throughout the United States. These scientists and the locations of their own laboratories include Henry Freimuth in Maryland; Leo Goldbaum at The Armed Forces Institute of Pathology; C.J. Umberger in New York; Irving Sunshine in Ohio; and Sidney Kaye in Puerto Rico (Eckert, 1980). These pioneers who had been trained by Gettler in turn trained a new generation of scientists, many of whom are active practitioners, who further disseminated the knowledge and special skills of forensic toxicology. Forensic toxicology truly is a young and continually developing scientific discipline in the United States.

1.4 FORENSIC TOXICOLOGY GROWING PAINS

Even though the pioneers of forensic toxicology were brilliant, perceptive men who laid the foundations of many of the present principles and concepts of forensic toxicology often found themselves enmeshed in controversy resulting from either the growing pains of the profession or their less than stellar behavior.

Alfred Swaine Taylor, 1806−1880, a renowned toxicologist of his time, has been called "the father of British forensic medicine" (Rosenfeld, 1985) and was "recognized as the leading medical jurist in England" (Coley, 1991). He wrote several texts on medical jurisprudence including the *Manual of Medical Jurisprudence* in 1846, more than one-third of which dealt with issues of toxicology. Taylor also was an early advocate of the Marsh test and gave the first course on medical jurisprudence in England (Rosenfeld, 1985). However, Taylor's reputation was sullied by his participation in two notable cases (Coley, 1991). In 1856, Dr William Palmer was accused of murdering J.P. Cook, a gambler and horse owner. His 1856 trial was one of the first of several "trials of the century" that were to occur throughout subsequent decades. The case hinged on two pieces of evidence: Cook had died while suffering severe convulsions and Taylor had failed to detect strychnine in Cook's stomach contents (Watson, 2006b). Taylor testified for the prosecution that in spite of his failure to detect strychnine, the convulsive symptoms were consistent with strychnine poisoning. This testimony was given even though he had written "In relation to external appearances, there are none indicative of poisoning upon which we can rely" (Burney, 2006). The several defense experts countered that there were several diseases that could cause the type of convulsions that Cook had displayed (Watson, 2010). However, despite the testimony of the defense experts, Palmer was convicted and sentenced to death. Interestingly, on the gallows his final words were "… I am innocent, of poisoning Cook by strychnine" not "I didn't kill Cook" (Anonymous, 1856). The Palmer case demonstrated the problems that may occur when there is an inconsistency between analytical results and signs and symptoms—such problems persist to this day.

Taylor again was in the center of controversy in the 1859 trial of the physician, Thomas Smethurst, who was accused of the murder of Isabella Bankes, the woman with whom he was living in an apparently bigamous relationship. Taylor was asked to analyze a sample obtained prior to Miss Bankes' death and he reported that he had detected arsenic by means of the Reinsch test. This finding led to the arrest of Dr Smethurst and he was subsequently convicted of murder. Because of defense testimony refuting Taylor's evidence and his admission that his result was a false-positive, due to the use of arsenic-contaminated copper foil in the analysis, Smethurst was granted a pardon on appeal; this pardon was apparently warranted since a modern opinion is that Miss Bankes was suffering from Crohn's disease (Fielding, 1985).

Even the great Orfila was not immune to ignominy. In 1818, he published a book on poisons intended for a nontechnical readership and was accused of plagiarism by Hector Chaussier who claimed that Orfila had taken ideas, "even in the errors," from Chaussier's earlier published book and included them in his own

(Bertomeu-Sanchez, 2009). However, a much greater discredit to his reputation awaited Orfila as a result of the trial of the viscount Bocarme and his wife. Prior to the trial, Orfila had obtained technical information from Stas concerning the method he had developed for the detection of nicotine. Orfila used it without attribution in a publication that was essentially a modification of Stas' work (Thomas, 1974). Additionally, Orfila published a *Memoir on nicotine* in which he applauded the work of Stas in the Bocarme case and presented data including the effects of nicotine in dogs, a description of methods for the detection of nicotine in various organs including several organs outside of the gastrointestinal tract (such findings were significant because they demonstrated the absorption of nicotine following oral administration), and a description of a method of detection of nicotine in putrefied samples. A review of Orfila's work by a panel of experts concluded that Stas was due the propriety claim for the significant findings presented by Orfila (Pasquier, 1852). These controversies cast a shadow on Orfila's reputation in the later years of his life.

Although the development of modern, or scientific, forensic toxicology was not without missteps, the pioneers in the discipline were able to successfully bring forth a new discipline through their brilliance, perseverance, and ingenuity. By incorporating the methodological and analytical techniques of chemistry, biology, and physiology into the structure and framework of the legal system, the forbearers of forensic toxicology created a set of principles and standards that directed the development of the discipline and that guide forensic toxicologists today. These principles and concepts as well as those developed more recently will be described and discussed throughout this text.

REVIEW QUESTIONS

1. Write your own definition of toxicology.
2. What is forensic toxicology?
3. What are the three main types of forensic toxicology, and what are the differences among these three branches of the field?
4. What were the most significant contributions of Orfila to the burgeoning field of forensic toxicology?
5. What is considered to be the landmark event in the development of forensic toxicology in the United States, and why was this event so important to the discipline?

APPLICATION QUESTIONS

1. Discuss the differences and similarities between a poison and a drug.
2. Classically, forensic toxicology was considered to be a purely retrospective discipline, whereas more recently the discipline has been acknowledged to include prospective aspects. Describe the differences between the retrospective functions and the prospective functions of forensic toxicology. Discuss the

societal and/or technological changes that have led to the development of the prospective functions of the discipline.

3. Select one person who was pivotal to the development of the discipline of forensic toxicology and describe his or her contributions to the field.

4. Select one legal proceeding that resulted in a technological or methodological advancement in the field of forensic toxicology. Describe the case and the advancement that resulted.

REFERENCES

Agren, H., 1984. Eastern and oriental sciences (book review). Ann. Sci. 41, 294–295.

Anonymous, 1752. The Tryal of Mary Blandy, Spinster; for the Murder of her Father, Francis Blandy, Gent. John and James Rivington, London.

Anonymous, 1830. Review of "a treatise on poisons, in relation to medical jurisprudence, physiology, and the practice of physic". Edinburgh Med. Surg. J. 32, 200–211.

Anonymous, 1856. Palmer's last words. Spectator 15.

Anonymous, 1882. Remarkable Trials of All Countries, vol. II. Peloubet & Company, New York.

Anonymous, 1885. JAMA 2, 473.

Ball, P., 2006. The Devils Doctor: Paracelsus and the World of Renaissance Magic and Science. Farrar Straus and Giroux, New York.

Bertomeu-Sanchez, J.R., 2009. Popularizing controversial science: a popular treatise on poisons by Mateu Orfila (1818). Med. Hist. 53, 351–378.

Borzelleca, J.F., 2001. The art, the science, and the seduction of toxicology: an evolutionary development. In: Hayes, A.W. (Ed.), Principles and Methods of Toxicology, fourth ed. Taylor & Francis, Philadelphia.

Burney, I.A., 2002. Testing testimony: toxicology and the law of evidence in early nineteenth-century England. Stud. Hist. Phil. Sci. 33, 289–314.

Burney, I.A., 2006. Poison, Detection and the Victorian Imagination. Manchester University Press, New York.

Campbell, W.A., 1965. Some landmarks in the history of arsenic testing. Chem. Br. 1, 198–202.

Caudill, D.S., 2009. Prefiguring the arsenic wars. Chem. Heritage 27.

Christison, R.C., 1829. A Treatise on Poisons in Relation to Medical Jurisprudence, Physiology and the Practice of Physic. Longman Rees Orme Brown & Green, London.

Coley, N.G., 1991. Alfred Swaine Taylor, MD, FRS (1806–1880): forensic toxicologist. Med. Hist. 35, 409–427.

Crowther, A., 2006. The toxicology of Robert Christison. In: Bertomeu-Sánchez, J.R., Nieto-Galan, A. (Eds.), Chemistry, Medicine, and Crime. Science History Publications, Sagamore Beach, MA.

Davis, A., 1993. Paracelsus: a quincentennial assessment. J. R. Soc. Med. 86, 657–660.

Eaton, D.L., Klaassen, C.D., 2001. Principles of toxicology. In: Klaassen, C.D. (Ed.), Casarett & Doull's Toxicology: The Basic Science of Poisons, sixth ed. McGraw-Hill, New York.

Eckert, W.H., 1980. Historical aspects of poisoning and toxicology. Am. J. Forensic Med. Pathol. 1, 261–264.

Ellenhorn, M.J., 1997. Ellenhorn's Medical Toxicology, second ed. Williams and Wilkins, Baltimore.

Emsley, J., 2005. The Elements of Murder. Oxford University Press, New York.

Farrell, M., 1994. Pioneer forensic toxicologists: Marsh, Orfila and their predecessors. Criminologist 18, 33—36.

Fielding, J.F., 1985. "Inflammatory" bowel disease. Br. Med. J. 290, 47—48.

Freimuth, H.C., 1983. Alexander O. Gettler (1883—1968). Am. J. For. Med. Path. 4. 303—305.

Freireich, A.W., 1969. In memoriam: Alexander O. Gettler, 1883—1968. J. For. Sci. 14, vii—ix.

Gaensslen, R.E., 1983. Sourcebook in Forensic Serology, Immunology and Biochemistry. National Institute of Justice, Washington, DC.

Gallo, M.A., 2001. History and scope of toxicology. In: Klaassen, C.D. (Ed.), Casarett & Doull's Toxicology: The Basic Science of Poisons, sixth ed. McGraw-Hill, New York.

Gettler, A.O., 1920. Critical study of methods for the detection of methyl alcohol. J. Biol. Chem. 42, 311—328.

Gettler, A.O., 1956. The historical development of toxicology. J. For. Sci. 1, 3—25.

Giles, H.A., 1924. The "Hsi Yuan Lu" or "instructions to coroners". Proc. R. Soc. Med. 17, 59—107.

Goldsmith, R.H., 1997. The search for arsenic. In: Gerber, S.M., Saferstein, R.W. (Eds.), More Chemistry and Crime: From Marsh Arsenic Test to DNA Profile. American Chemical Society, Washington, DC.

Haas, L.F., 1996. Pedanius Dioscorides (born about 40 AD, died about 90 AD) [Electronic version] J. Neurol. Neurosurg. Psychiatry 60 (4), 427.

Hayes, A.W., 2001. Principles and Methods in Toxicology, fourth ed. Taylor & Francis, Philadelphia.

Kemp, F., 1974. The future of forensic toxicology. In: Ballantyne, B. (Ed.), Forensic Toxicology. John Wright and Sons, Bristol, England.

Kiel, F.W., 1970. Forensic science in china — traditional and contemporary aspects. J. For. Sci. 15, 201—224.

Loomis, T.A., Hayes, A.W., 1996. Loomis's Essentials of Toxicology. Academic Press, New York.

Marsh, J., 1836. Account of a method of separating small quantities of arsenic from substances with which it may be mixed. Edinburgh New Phil. J. 21, 229—236.

McKean, E., 2005. The New Oxford American Dictionary, second ed. New York.

McKnight, B.E., 1981. The Washing Away of Wrongs: Forensic Medicine in Thirteenth Century China. The University of Michigan, Ann Arbor, Michigan.

Nieto-Galan, A., Bertomeu-Sanchez, J.R., 2006. Mateu Orfila and his biographers. In: Nieto-Galan, A., Bertomeu-Sanchez, J.R. (Eds.), Chemistry, Medicine, and Crime: Mateu J. B. Orfila (1787—1853) and his Times. Science History Publications, Sagamore Beach, MA.

Niyogi, S.K., 1980. Historic development of forensic toxicology in America up to 1978. Am. J. Forensic Med. Path. 1, 249—264.

Pasquier, 1852. Du rapport de la commission charge d'apprecier le differend qui s'est eleve entre sats et orfila a propos de la recherché de la nicotine dans le organs humains. Bull. R. Med. Belg. XII 990—997.

Plaa, G.L., 2007. Introduction to toxicology: occupational & environmental. In: Katzung, B.G. (Ed.), Basic & Clinical Pharmacology, tenth ed. McGraw-Hill, New York.

Reese, J.J., 1889. Textbook of Medical Jurisprudence and Toxicology. P. Blakiston, Son & Co, Philadelphia.

Reinsch, H., 1842. Uber das verhalten des metallischen kupfers zu einigen metallosungen about the behavior of the metal copper to some metal solutions. J. Pract. Chem. 24, 244.

Rosenfeld, L., 1985. Alfred Swaine Taylor (1806−1880), pioneer toxicologist−and a slight case of murder. Clin. Chem. 31, 1235−1236.

Saunders, E., 1952. The Mystery of Marie la Farge. William Morrow and Company, New York.

Severinghaus, J.W., 2003. Fire-air and dephlogistication. In: Roach, R.C., Wagner, P.D., Hackett, P.H. (Eds.), Hypoxia: Through the Lifecycle. Kluwer Academic/Plenum Publishers, New York.

Sigerist, H.E., 1951. A History of Medicine. Oxford University Press, New York.

Society of Toxicology, 2005. How Do You Define Toxicology? Retrieved February 3, 2014, 2012 from http://www.toxicology.org/AI/PUB/SI05/SI05_Define.asp.

SOFT/AAFS. 2006. Forensic Toxicology Laboratory Guidelines. Retrieved April 29, 2009 from http://www.soft-tox.org/files/Guidelines_2006_Final.pdf.

Stedman's Medical Dictionary, 28th ed., 2006. Lippincott Williams & Wilkins, Baltimore.

Thomas, F., 1974. Milestones in forensic science. J. For. Sci. 19, 241−254.

Thorwald, J., 1964. The Century of the Detective. Harcourt, Brace & World, New York.

Watson, K.D., 2006a. Criminal poisoning in England and the origins of the Marsh test for arsenic. In: Bertomeu-Sánchez, J.R., Nieto-Galan, A. (Eds.), Chemistry, Medicine, and Crime. Science History Publications, Sagamore Beach, MA.

Watson, K.D., 2006b. Medical and chemical expertise in English trials for criminal poisoning, 1750−1914. Med. Hist. 30, 373−390.

Watson, D., 2010. Forensic Medicine in Western Society. Rouledge, New York.

Weiner, D.B., 1959. Francois Vincent Raspail: Doctor and champion of the poor. Fr. Hist. Stud. 1, 149−171.

Wenning, R., 2009. Back to the roots of modern analytical toxicology: Jean Servais Stas and the Bocarmé murder case. Drug Test. Anal. 1, 153−155.

Wharton, F., Stillé, M., 1855. Treatise on Medical Jurisprudence, first ed. Kay and Brother, Philadelphia.

The Duties and Responsibilities of Forensic Toxicologists

2

This chapter introduces the core professional functions of forensic toxicologists—analysis, interpretation, and reporting. Each of these functions is the topic of an entire unit in the book and will be presented in greater detail in the chapters of those units.

The object of Toxicology then as a branch of Medical Jurisprudence is to embody all this information into one science. It ranges over the whole vast field of medical learning and draws together from a variety of quarters facts and principles which are seldom at any other time viewed in combination.

Robert Christison

The three basic functions of modern forensic toxicologists, established by the pioneers of this science, have remained essentially unchanged over the past 200 years or so. In summary, they are:

Analysis—the detection, identification, and frequently the quantitation of drugs and chemicals in biological samples, which generally are obtained from human subjects;
Interpretation—providing opinions as to the meaning of the presence of the detected substances, e.g., the effects that these drugs and chemicals may have produced on the subject; and
Reporting—the presentation of the analytical results and often the interpretation derived from them, either in written form, such as laboratory reports and written reports or as sworn testimony at deposition or trial (Figure 2.1).

These roles are common to all of the areas of forensic toxicology—postmortem forensic toxicology, human-performance forensic toxicology, and forensic urine drug testing.

The manner in which these roles are implemented and the standards employed to evaluate forensic toxicologists may be codified across the country as a result of the announcement in 2013 of the intent to establish a National Commission on Forensic Science as a collaborative action by the U.S. Department of Justice and the National Institute of Standards and technology (U.S. Department of Justice). The purpose of this commission is to propose to the Attorney General of the United States discipline-specific recommendations pertaining to the practices and policies

Forensic Toxicology. http://dx.doi.org/10.1016/B978-0-12-799967-8.00002-5

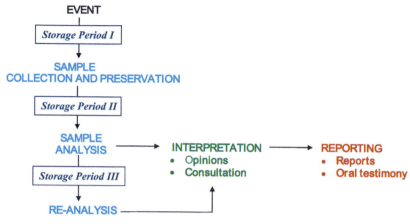

FIGURE 2.1

The Functions of Forensic Toxicologists.

of the forensic sciences in this country. The Commission includes members from various basic sciences, forensic sciences, and the legal and law enforcement communities. Although it is probable that the practice of forensic toxicology will be impacted by the actions of this Commission, it is unlikely that the traditional overall roles and responsibilities of forensic toxicologists will be meaningfully altered, if at all.

The scientific qualification of forensic toxicologists perhaps is best determined on the basis of whether they possess the knowledge and skills necessary to perform the three basic functions of the discipline. The remainder of this book is devoted to a detailed exposition of the many aspects of these three functions, including the other activities encompassed by each function such as on-scene investigation, consultation with pathologists, police and attorneys, the development of new methods of analysis and a better understanding of the interpretation of analytical results, and the education and training of future forensic toxicologists both in formal academic courses and in laboratory internships or entry-level employment (Winek, 1973). It is therefore sufficient at this juncture to briefly summarize what is required of forensic toxicologists in the execution of their duties of analysis, interpretation, and reporting.

2.1 ANALYSIS

Forensic toxicologists may be involved as experts in a variety of widely disparate events such as automobile accidents, undocumented deaths, therapeutic misadventures, preemployment physicals, and alleged parole violations. However dissimilar the events may be, the initial role of forensic toxicologists in each case is to determine whether any exogenous drugs or chemicals are present in samples obtained from individuals involved in the event.

The word "analysis" in this context should be considered to refer not only to the analytical methods that will be used to detect these substances, but also to the several procedures that occur between the event of interest and the completion of the last analysis to which the sample is subjected. As is seen in Figure 2.1, the first activity of forensic toxicologists is sample handling, which in this text refers to sample selection, identification, preservation, and transmittal. Since proper sample handling is essential for obtaining accurate results, all of the activities of which it is comprised should be considered components of the analysis. The selection, collection, and transmittal procedures all occur prior to the arrival of the samples in the forensic toxicology laboratory, whereas the preservation of samples begins with their collection and transmittal to the laboratory and continues until the samples have been discarded.

The methods of analysis that are employed to detect, identify, and quantitate drugs or chemicals present in biological samples will depend upon both the analytical strategy employed by the laboratory as well as any specific evidence that may indicate to which drugs or chemical subjects may have been exposed. Months or even years subsequent to the initial analyses, a reanalysis of one or more samples may be required as a result of several circumstances, e.g., the issuance of a court order allowing the defendant's expert to analyze the samples, the discovery of additional case information suggesting that drugs, which were not considered initially, may have been used by the subject, and the development and availability of improved methods allowing more sophisticated and informative analyses to be conducted.

All of the steps in the series of events that constitute the analysis—from sample handling through the final analysis—must be conducted appropriately in order to ensure that the results are accurate.

2.1.1 SAMPLE SELECTION

Generally, postmortem toxicologists have the ability to select samples required for the initial analysis and any reanalysis from among any in the body, except when the desired samples have been destroyed, e.g., as a result of incineration or putrefaction. Obviously, in the other areas of forensic toxicology, since the subjects usually are living, the samples that are available for analysis are limited usually to blood, urine, saliva, and hair.

With the exception of sample preservation, forensic toxicologists ordinarily are not directly involved in sample handling. However, they should be involved in establishing procedures for each of the steps of the process so that samples necessary for the analysis and interpretation of results are selected, collected, and transmitted in appropriate manners.

A reasonable description of an "ideal" sample is one that allows ease of analysis consistent with accurate results that may be interpreted to provide the required information. For example, the only information required is if the subject used a specific drug, then urine may be the sample of choice. However, if it is necessary to know the type or extent of effect that a drug had on a subject, then blood generally would be the preferred sample. In each instance, the samples collected are consistent with accurate and relatively easy analysis capable of generating results that allow for the necessary interpretation to be made. If the "ideal" samples are not available, then the collection and subsequent analysis of the so-called alternative samples, those not usually collected and analyzed, may be appropriate since the analysis of these samples may provide the desired information.

2.1.2 STORAGE PERIODS

Forensic toxicologists conduct analyses on samples that may have been stored for any or all of three different periods of time, identified in this text as storage periods I, II, and III (Figure 2.1). Ideally, there would be no change in the sample matrices or the detection or concentration of analytes as a result of these storage periods. However, frequently, as a result of the duration and conditions of sample storage, analyte concentrations may be altered. Obviously, if any such alterations occur, the interpretation of the analytical results becomes problematic. Therefore, forensic toxicologists must be aware of the changes that can occur during the three storage phases and take appropriate action when the samples are in their possession to minimize these alterations.

The Stage I storage period occurs between the time of the event and the time of sample collection. This period may be hours or days in length, or in some cases, centuries. During this storage period, drugs and chemicals may undergo metabolism, synthesis, nonmetabolic degradation, or redistribution from one anatomical site to another. Often, as a result of these events, the alterations of analyte concentrations that can occur are of sufficient magnitude to cause errors in interpretations.

Given that forensic toxicologists are not in possession of the samples during the Stage I storage period, they cannot institute measures that would prevent or minimize the alterations that may occur during this time. However, they must be aware of the events that can alter drug concentrations and the factors, such as heat, humidity, and putrefaction that may influence these events.

The Stage II storage period, the time between the collection and the initial analysis of the samples, usually is hours, days, or weeks in duration. During this period, the concentrations of drugs and chemicals in samples may be altered as a result of continuing metabolism, synthesis, nonenzymatic degradation, or redistribution within the sample. This storage period has two temporal components: the first is the transport time between the collection of the samples and their arrival at the forensic toxicology laboratory and the second is the time period between the arrival of the samples at the forensic toxicology laboratory and their analyses. During the transport of the samples to the forensic toxicology laboratory, the samples are in the custody of persons—phlebotomists, laboratory technicians, autopsy personnel, and police officers—who should be trained to employ appropriate methods so that any alterations of drug concentrations are minimized. Once in the forensic toxicology laboratory, the samples are under the control of forensic toxicologists who are expected to employ appropriate methods in order to minimize or prevent any further alterations in the sample matrices or concentrations of the analytes.

Stage III storage, a long-term storage of samples, is necessitated in anticipation of a future need either to repeat certain of the analyses because the results of the original analysis have been challenged or to conduct additional analyses because the continuing investigation has suggested the involvement of drugs or chemicals not considered at the time of the original analysis. Also, during a relatively long Stage III storage, new methods may be developed which will enable the detection of drugs which were undetectable at the time of the original analysis (Rejent, 1981). Generally, samples placed into long-term storage are those in which one or more drugs or exogenous chemicals have been detected. Since it is difficult to know how much time will be required to resolve the case—this is especially true in civil cases—there is no "industry standard" as to the proper length of the Stage III storage period. However, a storage period of several months would seem to be adequate especially in those cases in which litigation seems unlikely (a circumstance which becomes more uncommon with the passing years). For those cases in which litigation is either likely or ongoing, the most appropriate action would be to maintain the samples until the matter is resolved or for an infinite period, whichever occurs first! Since samples stored following the initial analysis are subject to similar alterations as those in the Stage II storage period, steps must be taken to stabilize the concentration of the analytes in the sample. The most common method of preservation of samples during this period is by freezing at greatly decreased temperatures.

From the time of their collection, throughout the three storage periods, samples must be handled in such a manner that not only the scientific integrity, but also the legal integrity of the samples is maintained. Although the scientific integrity is achieved by the storage of a sample in a manner that prevents or minimizes changes in both the structural nature of the sample and the analyte concentration, the legal integrity requires that the possibility of tampering is negated by the use of appropriate preventive measures and the maintenance of a chain of custody, i.e., a written record of who had control of the sample and where it was stored until its ultimate disposal. A component, the quality assurance/quality control program, of every laboratory should contain a statement identifying both the length of time samples should be stored and the manner by which they should be destroyed (Lemos, 2005).

2.1.3 ANALYTICAL STRATEGIES

Although the specific methods of analysis employed by forensic toxicologists may vary widely, the commonly accepted analytical strategy consists of two types of

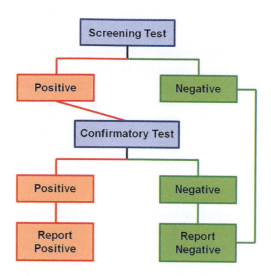

FIGURE 2.2

Interpretation of Presumptive and Confirmatory Tests.

analyses. The first is a presumptive or screening test designed to identify samples that do not require further analysis since the analytes of interest are not detected. Generally, the methods employed for presumptive analyses have very low detection limits, are easy to perform, inexpensive, and compatible with rapid, batch analysis. The second component of the analytical strategy is a confirmatory method that is used for the analysis of those samples in which one or more analytes have been presumptively identified. Confirmatory tests are more specific than the presumptive test and, ideally, have detection limits that are equal to or less than those of the presumptive tests. Positive results are reported only if both the presumptive and confirmatory tests are positive (Figure 2.2).

2.1.4 ANALYTICAL METHODS

The purposes of the analyses conducted by forensic toxicologists are to detect, identify, and often quantitate drugs and chemicals in ante- and postmortem samples.[1] This requires forensic toxicologists to be competent analytical chemists who are knowledgeable about the modern methods of immunological and instrumental analysis. In addition, because forensic toxicologists are confronted with problems unique to the samples that they analyze, e.g., interference from postmortem putrefactive

---

[1]Although these samples are generally human, forensic toxicologists may be called upon to analyze nonhuman samples, e.g., from dogs and cats, in cases of suspected animal poisoning or horses in sporting events.

products, alterations in concentrations of drugs due to their postmortem synthesis or degradation, detection of submicrogram quantities of drugs in extremely complex matrices such as liver and brain, they have developed new methods and modified existing methods to meet their specific needs and to overcome these specific problems with which they are confronted.

The analytical competence of forensic toxicologists should range from chemical methods such as the relatively undemanding color tests, through immunological methods of analysis to the sophisticated and continually increasing hyphenated mass spectrometry methods such as LC-MS-MS. In practice, due to the complexity and sophistication of modern analytical methods, no forensic toxicologist possesses, nor should be expected to possess, expertise in all methods that have an application in forensic toxicology. However, they should possess a thorough understanding of the theory and practical aspects of the methods that they use on a regular basis. To expect more is not appropriate since it might compel forensic toxicologists to expand their analytical activities into areas in which they lack the necessary competence. Thus, the qualification of forensic toxicologists should not be a "blanket" endorsement of them as "analysts," but rather recognition that they possess the ability to perform specific methods of analysis proficiently.

2.2 INTERPRETATION

Analyses by forensic toxicologists are performed in an attempt to answer many varied and wide-ranging questions such as: Was the sudden death of a 75-year-old man in his bedroom consistent with an overdose of Viagra®? Was the driver of a car involved in an automobile accident under the influence of cocaine? Does the detection of marihuana metabolite in the urine of a 22-year-old parolee indicate "recent" use of marihuana? The answers to these and numerous other questions are not based on analytical results alone, but rather in the consideration of nonanalytical evidence obtained from police investigations, medical history, eyewitness testimony, and autopsy findings. Consideration of nontoxicological evidence may allow for conclusions to be drawn that may be difficult to draw based upon analytical results alone. Additional consideration must be given to evidence pertaining to specific subjects including gender, age, existing pathology, tolerance, and postmortem redistribution—all factors that may influence the interpretations of analytical results. In order to formulate accurate interpretations of analytical results, forensic toxicologists must have an understanding of the relevant concepts of pharmacology, biochemistry, physiology, and pathology, and especially an understanding of the events of drug disposition—absorption, distribution, metabolism, and excretion, the rates at which they occur and the conditions that may alter them. It is most likely that forensic toxicologists will be able to provide reliable answers to questions posed when both accurate analytical results and relevant nonanalytical evidence are available; in the absence of both reliable results and

---

OF INTEREST 2.1 CAVEAT TOXICOLOGIST!

At a meeting of forensic toxicologists at which problems of interpretation were being discussed, a respected toxicologist of national renown relayed an event that occurred early in his career and which demonstrated that determining the cause of death is the function of the medical examiner.

The toxicologist had detected a rather high morphine concentration in the blood of a young man who had been found near railroad tracks. When the medical examiner called and asked how the morphine level should be interpreted, the young toxicologist replied that he was convinced the decedent had died from a morphine or heroin overdose. The medical examiner responded that this was a very interesting conclusion considering that the decedent had been decapitated!

---

nonanalytical evidence, it may be difficult or impossible to generate reliable conclusions. It is important to note, however, that forensic toxicologists must not make interpretations or draw conclusions that are out of the purview of their expertise. This includes conclusions opining as to the cause of death, since toxicology results are only one piece of information in a death case. The ultimate conclusion as to the cause and manner of death is made by the medical examiner who has not only the toxicology results, but also the results of all other examinations and investigations (Of Interest 2.1).

2.3 REPORTING

Finally, forensic toxicologists must be able to present reports of their findings and interpretations both in laboratory reports and opinion reports and as sworn oral testimony at deposition or at trial. These findings must be presented in a clear, unambiguous, and impartial manner, which is both scientifically sound and comprehensible to experts (reports) as well as nonexperts (testimony).

The results of forensic toxicological analyses, presented in an official laboratory report, become a component of the official report of the case. Generally, these laboratory reports are a "bare bones" presentation including little more than a summary of the results, but lacking the details of the analyses, such as the site of sample collection, the method of analysis, and the interpretation of results. Forensic toxicologists may also be asked to prepare written reports in which they review the toxicologically relevant evidence and state the opinions that they have formulated based on that evidence.

Forensic toxicologists present sworn oral testimony at pretrial depositions (usually in civil cases) and at trial. Forensic toxicologists in these circumstances are presented as expert witnesses and, when accepted by the court as such, are allowed to testify not only to the facts of which they are aware, e.g., the results of the analyses that they conducted, but also to their opinions, e.g., the interpretation of the results and the conclusion that, in their opinion, are supported by these results.

2.4 RESEARCH

In addition to the case-related duties of analysis, interpretation, and reporting, forensic toxicologists frequently are involved in research related to their work. Traditionally, forensic toxicology research has consisted largely of the development and application of analytical methods or case reports of the drug and chemical concentrations that have been determined in various postmortem tissues and fluids. Case reports were, and continue to be, important as they provide information on important topics such as the detection of an increased abuse of specific drugs in local areas, the identification of problems of sample handling and analytical methodologies, the description of postmortem drug distribution and redistribution, the estimation of therapeutic and toxic tissue concentrations in antemortem clinical cases, and lethal drug concentrations in postmortem cases. Method development and application are of obvious importance and over the past half century have lead to meaningful advances in both the sensitivity and specificity of analytical methodology in forensic toxicology.

A vision of future research in forensic toxicology may be seen in the recommendations of the Scientific Working Group for Forensic Toxicology (SWGTOX) (2013), which has proposed several specific priority research areas in forensic toxicology including chemical terrorism, drug interactions, emerging drugs of abuse, nanotechnology, population-based toxicology (e.g., sex, race, disease states, pregnancy, elderly, pediatric, toxic concentration ranges), pharmacodynamics, toxicodynamics, pharmacokinetics, toxicokinetics, pharmacogenetics, and pharmacogenomics. As these proposed research areas demonstrate, it is necessary that forensic toxicologists are knowledgeable in areas other than analytical and instrumental analyses.

2.5 ETHICS

The placement of a discussion of ethics at the end of this chapter should not signal that it is of minimal importance. To the contrary, it is the most important section of this chapter. Without the establishment of and compliance with standards of ethical behavior, all that forensic scientists do is rendered worthless. Moreover, unethical forensic toxicologists who fail to function in an impartial and honest manner by misrepresenting their qualifications, what they have done, or the meaning of their findings are a danger to our profession, our legal system, and our society.

Therefore, the ethical behavior of forensic toxicologists and all other forensic scientists must be of the highest caliber. They must not have a "dog in the fight" in legal cases in which they are involved and must function as disinterested third parties who have neither a professional nor personal interest either in the results they obtain or in the interpretations they make. Forensic toxicologists must not have an opinion about either the guilt or innocence of a defendant in a criminal case or the outcome of a civil case. Their only concern and responsibility is to provide an accurate and objective report of findings and interpretations that will assist the trier of fact in arriving at a decision, e.g., a jury's decision as to guilt or innocence. The actor and eponymous restaurateur Arthur Treacher when asked for his philosophy of acting replied: "Say the words take the money and go home." When applied to forensic scientists, including forensic toxicologists, this may be construed as: Provide ethical and accurate opinions, receive payment for your efforts and the application of your skills, and have no professional or personal opinions as to the outcome of the cases in which you are involved.

The behavior that is appropriate for forensic scientists generally and forensic toxicologists specifically has been codified by several regional, national, and international professional organizations. Although the specific language of these and other organizational codes varies, the recurrent principles of ethical behavior require forensic toxicologists to perform their functions with the highest levels of honesty, morality, impartiality, objectivity, and responsibility (Saady, 2001). In addition to those general principles of ethical behavior, the following specific examples are widely agreed upon: forensic toxicologists should possess competence in the analysis and interpretation that they conduct and this competence should be maintained by continuing study and education; forensic toxicologists should maintain confidentiality about their work and not divulge either the names or personal information of persons from whom samples have been obtained or the results of any analyses, except to authorized persons or as a result of judicial proceedings; forensic toxicologists should disclose all probative information to both parties in a litigated matter when required to do so by appropriate legal authority.

These ethical requirements apply not only to forensic toxicologists employed by governmental agencies, but also to the many forensic toxicologists who are employed in private laboratories and those who are independent consultants. An additional and extremely important stricture for nongovernmental scientists is that any fees that they receive for their services must be independent of their findings. That is, they cannot be paid on a contingent fee basis, which is an arrangement by which a fee for services is based on the legal outcome of a case, e.g., the fee is a percentage of a court award in a civil case. This prohibition against contingent fees is essential since it safeguards forensic scientists against a financial temptation as well as an appearance of bias, both of which would diminish the validity of their opinions.

The codes of ethics of the American Board of Forensic Toxicology, the Society of Forensic Toxicologists, and The International Association of Forensic Toxicologists are presented in Of Interest 2.2.

OF INTEREST 2.2 CODES OF ETHICS

American Board of Forensic Toxicology

Code of Ethics

(American Board of Forensic Toxicologists (2011))

The process of certification of Diplomates and Forensic Toxicology Specialists has always required a minimum of three references from peers, who testify to the moral and ethical behavior of the applicant. However, in February 2000, the ABFT drafted and adopted a Code of Ethics of its own. The ABFT is in the process of sending that Code to all its certificants. All new applicants will have to agree in writing to abide by that Code, as will all subsequent applicants for recertification starting with the 2001 cycle.

Guide to Ethics The American Board of Forensic Toxicology expects all persons holding a Certificate of Qualification from this Board to maintain the good moral character, high integrity, good repute, and high ethical and professional standing which are initial and continuing qualifications for recognition by this Board, and to conform to the following principles of ethical conduct:

- Conduct themselves with honesty and integrity at all times.
- Perform all professional activities in forensic toxicology with honesty and integrity and refrain from any knowing misrepresentation of their professional qualifications, knowledge and competence, evidence and results of examinations, or other material facts.
- Hold in proper confidence all information obtained or received in the course of their professional practice and refrain from misuse of any such information.
- Strive to be aware of and alert to any actual or potential conflicts of interest and strive to avoid or appropriately resolve any such conflicts.
- Maintain and enhance their qualifications and competence for the practice of forensic toxicology, to the best of their ability.
- Act in accordance with the long-standing precepts for ethical practice of the profession of forensic toxicology and refrain from any action or activity, which would tend to bring disrepute upon or otherwise harm the profession of forensic toxicology or the American Board of Forensic Toxicology.

Society of Forensic Toxicologists

Code of Ethics

(Society of Forensic Toxicologists)

As a Member of the Society of Forensic Toxicologists (SOFT), I agree to conduct myself in a professional manner, in accordance with the following ethical principles of the SOFT.
I understand if I behave in a manner detrimental to the organization or the profession of forensic toxicology in general, I may be censured or expelled from membership.

Members agree to:

1. Perform professional activities with honesty, integrity, and objectivity.
2. Refrain from knowingly misrepresenting professional qualifications including, but not limited to: education, training, experience, certification, area of expertise, and professional memberships.
3. Hold in confidence and refrain from misuse of information obtained or received in the course of professional activities.
4. Provide expert advice and opinions within the limits of individual competence and generally accepted scientific principles.
5. Render testimony in a truthful manner without bias or misrepresentation.

The International Association of Forensic Toxicologists

Code of Conduct

(Wenning et al.)

Introduction TIAFT is an international organization of forensic toxicologists founded in 1963 in London, UK. As forensic toxicological investigations may have important medical, social, and legal implications, all members of TIAFT should have a high sense of professional responsibility

Continued

OF INTEREST 2.2 CODES OF ETHICS—cont'd

and high ethical standards. Because of the importance of these high standards, TIAFT members should be asked to sign a declaration promising to adhere to them.

General All TIAFT members should treat their peers and colleagues with honesty and respect. Membership in TIAFT should not be regarded as a qualification, e.g., not used on letterhead, business cards. TIAFT members should not misrepresent their academic and professional qualifications. TIAFT publications should not be used for advertising personal professional services.

The highest standards of integrity are required when writing and submitting scientific papers for publication. The same high standards should apply to press and broadcast interviews as well as other forms of communication such as books, lectures, and contributions to electronic media.

Privacy and dignity of persons (living or dead) should be respected.

Research TIAFT members should strive to present and publish their research findings in suitable scientific media such as journals and at appropriate scientific meetings.

Authors should be aware of intellectual property laws governing copyright. In particular, they should guard against wrongful disclosure of confidential information, especially that relating to current research and development work. In case of any doubt, specific written approval from the appropriate organization or individual should be obtained.

Research results should be presented in an unequivocal manner and as completely as practical to avoid misinterpretation. It is unethical to manipulate analytical or experimental data in an effort to bias interpretation. Results or data obtained from another source or results already published should be properly cited or acknowledged.

Experiments with human volunteers must conform to the recommended guidelines for biomedical research involving human subjects published by the World Medical Association's Declaration of Helsinki and subsequent amendments, in addition to any local guidelines or legislation.

All experiments with human volunteers or laboratory animals should be approved by a local ethics committee.

In planning research projects, great care must be taken to minimize risk to those involved. Animal experiments should be minimized and any stress, pain, and privations kept to a minimum.

Continuing Education TIAFT members should strive to remain current in the field of forensic toxicology and related fields. In order to assist in promoting a high level of professional competence, TIAFT members should try to participate in scientific meetings, seminars, and workshops, including TIAFT conferences.

Competence Where TIAFT members are directly involved in analytical work, demonstration and documentation of competence through participation in quality assurance and proficiency testing programmes is strongly recommended. TIAFT members should only provide expert opinions and services for which they have sufficient professional competence.

Safety and Environmental Awareness Daily laboratory work should be undertaken with proper regard for accepted safety standards. The materials and procedures used should minimize hazards to the environment.

Expert Opinions The function of an expert witness is to assist courts in arriving at a verdict by explaining and interpreting the technical and scientific facts on which a lawsuit may depend. Opinions should be given with a conscientious, objective, and neutral manner, with proper regard for the serious nature of the matter at hand. The same considerations apply when evidence is presented at other hearings and committees.

Data Protection and Professional Discretion Personal data must be protected. Where cases are published, it should not be possible to discover the identity of the subject. Results of investigations should be disclosed only to authorized persons or agencies.

TIAFT Meetings TIAFT meetings should not be organized with the goal of personal financial gain.

REVIEW QUESTIONS

1. What are the three core professional functions of a forensic toxicologist? Briefly describe each function.
2. What is the planned function of the National Commission of Forensic Science?
3. What are the major mechanisms by which forensic toxicologists report their findings and interpretations?
4. To effectively perform toxicological analyses, a forensic toxicologist must have a working knowledge of several scientific disciplines, what are the major disciplines with which a toxicologist must be familiar?
5. Describe the ethical standards that forensic toxicologists must adhere to; what are some ethical considerations of importance to forensic toxicologists?

APPLICATION QUESTIONS

1. Discuss the major factors that must be considered when planning an analytical strategy in a forensic toxicology laboratory.
2. Forensic toxicologists conduct analyses on samples that have been stored for varying lengths of time, defined as storage periods I, II, and III. Are there any special considerations that you, as a forensic toxicologist, must be aware of if analyzing a sample that has been stored for storage period I, II, and/or III? Discuss.
3. The interpretations performed by forensic toxicologists are generally not based on analytical data alone. Describe the types of nonanalytical evidence that are frequently of importance to forensic toxicologists.
4. It is important to the discipline of forensic toxicology that the scientists working within the field regularly participate in original scientific research projects. Describe a research project that would be of interest to a forensic toxicologist.

REFERENCES

American Board of Forensic Toxicologists, 2011. Code of Ethics. Retrieved December 5, 2014 from: http://www.abft.org/index.php?option=com_content&view=article&id=56&Itemid=65.

Lemos, N.P., 2005. Postcard from America—post-mortem forensic toxicology [Electronic version]. Med. Sci. Law 45 (3), 185–186.

Rejent, T.A., 1981. Collection and storage of evidence. In: Cravey, R.H., Baselt, R.C. (Eds.), Introduction to Forensic Toxicology. Biomedical Publications, Davis, CA.

Saady, J.J., 2001. Ethics for toxicologists: an examination of conscience. J. Anal. Toxicol. 25, 390–392.

Scientific Working Group for Forensic Toxicology (SWGTOX), 2013. Recommendations of the research, development, testing and evaluation committee. J. Anal. Toxicol. 37, 187–191.

Society of Forensic Toxicologists. Code of Ethics. Retrieved December 5, 2014 from: http://www.soft-tox.org/ethics.

U.S. Department of Justice. National Commission on Forensic Science, 2013. Retrieved December 6, 2014 from: http://www.justice.gov/ncfs.

Wenning, R., Uges, D., Pierce, A., Rivier, L., Lewis, J., Jones, G. Code of Conduct for TIAFT Members. Retrieved August 5, 2012 from: http://www.tiaft.org/node/46.

Winek, C.L., 1973. The adversary system: role of the forensic toxicologist. J. For. Sci. 18, 178−183.

Forensic Toxicology Resources

Knowledge is of two kinds. We know a subject ourselves, or we know where we can find information upon it. When we inquire into any subject, the first thing we have to do is to know what books have treated it.
Samuel Johnson

This chapter is a compilation of selected books, journals, online resources, and organizations from which information of direct or ancillary importance to forensic toxicology may be found.

Maintaining competence is of obvious importance to forensic toxicologists. This can be achieved by attending symposia, professional meetings, continuing education courses, academic courses, and by reading the relevant literature in forensic toxicology. Fortunately, there is a wealth of resources that may be used to achieve this goal.

A rapid development of analytical methods, especially immunological and instrumental methods, occurred in the second half of the twentieth century. Concurrently, there were advances in the understanding of drug disposition, pharmacodynamics, pharmacogenomics, and toxicogenomics, all of which improved the interpretation of analytical results. Such advances have been the foundation of the development and progress that has occurred in forensic toxicology over the same period. The resulting increase in the body of knowledge in forensic toxicology has spurred the creation of professional organizations and the publication of books and journals devoted largely or exclusively to forensic toxicology. These organizations and printed materials provide a mechanism for a more rapid and widespread dissemination of information of value to the increasing number of forensic toxicologists.

The expert or peer review of the publications in forensic toxicology, the bulwark of reliability, requires that persons withstanding in their professions opine whether material presented for publication is reliable by assessing "... whether the measurements are reasonable, whether the data make sense and whether the data presented support the conclusions the authors want to draw" (Gaennslen, 2001).

Although books and journals arguably remain the mainstay of the record in forensic toxicology, the means of transmitting the knowledge contained in these volumes has undergone a transformation with the advent of the internet. Accordingly, the internet allows forensic toxicologists to seek out information on a topic

Forensic Toxicology. http://dx.doi.org/10.1016/B978-0-12-799967-8.00003-7

of interest by the use of searchable databases that catalog articles published in many hundreds of journals worldwide. The internet has allowed rapid dissemination of research findings as articles from many journals are available online prior to, or shortly after, their print publication. In addition, archival materials extending back many decades, as well as journals that appear exclusively online without a print version, are also available. Thorough literature searches, which previously required hours or days of work examining many volumes of printed databases, now may be completed entirely online in a fraction of the time. Not only can such a search be completed in a matter of minutes rather than days, but the desired articles may be obtained online and printed at the desk. This process remains somewhat a miracle to those of us who wrestled with the monthly and yearly volumes of *Index Medicus* and stalked the library stacks in search of elusive articles, which when located had to be carried to the copier to produce copies to take back to our offices. All of this, in addition to walking barefoot in the snow uphill both ways! The internet has become so dominant for the dissemination and retrieval of information that many libraries have decreased their subscriptions of print journals and rely exclusively on the online versions of publications. Unfortunately, as a wise man once said "There is no free lunch" and, therefore, accompanying the advantages provided by the internet is the problem of reliability. Since there is much material posted directly on the internet without first having been subjected to the checks and balances of peer review, a great deal of potentially unreliable information is now available in the public forum where it may be accepted as reliable by the uncritical.

What follows is a compilation of resources that is not meant to be, and cannot be, exhaustive, but rather is intended to provide an introduction to the resources that are available to forensic toxicologists. Many of the books and journals listed are available online by subscription.

3.1 BOOKS

Forensic toxicology has been nurtured by the publication of books and journals dedicated to issues of specific interest and importance to forensic toxicologists. These materials have become the body of knowledge of forensic toxicology that has grown virtually exponentially during the mid-twentieth century and into the twenty-first century. What follows is only a sampling of the many books that are of value to forensic toxicologists.

3.1.1 HISTORICAL CLASSICS

These books present a fascinating and informative look at the formative years of a science, the men who created this science and their thought processes. The brilliance, creativity, and personalities of these men who founded and nurtured forensic toxicology through its infancy are readily apparent. Fortunately, several of the historical works in forensic toxicology, such as the works of Orfila and Christison, are now available online. Both practitioners and students of forensic toxicology would benefit from reading as much of these works as possible in order to gain an appreciation for the patience and skill of the scientists who performed the tedious and laborious methods of analysis and who wrestled with the problems of interpretation in the early days of the discipline; their accomplishments are the foundation of modern forensic toxicology. Much of the content of these historical and modern classics is relevant to us in the twenty-first century, and learning about the history of the science is a rewarding experience that should be a component of the training of all forensic toxicologists.

- Orfila, M.P., 1817. *A General System of Toxicology or a Treatise on Poisons Found in the Mineral Vegetable and Animal Kingdoms Considered in Their Relations with Physiology Pathology and Medical Jurisprudence (Abridged and partly translated by J.G. Nancrede)*, Philadelphia: M. Carey and Son. Available at http://books.google.com/books?id=a34XAQAAMAAJ&pg=PA461&lpg= PA461&dq=m+AND+toxicology+fodere&source=bl&ots=XCB6oGgEBP& sig=X1nFL0Q0GqCqMy1ZQu-BNiLB8Jw&hl=en&sa=X&ei=4QcMUNPv FMXs0gGE_83tAw&ved=0CDMQ6AEwAQ#v=onepage&q=m%20AND% 20toxicology%20fodere&f=false
- Christison, R., 1829. *A Treatise on Poisons in Relation to Medical Jurisprudence, Physiology and the Practice of Physic, 3rd ed.*, Edinburgh: Adam Black. Available at http://books.google.com/books?id=mQEAAAAAQAAJ&printsec =frontcover&source=gbs_ge_summary_r&cad=0#v=onepage&q=reinsch& f=false
- Otto, F.J., 1857. *A Manual of the Detection of Poisons, by Medico-chemical Analysis*, New York: H. Baillier. Available at http://books.google.com/books? id=Ho5n8eT3hPYC&printsec=frontcover&dq=%22friedrich+julius+otto% 22&source=bl&ots=vt4Z4UkZuA&sig=7KttvOL6KiSVniiiMAVjw5V5CTQ &hl=en&ei=9u5zTL7aNoL-8Aav7PmFCQ&sa=X&oi=book_result&ct= result&resnum=6&ved=0CCUQ6AEwBQ#v=onepage&q=Stas&f=false
- Wharton, F. and Stillé, M., 1855. *A Treatise on medical jurisprudence, 2nd ed.*, Philadelphia: Kay and Brother. Available at http://books.google.com/books? id=pOrXtaqL9n0C&printsec=frontcover&source=gbs_gesummary_r&cad= 0#v=onepage&q&f=false
- Wormley, T., 1867. *Micro-Chemistry of Poisons, Including Their Physiological, Pathological, and Legal Relations, Adapted to the Use of the Medical Jurist, Physician, and General Chemist*, New York: Baillier Brothers. Available at https://play.google.com/books/reader?id=Vgg1AQAAMAAJ&printsec= frontcover&output=reader&authuser=0&hl=en
- Taylor, A.S., 1848. *On Poisons in Relation to Medical Jurisprudence and Medicine (Edited and with additions by R.E. Griffith), 2nd ed.*, Philadelphia: Lea & Blanchard. Available at http://books.google.com/books?id=WLQ0AA AAIAAJ&printsec=frontcover&source=gbs_ge_summary_r&cad=0#v=one page&q&f=false

- Reese, J.J., 1874. *A Manual of Toxicology, Including the Consideration of the Nature, Properties, Effects, and Means of Detection of Poisons, More Especially in Their Medico-legal Relations*, Philadelphia: J.B. Lippincott & Co. Available at http://www.archive.org/stream/manualoftoxicolo00reesiala/manualoftoxicolo00reesiala_djvu.txt
- Stas, J.S., 1894. **Oeuvres Completes**, Brussels. Available at http://archive.org/stream/oeuvrescomplte02stasuoft#page/n7/mode/2up
- Stewart, C.P. and Stolman, A., eds., 1960. *Toxicology: Mechanisms and Analytical Methods, vols. 1 and 2.* New York: Academic Press. This book was perhaps the authoritative analytical toxicology treatise of its time. It contained chapters dealing with the disposition and mechanism of action of a number of substances including drugs, metals, and gases as well as descriptions of the modern methods of analysis of the time such as liquid–liquid extraction methods, UV spectrophotometry, paper chromatography, and microdiffusion.
- Stolman, A., ed. 1963–1974. *Progress in Chemical Toxicology, vols. 1–5.* New York: Academic Press. This series expanded on *Toxicology: Mechanisms and Analytical Methods* and presented the decade-long progress in disposition, analysis, and interpretation.
- Curry, A.S., 1972. *Advances in Forensic and Clinical Toxicology.* Cleveland: CRC Press. This is a thorough review of the literature of the time pertaining to methods of detection and interpretation of results for a wide variety of substances including drugs of abuse, metals, plant, and animal poisons.

3.1.2 FORENSIC AND ANALYTICAL TOXICOLOGY

Collectively, these books along with those in Sections 3.1.3 and 3.1.4 can serve as a core of the library of the modern forensic toxicologist.

- Baselt, R.C., 2014. *Disposition of Toxic Drugs and Chemicals in Man, 10th ed.*, Seal Beach, CA: Biomedical Publications. This reference, which was first published in 1977, contains monographs of hundreds of drugs and chemicals providing a summary of the disposition including tissue and fluid concentrations, e.g., blood, urine, and liver, consistent with therapy and toxicity in both antemortem and postmortem cases. This work has become a standard reference book for forensic toxicologists, often serving as the first stop in a literature search.
- Cravey, R.H. and Baselt, R.C., eds., 1981. *Introduction to Forensic Toxicology.* Davis, California: Biomedical Publications. This book is true to its title as it serves as an introduction to the theory and practice of forensic toxicology. The chapters cover the pharmacological, toxicological, pathological, and analytical foundations of forensic toxicology as well as the roles and functions of forensic toxicologists.
- Drummer, O.H., 2001. *The Forensic Pharmacology of Drugs of Abuse.* London: Arnold. As the name suggests, this book is a description of the pharmacokinetics

and pharmacodynamics of several of the most common drugs of abuse. Case reports demonstrating the application of these concepts to forensic toxicology are included.

- Flanagan, R.J., Taylor, A., Watson, I.D. and Whelpton, R., 2007. *Fundamentals of Analytical Toxicology.* Hoboken, New Jersey: John Wiley and Sons, Ltd. This book provides a thorough description of the principles of analytical toxicology from sample collection to the most common methods of analysis that are used. Also included are chapters on drug disposition and interpretation of analytical results. Although directed largely at the clinical analytical toxicologist, there is much here for the forensic toxicologist.

- Levine, B., ed. 2010. *Principles of Forensic Toxicology, 3rd ed.*, Washington, DC: American Association for Clinical Chemistry. This book is divided into three sections: Introduction, Methodologies, and Analytes and summarizes the widely used methods of analytical toxicology and the toxicology of common drugs of abuse.

- Moffat, A.C., Osselton, M.D., Widdop, B. and Watts, J., eds., 2011. *Clarke's Analysis of Drugs and Poisons, 4th ed.*, London: The Pharmaceutical Press. Originally published as *Clarke's Isolation and Identification of Drugs* in 1969, this is an extensive presentation of toxicological information and methods of analysis for hundreds of compounds. The latest edition, approximately 2500 pages in 2 volumes, contains more than 2000 drug monographs as well as chapters on modern methods of analysis. In addition, there is an abbreviated version published as *Clarke's Analytical Forensic Toxicology* that is more suitable in content and price for students.

- Caplan, Y.H. and Goldberger, B.A. (eds.), 2014. *Garriott's Medicolegal Aspects of Alcohol, 6th ed.*, Tucson, Arizona: Lawyers & Judges Publishing Company.

3.1.3 PHARMACOLOGY AND TOXICOLOGY

In addition to the above listed books that are specifically intended for the forensic toxicologist, texts in the foundational disciplines of pharmacology, general toxicology, medicinal chemistry, and pathology should be included in the libraries of forensic toxicologists.

- L. Brunton et al., ed. 2010. *Goodman and Gilman's The Pharmacological Basis of Therapeutics, 12th ed.*, New York: McGraw-Hill. This book, the first edition of which was published more than 70 years ago, is often referred to as the "bible of pharmacology." The basic and clinical pharmacology of virtually all drugs of clinical and forensic interest are presented.

- Klaasen, C.D., ed. 2008. *Casarett and Doull's Toxicology: The Basic Science of Poisons, 7th ed.*, New York: McGraw-Hill. This one-volume text of general toxicology including toxicokinetics, mechanisms of toxicity, organ, and nonorgan-based toxicity is an excellent introduction to the science of toxicology.

- Karch, S.B., 2006. *Drug Abuse Handbook, 2nd ed.*, Boca Raton, FL: CRC Press. A wide-ranging presentation of the pharmacokinetics, pharmacodynamics, pathology, and forensic considerations of drugs of abuse.
- Karch, S.B. and Drummer, O., 2012. *Karsh's Pathology of Drug Abuse.* Boca Raton, FL: CRC Press. A presentation of the pathology and toxicology of several classes of abused drugs, including the investigation of drug-related deaths.
- Advokat, C.D., Comaty, J.E. and Julien, R.M., 2014. *A Primer of Drug Action, 13th ed.*, New York: Worth Publishers.
- R.E. Ferner, 1996. *Forensic Pharmacology*, New York: Oxford University Press.

3.1.4 CLINICAL PHARMACOLOGY AND TOXICOLOGY

These sources contain information on overdoses including the mechanisms of toxicity, toxic doses, signs and symptoms of toxicity, and interpretation of drug concentrations.

- Barceloux, D.G., 2012. *Medical Toxicology of Drug Abuse: Synthesized Chemicals and Psychoactive Plants.* New York: John Wiley & Sons Inc.
- Ellenhorn, M.J., 1997. *Ellenhorn's Medical Toxicology: Diagnosis and Treatment of Human Poisoning, 2nd ed.*, Baltimore: Williams and Wilkins. This valuable companion to *Goodman and Gilman* is an exhaustive presentation of the clinical toxicology of therapeutic and abused drugs as well as natural toxins, biological and chemical warfare agents, metals, and industrial chemicals.
- Ford, R., ed. 2001. *Clinical Toxicology.* Philadelphia: W. B. Saunders Company.
- Olson, K.R., ed. 2007. *Poisoning & Drug Overdose, 5th ed.*, New York: McGraw-Hill.

3.1.5 MISCELLANEOUS TOPICS

- Dimaio, D.J. and Dimaio, V.J.M. 1993. *Forensic Pathology.* Boca Raton, FL: CRC Press.
- Nogrady, T. and Weaver, D.F. 2005. *Medicinal Chemistry: A Molecular and Biochemical Approach, 3rd ed.,* New York: Oxford University Press.
- Jablonski, S. 2009. *Dictionary of Medical Acronyms & Abbreviations*, 6th ed., Philadelphia, PA: Saunders Elsevier.
- Williamson, M.A. and Snyder, L.M. 2005. *Wallach's Interpretation of Diagnostic Tests, 10th ed.*, Philadelphia, PA: Wolters Kluwer.

3.2 JOURNALS

There are many refereed journals that publish articles of specific interest to forensic toxicologists, whereas others publish articles of widespread forensic interest, including forensic toxicology as well as other forensic disciplines. These journals are available in print and also online, generally to subscribers or members of the organizations that publish them.

- *The Journal of Analytical Toxicology*: This journal publishes articles dealing with methods of toxicological analysis and interpretation of analytical results. It has become a "go to" journal for forensic toxicologists
- *Journal of the American Academy of Forensic Sciences*: This is the official publication of the American Academy of Forensic Sciences
- *Science and Law*: This publication of the Forensic Science Society of Great Britain was formerly published as *The Journal of the Forensic Science Society*
- *Canadian Society of Forensic Science Journal:* This is the official publication of the Canadian Society of Forensic Science
- *Forensic Science International*: This journal formerly was published as *Forensic Science*
- *The American Journal of Clinical and Forensic Pathology*
- *The International Journal of Legal Medicine*
- *Legal Medicine*
- *Drug Testing and Analysis*

3.3 WEB RESOURCES

- *PubMed* (http://www.ncbi.nlm.nih.gov/pubmed): This search engine, which is a service of the National Center for Biotechnology Information (NCBI), at the U.S. National Library of Medicine (NLM), located at the National Institutes of Health (NIH), is the premier search site for biomedical literature, including numerous journals of interest to forensic toxicologists. PubMed allows keyword access to more than 20 million citations from MedLine. These citations may contain abstracts, links to additional citations on the same topic, and links to full text articles. By means of the My NCBI feature, alerts of newly published articles on requested topics are sent by e-mail and may be saved in desired categories.
- *Web of Science* (http://thomsonreuters.com/products_services/science/science_products/a-z/web_of_science): The Web of Science provides a number of search services for the retrieval of literature information. For example, searches made for a specific published article will provide the following: the number of times and the articles in which the citation has been cited, the references cited in the citation, and other journal articles and books related to those references. This information allows for the easy identification of articles related to the topic of the article being searched and of relevant articles published since the publication of the cited article, allowing the search to be brought up to date from the date of the searched article's publication.
- *Government Sites:* The U.S. government maintains a number of sites containing a wealth of information about the disposition, pharmacology, and animal and

human toxicity studies of an extensive number of drugs and chemicals. This information is presented in the form of various types of publications including data sheets, including monographs. There are also links to other databases inside and outside the agency. These sites include:

- The Occupational Health and Safety administration (OSHA) http://www.osha.gov
- The National Institute for Occupation Safety and Health (NIOSH) http://www.cdc.gov/niosh/
- Toxicology Data Network (ToxNet) http://toxnet.nlm.nih.gov/
- Agency for Toxic Substances and Disease Registry (ATSDR) http://www.atsdr.cdc.gov/

- *RTI Training Programs* (https://www.forensiced.org/index.cfm): RTI International Center for Forensic Sciences provides Web-based training programs in forensic toxicology and related areas. Registration is required to receive free live and on-demand programs.

3.4 PROFESSIONAL ORGANIZATIONS

Several organizations that are devoted to forensic toxicology and forensic toxicologists have been established to serve the needs of the profession. In addition, organizations that advance the needs of all forensic scientists include sections devoted exclusively to forensic toxicologists. These organizations offer many services to their members including hosting meetings, publishing bulletins and monographs, sponsoring research and training grants, and maintaining employment information. These organizations and their own statements describing their purposes and functions are presented below.

- *The American Academy of Forensic Sciences (AAFS):* "The American Academy of Forensic Sciences is a multi-disciplinary professional organization that provides leadership to advance science and its application to the legal system. The objectives of the Academy are to promote professionalism, integrity, competency, education, foster research, improve practice, and encourage collaboration in the forensic sciences" (The American Academy of Forensic Sciences, accessed 23.08.12).
- *The International Association of Forensic Toxicologists (TIAFT):* The aims of this association are as follows: "To provide an organization of professionals engaged or interested in the field of forensic toxicology or related areas of analytical toxicology, including the interpretation of the results of these analyses. To promote cooperation and coordination of effort among members. To encourage research in and the practice of forensic toxicology and related areas of analytical toxicology. To provide a forum for the discussion and

exchange of professional experiences in forensic toxicology and related areas of analytical toxicology between forensic toxicologists and all other interested parties. To promote education and training in forensic toxicology and related areas of analytical toxicology" (The International Association of Forensic Toxicologists, accessed August 23, 2012).

- *The Society of Forensic Toxicologists (SOFT):* "The Society of Forensic Toxicologists, Inc. is an organization composed of practicing forensic toxicologists and those interested in the discipline for the purpose of promoting and developing forensic toxicology. Through its annual meetings, the Society provides a forum for the exchange of information and ideas among toxicology professionals in a friendly, relaxed atmosphere. SOFT-sponsored programs such as workshops, newsletters, proficiency testing and SOFT-sponsored technical publications constantly improve the forensic toxicologists' skills and knowledge. The Society fosters friendship and cooperation among toxicologists and advocates a high level of professionalism by sponsoring certification programs for its members" (Society of Forensic Toxicologists).

- *The American Board of Forensic Toxicology (ABFT):* "The purpose of the American Board of Forensic Toxicology is to establish and enhance voluntary standards for the practice of forensic toxicology and for the examination and recognition of scientists and laboratories providing forensic toxicology services" (The American Board of Forensic Toxicology, accessed August 23, 2012). ABFT offers certifications for forensic toxicologists and forensic toxicology laboratories.

- *The Forensic Sciences Foundation:* "The Forensic Sciences Foundation, Inc., founded in 1969, is a nonprofit organization studying the application of science to the resolution of social and legal issues. The overall objectives of the Foundation are: to develop and conduct education and training programs; to develop new ways to improve the forensic sciences; to promote public education concerning all disciplines in the forensic sciences; and to support research in fields relating to the forensic sciences" (The Forensic Sciences Foundation, accessed August 23, 2012).

REVIEW QUESTIONS

1. What are some ways in which forensic toxicologists can stay current within the field?
2. What are the major types of resources of use to a forensic toxicologist?
3. What are the professional organizations to which a forensic toxicologist might typically belong? What are the advantages of being a member of a professional organization?
4. What governmental organizations provide resources to forensic toxicologists?

APPLICATION QUESTIONS

1. Discuss why peer review is considered to be the standard of reliability within the scientific literature. What are some key elements of peer review that make it a valuable process? Describe some alternative methods of publication, which do not employ peer review; what are the advantages and disadvantages of these mechanism?

2. Select a book of relevance to a forensic toxicologist and describe the significance of the volume. What topics does the book cover? Why would the book be of value to a forensic toxicologist?

3. Describe several online resources that you, as a forensic toxicologist, might find useful. What are some advantages and disadvantages of utilizing Web-based resources? Are there any special considerations that must be acknowledged when using online resources?

REFERENCES

Gaennslen, R., 2001. Informatics and scientific information exchange in forensic toxicology. J. For. Sci. 25, 386—389.

Society of Forensic Toxicologists. Code of Ethics. Retrieved December 5, 2014 from: http://www.soft-tox.org/ethics.

The American Academy of Forensic Sciences. From: http://www.aafs.org (accessed 23.08.12).

The American Board of Forensic Toxicology. From: http://www.abft.org (accessed 23.08.12).

The Forensic Sciences Foundation. From: http://www.forensicsciencesfoundation.org/FP.htm (accessed 23.08.12).

The International Association of Forensic Toxicologists. From: http://www.tiaft.org/documents/tiaft_brochure.pdf (accessed 23.08.12).

The Laboratory

4

Ideally, public forensic science laboratories should be independent of or autonomous within law enforcement agencies.
National Academy of Sciences, 2009

The goals of analyses that are conducted in forensic toxicology laboratories are the detection, identification, and/or quantitation of any drugs and exogenous chemicals that are present in the samples collected. These analyses must be conducted in appropriately staffed and equipped forensic toxicology laboratories in which validated procedures and methods are employed.

4.1 ADMINISTRATIVE LOCATION OF THE LABORATORY

Generally, the analyses associated with each branch of forensic toxicology are conducted in different characteristic types of laboratories: postmortem toxicology for the detection of drugs in urine, blood, and semisolid tissues is conducted in laboratories affiliated with medical examiner's and coroner's offices, whereas the detection of drugs in urine, saliva, hair, and oral fluid collected from living subjects for purposes of human-performance toxicology including preemployment testing, forcause testing after an accident, and parole monitoring are often performed in private commercial laboratories, hospital laboratories, and forensic laboratories not administratively affiliated with medical examiner or coroners' offices. In 2009, publicly funded forensic toxicology laboratories received approximately 600,000 requests for analyses of which the majority were for the analyses of antemortem samples for ethanol and other drugs, and 40% for the analyses of postmortem samples (Durose et al., 2012).

Many publically funded forensic science laboratories, including a number of forensic toxicology laboratories, are under the administrative control of law enforcement agencies or prosecutorial offices of the executive branch of government. This is an undesirable situation as it conveys the impression that forensic scientists are a component of the prosecution, rather than a nonprosecutorial scientific agency. Although forensic toxicology laboratories are less likely to be administered in this manner, there often is a very close working relationship between the forensic toxicology laboratory and these prosecutorial agencies. It is of great concern that

Forensic Toxicology. http://dx.doi.org/10.1016/B978-0-12-799967-8.00004-9

forensic scientists working under the purview of governmental agencies sense or are under pressure to enhance the interpretation of their findings in order to support the prosecution of a case and as a result may have their objectivity compromised. Because the prosecution of a case is the duty of the prosecutor, not the forensic toxicologist, it is essential that forensic toxicologists are free to present all scientific findings that may have probative value, whether they are of value to the prosecution or not. In recognition of this inherent problem of a potential conflict of interest, the National Research Council has suggested that the federal government should provide funds to be used for removing forensic laboratories from the organizational management of police or prosecutors' offices (Of Interest 4.1).

The problem of administrative control has been addressed in jurisdictions in which forensic science laboratories currently are administered by nonprosecutorial offices in the executive branch of government. For example, in Washington, DC, administration of the new Consolidated Forensic Laboratory, which includes the medical examiner's toxicology laboratory, is not under the administrative control of the police or prosecutors—instead, the laboratory director of the Consolidated Forensic Laboratory reports directly to the mayor (Hamilton and Alexander, 2012). In Virginia, the Department of Forensic Sciences is one of the 14 separate state agencies within the office of the Secretary of Public Safety, which also includes agencies with law enforcement and prosecutorial functions (Virginia.gov).

OF INTEREST 4.1 THE NATIONAL RESEARCH COUNCIL REPORT

"Strengthening Forensic Science in the United States: A Path Forward" was the result of an exhaustive study by a committee of The National Research Council Report of several problems facing the forensic sciences. This committee was composed of forensic scientists, attorneys, and statisticians who heard testimony from numerous forensic science stakeholders. The report contains a detailed analysis of the problems facing the forensic sciences as well as recommendations for the solution of those problems.

The independence of forensic science laboratories and a related recommendation were addressed by the committee and are presented below.

Independence of Forensic Science Laboratories

"The majority of forensic science laboratories are administered by law enforcement agencies, such as police departments, where the laboratory administrator reports to the head of the agency. This system leads to significant concerns related to the independence of the laboratory and its budget. Ideally, public forensic science laboratories should be independent of or autonomous within law enforcement agencies. In these contexts, the director would have an equal voice with others in the justice system on matters involving the laboratory and other agencies. The laboratory also would be able to set its own priorities with respect to cases, expenditures, and other important issues. Cultural pressures caused by the different missions of scientific laboratories vis-a-vis law enforcement agencies would be largely resolved. Finally, the forensic science laboratories would be able to set their own budget priorities and not have to compete with the parent law enforcement agencies."

Recommendation of the Committee

"To improve the scientific bases of forensic science examinations and to maximize independence from or autonomy within the law enforcement community, Congress should authorize and appropriate incentive funds to the National Institute of Forensic Science (NIFS) for allocation to state and local jurisdictions for the purpose of removing all public forensic laboratories and facilities from the administrative control of law enforcement agencies or prosecutors' offices."

An alternative to the control of forensic laboratories, including forensic toxicology laboratories, by the executive branch of government is the control by the legislative branch (an unpleasant thought and a situation that would be fraught with the potential for political machinations) or the judicial branch. Forensic laboratories under the administrative control of the judicial branch of government would be independent of prosecutorial and law enforcement agencies. It is reasonable to consider that such a situation would free forensic scientists from any pressure (real or perceived) to act in a manner supportive of the prosecutorial team. The laboratories could freely conduct analyses that are scientifically appropriate and provide the results to all parties on an equal basis. Forensic scientists would perform analyses, write reports submitted to both of the parties in a case, and then meet with both parties simultaneously to provide equal access to the information of the laboratory. Forensic scientists would perform the same functions, at the same level, as they do presently; however, their entire work product—analyses conducted, results, interpretations, comments, written or oral reports, etc.—would be made available equally, completely, and simultaneously to both the prosecution and defense. Any information transmitted to one party would be transmitted to the other without the need for subpoena. In addition to the information provided by the judicial forensic scientist, either party would have the option of obtaining its own additional and confidential experts, although it might be anticipated that due to the complete transparency of the system, this option would not be exercised extensively. The location of the forensic laboratory in the judicial branch could reasonably be expected to increase the likelihood of greater impartiality of forensic scientists, including forensic toxicologists. In short, such a placement of forensic laboratories would presumably serve to retain forensic scientists as important impartial components of the legal system, but not as adversaries. Regardless of the administrative control under which a forensic toxicology laboratory is placed, however, the internal structure of the laboratory must possess several key organizational components as described below.

4.2 PERSONNEL

Central to the successful administration of a forensic toxicology laboratory is the clear and transparent description and monitoring of personnel duties and responsibilities. The various personnel positions in forensic toxicology laboratories and the specific duties and authority associated with each position must be described in detail to the individual members of the laboratory staff and to position applicants. Well-defined job descriptions, including educational and experiential requirements, should be established for each of the laboratory positions. Furthermore, the training, periodic evaluation, and continuing education requirements of personnel should be explicitly described, administered, and monitored in a systematic manner. Certification as a diplomate of the Board (ABFT 1) or specialist in forensic toxicology (ABFT 2) may be obtained from the American Board of Forensic Toxicology and may be required in some laboratories. Both certifications require 3 years of full-time professional experience or the equivalent and successful performance on a written examination. In addition, the requirements for certification as a diplomate of the American Board of Forensic Toxicology (DABFT) or as a specialist in forensic toxicology include a doctor of philosophy (or doctor of science) or a bachelor's degree, respectively.

It is apparent that forensic toxicologists in the twenty-first century begin their professional careers with more formal education in forensic toxicology than was the case in the past when it was common that chemists and biologists learned virtually all of their forensic toxicology "at the bench." Although this bench training continues to be essential, it no longer constitutes the major form of education or training for new forensic toxicologists since several colleges and universities offer both academic courses and programs in forensic toxicology at the undergraduate and graduate levels. These educational opportunities enable new forensic toxicologists to develop an understanding of the principles and concepts of forensic toxicology and often to gain some practical experience as interns in forensic toxicology laboratories, before beginning their careers.

Although the duties and functions required of the personnel in all well-run forensic toxicology laboratories are the same, there may be differences in the titles of the positions depending upon the type of forensic toxicology laboratory and the size of the staff.

4.2.1 CHIEF TOXICOLOGIST[1]

Chief toxicologists, also designated as laboratory directors, are the administrative and scientific directors of forensic toxicology laboratories. Since chief toxicologists direct the overall operation of all aspects of the laboratory, they ultimately are accountable for the successes, as well as the failures, of the laboratory.

Generally, the requirements for this position include either a master's degree or doctorate, usually in an appropriate science such as forensic science, toxicology, or analytical chemistry. Additionally, several years of bench and supervisory laboratory experience are commonly required. Training and education in areas such as personnel or organizational management also would be beneficial for chief toxicologists.

The roles of chief toxicologists require that they develop, as well as directly manage and administer, several diverse laboratory functions, which are summarized below.

- **Hiring and training of the laboratory staff**: Hiring staff members is one of the most important functions of chief toxicologists because a well-educated and skilled staff is essential if laboratories are to provide accurate results and

---

[1]In human-performance toxicology and forensic drug-testing laboratories, several of the functions of the Chief Toxicologist, e.g., review of analytical results, interpretation of results, and testifying, may be within the purview of the medical review officer.

interpretations with competence, efficiency, and professionalism. Chief toxicologists should establish programs of continuing education, training, and periodic evaluation of the staff, both of which should be clearly described and conducted in a systematic manner. These programs will serve to maintain the skill of the staff at high level consistent with technical advances and to identify and correct any deficiencies of performance. Staff members must possess the appropriate education and experience and be provided with any additional training required for them to perform their specific and well-defined duties successfully if the laboratory is to achieve the goals of providing dependable results and interpretations.

- **Development and implementation of analytical methods**: The detection of drugs in biological materials is a continually evolving and improving process due to both the continual development and availability of new therapeutic and abused drugs and the rapidly increasing advances in analytical and instrumental chemistry. Therefore, it is necessary that existing analytical methods are altered or new methods are adopted as needed to ensure that laboratories keep pace with new developments in drug development and analytical toxicology.

- **Design and implementation of quality control (QC) and quality assurance (QA) programs**: The proper operation of a modern forensic toxicology laboratory necessitates that the work products of the laboratory, i.e., analytical results, are of the highest degree of accuracy that the laboratory can provide. In order to achieve this, the laboratory must have a quality QC/QA program in place. QC/QA programs are managed by chief toxicologists, or designated members of the staff who report directly to them. In summary, QC/QA programs should include well-described methods for the establishment of a standard operating manual (SOP); control charts; instrument calibration and maintenance; validation methods; and complete and thorough record keeping, including instrument logs, methods of reagent preparation, and custody of analytical results. QC/QA programs are discussed in greater detail in Chapter 11.

- **Review of analytical results and approval of official reports**: Chief toxicologists have the ultimate responsibility for the accuracy of all laboratory results and, therefore, they, or a designated member of the staff, sign all official laboratory reports after they have been reviewed to ensure that the results are consistent with the QC/QA criteria.

- **Rendering of interpretations and opinions**: Generally, chief toxicologists confer with other members of the medical investigative team, especially the medical examiner, and offer opinions based on the analytical results obtained by the forensic toxicology laboratory. This duty requires that chief toxicologists have knowledge not only of the analytical methods employed, including their limitations, but also of the pharmacology and toxicology of the drugs involved.

Historically, it has been customary that chief toxicologists have had the responsibility of appearing in court to testify as to the results of toxicological analyses performed in their laboratories as well as to the meaning and significance of these results. However, in light of recent Supreme Court decisions, this practice has changed (Chapter 15), and the staff toxicologist who performed the analysis may now be required to present this testimony instead of the chief toxicologist. This change in protocol has necessitated that staff members receive additional training to prepare them for the presentation of sworn testimony.

4.2.2 ASSISTANT CHIEF TOXICOLOGIST

The assistant chief toxicologist position is a supervisory position held by an upper level scientist whose duties include management of the day-to-day operation of the laboratory, personnel training, methods review, development and validation of analytical methods, performance of special or nonroutine analyses, and administration of QC measures including the design of internal proficiency evaluation programs and the participation in external proficiency evaluation programs. Assistant chief toxicologists, who frequently have advanced degrees, commonly will assist the chief toxicologist in the development of the specific components of the described activities and will oversee their implementation.

4.2.3 TOXICOLOGIST I AND II

Usually the toxicologist I position is an entry-level position and requires a bachelor's or master's degree. The duties of these toxicologists include performing specific routine analyses such as presumptive (screening) testing, maintaining instruments, and record keeping. The toxicologist II position generally requires similar educational requirements as the toxicologist I positions, but in addition requires relevant experience in a forensic toxicology laboratory. The analytical duties of forensic toxicologists II include performing more sophisticated methods of analysis such as confirmatory methods. Toxicologists II may also participate in the development and validation of new analytical methods.

4.2.4 TECHNICIANS

Technician positions are generally support positions consisting of routine, nonanalytical duties such as the preparation of solutions and reagents, maintenance of reagent and chemical inventories, and care of noninstrumental materials. Unlike other staff members, technicians do not handle samples or conduct analyses and therefore, they do not testify as to analytical results or their interpretations.

4.3 LABORATORY DESIGN (NATIONAL INSTITUTE OF JUSTICE, 1998)

Forensic toxicology laboratories must be designed so that the functions and responsibilities of the laboratory are accomplished accurately, safely, and efficiently. In a well-designed laboratory, space will be divided and allocated for purposes of analytical operations and administrative functions. Of course, the specific areas located within the laboratory, as well as the size of each area, will vary dependent on the size of the case load, number of employees, and analytical responsibilities of the laboratory.

4.3.1 ANALYTICAL SPACE

All of the analytical functions of forensic toxicology laboratories should not be conducted in a single space, but rather in separate, dedicated, laboratories designed and equipped with the equipment necessary for the specific types of analyses conducted therein. The space allotted for analytical procedures should be separated on the basis of the type of procedures being conducted. For example, there should be a wet chemistry laboratory in which sample preparation, including procedures such as protein precipitations, liquid—liquid extractions, and solid-phase extractions are performed. In this same space, analyses such as color tests and immunoassays may be conducted. A separate laboratory would house analytical instrumentation such as gas chromatographs (GCs), liquid chromatographs (LCs), and mass spectrometers (MSs).

4.3.2 ADMINISTRATIVE SPACE

The administrative area should include office space for the chief and assistant chief forensic toxicologists as well as work space that can be used by other members of the laboratory staff to perform necessary case-related "paper work" such as reviewing results, completing lab reports, and entering data into case files. In addition, laboratory administrative space should include a conference room in which the staff can meet for discussions pertaining to laboratory operations and specific cases. The conference room may double as a library in which relevant reference books and journals in forensic toxicology, pharmacology, physiology, biochemistry, instrumental analysis, and standard operating manuals and operation manuals for the instruments in the laboratory are available. In laboratories with a large case load, there may be need for specific space designated for the receipt and processing of incoming samples.

4.3.3 MISCELLANEOUS SPACE

The successful functioning of a forensic toxicology laboratory is also dependent on the inclusion of lab space that is allocated to the miscellaneous functions of the laboratory, including functions such as reagent preparation and sample storage. Reagents should be prepared apart from the analytical spaces in a suitably large area that is equipped with the necessary materials and equipment, for example, fume hoods, balances, and glassware. Space sufficient for the accommodation of large walk-in refrigerators and freezers must be available for the long-term storage of samples.

4.4 LABORATORY EQUIPMENT

A forensic toxicology laboratory must possess the equipment necessary to perform three basic and distinct, but interrelated functions: analysis, storage, and safety. The type, number, and capacity of the equipment will depend upon the size of the laboratory and number of analyses performed. Although appropriate instrumentation is essential to the proper functioning of a forensic toxicology laboratory, only 37% of forensic toxicology laboratories within medical examiner/coroner's offices possess the requisite in-house analytical capabilities, necessitating costly analyses by external, often commercial, laboratories or even more undesirably, the failure to have the necessary analyses conducted (National Research Council, 2009). All laboratory equipment must be kept in proper operating condition by means of regularly scheduled maintenance. Records must be kept of the dates of any maintenance conducted, repairs completed, and calibrations performed to ensure the reliability of analytical results. All records of the dates of use, names of users, the purpose of use, and any comments concerning the functioning of a specific instrument must be maintained in a log book for each instrument.

The basic analytical instruments found in a typical forensic toxicology laboratory include GCs and LCs, as standalone instruments as well as coupled to various detectors including single or tandem MSs. MSs require a computer-based library containing spectra of compounds of interest including their metabolites and postmortem products and analytical artifacts. Certain of these instruments may be of research quality for special analyses and research projects, whereas others may be dedicated for specific analyses. For example, GCs may be dedicated for the detection and quantitation of volatiles, including ethanol, by headspace analysis. The detection and identification of elements, especially metals, may be achieved by atomic absorption spectroscopy or if greater speed and lower detection limits are required, by inductively coupled plasma mass spectrometry. The type of instruments used for immunoassays will vary depending upon the immunoassay being employed.

Fume hoods and ventilation equipment are especially important since a number of potentially harmful volatile organic compounds are used routinely for the extraction of drugs from samples. Specially designed cabinets and closets must be used for the storage of volatile and corrosive chemicals in a safe manner. There should be several refrigerators in the laboratory large enough to accommodate the samples from active cases. Ideally, these refrigerators should be explosion-proof, designed so that points of potential ignition are shielded, thus minimizing the likelihood of a fire or explosion resulting from the ignition of a flammable or explosive material. Laboratories should possess freezers that are capable of maintaining temperatures of approximately $-20°C$ for routine sample and reagent storage and also possibly additional freezers capable of maintaining temperatures of approximately -40 to $-85°C$ for the long-term storage of samples that have been analyzed. The security of all refrigerators and freezers must be maintained with limited access to authorized personnel. Refrigerators and freezers should be outfitted with a system that monitors temperatures and users and have a malfunction alarm.

4.5 LABORATORY SAFETY

The work being done in forensic toxicology laboratories is important, but not sufficiently important so as to endanger the health or well-being of the staff, which must be of the paramount importance. Although all risks and dangers cannot be eliminated completely, laboratories must establish the necessary policies and procedures and possess the appropriate safety materials and equipment in order to minimize the risks of working in the potentially dangerous environment of the laboratory and to protect the health and lives of the staff.

The two most common sources of danger in the forensic toxicology laboratory are the chemical reagents, such as volatile organic solvents and corrosive acids and bases, which are utilized routinely in forensic analyses, and the biological samples that are analyzed, which may contain infective agents such as tuberculosis, hepatitis B, and/or human immunodeficiency virus—this is especially true for samples that have been obtained from drug abusers (Flanagan et al., 2007, p. 21).

A safety manual, which must be available in the laboratory and kept up-to-date, is the mandatory reading by all members of the staff. In this manual, safety policies and procedures must be described including, at a minimum, procedures for the following: the proper handling and disposal of reagents and samples including infectious biological samples; the emergency remedies for biological and chemical spills; the response to personal injuries; and the operation of the safety equipment and materials.

Required safety equipment includes eyewash stations, overhead showers for chemical spills, fire extinguishers, fire blankets, absorbents, and neutralizers for chemical spills. The locations of this equipment as well as laboratory exits should be clearly marked with appropriate signs. Members of the staff should be provided with, and should wear, appropriate personal clothing and equipment such as lab coats, gloves, and goggles for protection against impact and chemicals splashes and spills. A member of the staff should be assigned the duty of ensuring that members of the laboratory staff are using the proper personal protective clothing and that the safety equipment are available, located in the proper location, and in proper working order.

Forensic toxicology laboratories must adhere to/comply with all relevant local, state, and federal regulations pertaining to laboratory safety and must take the necessary actions to insure that the functions of the laboratory may be performed in the safest possible manner. A summary of basic safety measures and sources for more extensive information concerning laboratory safety are presented in Tables 4.1 and 4.2, respectively.

Table 4.1 Safety Precautions *(Not listed in order of importance)*

- Wear laboratory coats and goggles while in the laboratory.
- Use other appropriate equipment, such as respirators, as appropriate.
- Familiarize yourself with the location and proper use of safety equipment, e.g., fire blanket, fire extinguisher, safety shower, eyewash station.
- Familiarize yourself with the hazards associated with any chemicals that you use. Material safety data sheets will provide this information for you.
- Treat biological samples as though they contain infectious agents.
- Always wear disposable plastic gloves when handling all biological materials.
- Wash hands thoroughly after handling any biological material and before leaving the laboratory.
- Do not pipette biological samples by mouth.
- Clean and/or disinfect, as appropriate, all bench tops, hoods, sinks, and all other work areas following each use.
- Clean any area contaminated with biological material with Clorox.
- Soak all glassware in a 1% hypochlorite solution prior to washing or disposal.
- Discard all disposable items that have been in contact with biological materials in sealed plastic bags.
- Flush all wastes that are discarded in a sink with a copious amount of cold water.
- Clean all spills of acids, bases, or volatile material immediately with appropriate kits provided for this purpose.
- Store all volatile solvents and reagents in appropriate containers in a solvent storage cabinet.
- Refrigerate volatile solvents and reagents only in an explosion-proof refrigerator.
- Use all volatile solvents in or near a hood, away from heat or flames.
- Carefully vent separatory funnels and other extraction vessels before continuing the extraction.
- Notify the appropriate person of all laboratory accidents. http://chemlabs.uoregon.edu/Safety/GeneralInstructions.html

Table 4.2 Guidelines for Laboratory Safety

Guidelines describing the appropriate laboratory safety protocols and procedures to be employed in a forensic toxicology laboratory may be found in the following resources:

1. Occupational and Safety Administration (OSHA): http://www.osha.gov/SLTC/healthguidelines/index.html
2. National Research Council: http://www.nap.edu/openbook.php?record%20id=12654&page=R1
3. The Laboratory Safety Institute: http://www.osha.gov/SLTC/laboratories/index.html
4. The American Board of Forensic Toxicology (ABFT): http://www.abft.org/files/ABFTLaboratoryManual.pdf
5. The Federal Bureau of Investigation: http://www.fbi.gov/about-us/forensic-science-sommunications/fsc/april2003/swgdamsafety.htm

The additional laboratory functions of sample acquisition, chain of custody maintenance, and laboratory accreditation are discussed in Chapters 6 and 11, respectively.

4.6 LABORATORY SECURITY

Because of the confidential nature of the analyses being conducted and due to the legal requirements to protect samples against the possibility of tampering, steps must be taken to ensure the security of the laboratory. At a minimum, access to laboratories should be restricted to authorized personnel with access controlled by means of coded locks or ID cards. All refrigerators and freezers should be locked, and access should be limited to specifically designated persons. An alarm system capable of detecting unauthorized entry to the laboratory should be in place.

All drug standards should be stored in a locked safe together with a record for each drug that includes the amount of drug received, the name and address of the supplier, the date the sample is received, the names of persons using the standard, the dates on which the standards were used, the purpose for which the standards were used, and the quantities of the standards used. Controlled substances should be ordered by one person, who has the only authorized signature, and stored in a safe to which another person has the combination. This protocol ensures that a single person cannot both order and have access to the controlled substances.

Furthermore, steps should be taken to minimize the possibility that the security measures can be circumvented easily, and protocols must be established that would allow the detection of any security breaches.

REVIEW QUESTIONS

1. What office or agency is typically responsible for the oversight and administration of a forensic toxicology laboratory?
2. What educational and/or training experiences are typically required of a chief toxicologist, an assistant chief toxicologist, and a toxicologist (I or II)?
3. What are the key physical elements that should be found in every forensic toxicology laboratory space?
4. What are the fundamental pieces of analytical instrumentation that are found in most forensic toxicology laboratories?
5. What measures should laboratory personnel take to monitor and protect their safety while working in a forensic toxicology laboratory?

APPLICATION QUESTIONS

1. Discuss the most significant issues (real or perceived) facing scientists working in a forensic toxicology laboratory that is affiliated with a prosecutorial agency.

How would you, as a toxicologist working within such a laboratory, handle these issues?

2. Compare and contrast the duties and responsibilities of a chief toxicologist, an assistant chief toxicologist, and a toxicologist (I or II). What interactions do the personnel in the various laboratory positions have with each other? Is there a system of checks and balances within a forensic toxicology laboratory?

3. Describe several ways in which a chief toxicologist may ensure that the skills and competencies of the laboratory personnel under his administration are current and relevant. How would you, as a chief toxicologist, manage an employee who does not demonstrate the required competencies for his/her position?

4. Discuss the precautions that must be taken in order to ensure the security of biological samples (collected for analysis) within a forensic toxicology laboratory. Formulate an appropriate course of action that you, as a chief toxicologist, would take if a security breach occurred at your laboratory.

REFERENCES

ABFT 1.Certification as a Diplomate of the Board. Retrieved October 5, 2012, from: http://abft.org/index.php?option=com_content&view=article&id=46&Itemid=2.

ABFT 2.Certification as a Forensic Toxicology Specialist. Retrieved October 5, 2012, from: http://abft.org/index.php?option=com_content&view=article&id=47&Itemid=2.

Durose, M.R., Walsh, K.A., Burch, A.M., 2012. Census of Publicly Funded Forensic Crime Laboratories, 2009. Bureau of Justice Statistics, Washington, DC.

Flanagan, R.J., Taylor, A., Watson, I.D., Whelton, R., 2007. Fundamentals of Analytical Toxicology. John Wiley & Sons, Hoboken, NJ.

Hamilton, P., Alexander, K.L., September 21, 2012. DC Police Crime Lab Technicians Ordered Transferred; to be Replaced by Civilians. The Washington Post.

National Institute of Justice, 1998. Forensic Laboratories: Handbook for Facility Planning, Design, Construction, and Moving. U.S. Department of Justice, Washington, DC.

National Research Council, 2009. Strengthening Forensic Science in the United States: A Path Forward. The National Academies Press, Washington, DC.

Virginia.gov. Agency information. Retrieved October 12, 2012, from: http://www.publicsafety.virginia.gov/Agencies/index.htm.

Analytical Strategy

5

The three major tasks in analytical toxicology are to detect, identify and quantitate potentially harmful substances in biological or other relevant specimens.

Rokus A. de Zeeuw

Analysis is the first in the sequence of the three principal functions of forensic toxicologists—analysis, interpretation, and reporting—and is the foundation of appropriate and accurate interpretations and reporting. In the broadest sense, the goals of analytical toxicology are the detection, identification, and quantitation of specific drugs and their metabolites in various types of samples. Analytical results are used to answer the several questions asked of forensic toxicologists from the relatively simple—Is a specific drug in the body of the deceased?—to the more complex—Is the presence of two drugs in blood, each at a concentration consistent with therapeutic use, sufficient to have caused the death of the deceased?

In order to obtain the results necessary to answer the various questions posed to them, forensic toxicologists must develop and implement appropriate analytical strategies to direct the handling of samples and the use of analytical methods for the detection, identification and, when required, quantitation of selected analytes in relevant samples.

5.1 TYPES OF ANALYTICAL STRATEGIES

Because of the large number of analytes of potential interest in forensic toxicology, analytical strategies developed and employed in a forensic toxicology laboratory are designed not only for the detection of those drugs and chemicals that are commonly encountered, but also for substances that are rarely or only occasionally encountered. Regardless of the strategy employed, determining whether *any drugs* are present in a sample is an ideal that cannot be realized since there exists a seemingly infinite number of drugs and chemicals to which individuals may be exposed—prescription drugs, over-the-counter preparations, abused substances, industrial and commercial materials, and environmental chemicals. It has been suggested that forensic toxicologists may be called upon "… to find the well-known needle in a haystack without knowing what the needle looks like!" (Van Boexlaer, 2005)

Forensic Toxicology. http://dx.doi.org/10.1016/B978-0-12-799967-8.00005-0

or it might be added—to determine whether the needle is present. Thus, the analytical strategies established by forensic toxicologists must be formulated to determine whether any needles are present, and if so, to identify them and, if necessary, determine the concentration(s) at which they are present.

Although there are similarities in the approaches commonly employed by laboratories for achieving these analytical goals, the development and implementation of a specific analytical strategy is dependent on the expertise of the laboratory personnel, the operating budget of the laboratory, the availability of equipment, the circumstances of the case, the specific goals of the analyses, and the case load of the laboratory. Thus, the analytical strategies of laboratories are based on the determination of how the capabilities of the laboratories and the time and efforts of their staffs can be allocated most efficiently. Due to a variation of these factors, analytical strategies vary among laboratories, from narrowly limited to broadly based approaches.

At one extreme is the analytical strategy by which the only analyses conducted are those intended to detect exogenous substances that are reasonably suspected of being present in the sample based on the information collected from the nonanalytical investigation of the case, including police reports, eyewitness testimony, and medical and autopsy reports. This strategy is the so-called directed search (Hartstra et al., 2000). For example, in a fatality, the nonanalytical investigative information that may commonly direct toxicological analyses toward a search for specific drugs and chemicals in a sample include a description of the site and circumstances of the death, the collection and identification of drug-related materials collected during a police investigation (such as partially filled drug containers and drug paraphernalia found at the death scene), the medical history of the subject (obtained by investigators of the Office of the Chief Medical Examiner, including the identification and description of preexisting diseases and prior therapeutic or abusive drug use), and drug-related abnormalities detected on autopsy (such as "narcotic lung" and track marks). The strategy of the directed search was advocated in the developing period of forensic toxicology by Reese (1874, p.74) who stated in his text *A Manual of Toxicology*:

> *... it is desirable that the toxicologist should inform himself, as far as possible, of the nature of the symptoms and (in a fatal case) of the post-mortem appearances observed in the suspected case. Such a knowledge will generally serve at least to put him on the proper track, by indicating to what particular class of poisons he should direct his researches.*

In agreement, Sunshine (1977) wrote of the "artful approach" and was of the opinion that "... a complete toxicological analysis for any exogenous substance—a general unknown—is seldom performed and seldom required. Each case under investigation is peculiar unto itself—the toxicological support required for its resolution should be designed appropriately."

The other extreme of analytical strategies, general unknown screening (GUS), is "... the analytical process that takes place when no prior information about possible toxic agents is available" (Gergov et al., 2015). The essence of this approach "… comprises the logical search for a potentially harmful substance whose presence is uncertain and its identity unknown" (Bogusz et al., 1983). In the earlier literature of the modern era, the implementation of a GUS procedure relied extensively on the use of laborious and time-consuming steam distillations and multiple liquid—liquid extractions for the separation of drugs from the biological matrix[1] (Curry, 1960, 1961). Extracts thus produced were subjected to detection methods including spot tests, crystal tests,[2] and paper- and thin-layer chromatography (TLC) and to a lesser extent ultraviolet spectrophotometry. In subsequent years, although the methods of analysis employed frequently maintained a reliance on similar extraction methods, the methods of detection, identification, and quantitation employed were replaced largely by ultraviolet spectrophotometry and gas—liquid chromatography (GC-LC) (Goldbaum and Domanski, 1965; Stolman, 1965; Anders and Mannering, 1967; Goldbaum and Dominguez, 1974; Stajic, 1981; Wu Chen et al., 1983). Because of the limitations of the methods employed in GUS, it was considered an inefficient shot-in-the-dark method requiring more time, labor, and/or expense than a more directed approach of analysis and, therefore, should be conducted only as a "last resort" in those cases in which evidence is lacking as to the potential presence of specific drugs or chemicals (Stajic, 1981).

In the modern forensic toxicology laboratory, GUS is achieved by an analytical strategy known as the systematic toxicological analysis (STA). STA is "a comprehensive and systematic analysis of specimens, for the presence of chemicals of toxicological importance" (Drummer, 1999) that includes methods for "… sampling, sample preparation (isolation), differentiation, detection, as well as identification" (Gergov et al., 2015).

A typical STA includes a predetermined battery of methods based on several principles of detection including immunoassays, GC/MS (MS), and LC/MS (MS). The STA is designed to detect or identify a wide range of analytes, such as commonly used and abused drugs, in the most efficient manner. The STA strategy is commonplace and enables the rapid detection and identification of dozens or hundreds of analytes at low concentrations, even in cases in which the presence of specific drugs and chemicals is not indicated by investigation (Drummer and Gerastamoulos, 2002; Drummer, 2007, 2010; Maurer, 2010a).

The most widely employed analytical strategy in forensic toxicology laboratories is neither a directed search nor an STA, but a strategy that combines both of these strategies.

---

[1]For example, a "systematic search" proposed by Curry in 1960 (Curry, 1961) consisted of more than 20 procedures including distillation, dialysis, and liquid—liquid extractions, all prior to application of the method of detection.

[2]Farmilo and Genest (1961) devoted more than 100 pages to tables describing the crystals produced from numerous drugs!

5.2 THE COMMON STRATEGY

In the mid-eighteenth century, several prominent forensic toxicologists understood that relying on results obtained from the use of a single analytical method was inappropriate because most of the methods available were not sufficiently specific and often resulted in false-positive results. Therefore, it was their judgment that the reliance on results obtained from a single method of analysis, and the subsequent interpretations based on these results, was not sound scientific practice due to the likelihood of obtaining inaccurate results. These early toxicologists concluded that this problem of specificity could be minimized and possibly prevented if several different methods of analysis, each based on a different principle of detection, were used. This approach was employed in an attempt to reduce the occurrence of errors, as errors resulting from the use of a single method likely would not occur in all of the methods (Burney, 2002).

This two-stage approach to analysis is widely recognized as a requirement of modern forensic toxicology. Regardless of the specific analytes designed to be detected by either the directed search or STA components of the analytical strategy, the common strategy consists of two stages. The first stage consists of one or more, usually qualitative presumptive analyses, also commonly known as screening tests, by which several analytes or analyte classes may be detected. The second stage consists of confirmatory methods that are of greater specificity than the presumptive analyses and that are based on a different analytical principle than the presumptive methods by which the analytes were detected. The purpose of the second-stage analyses is the identification and, if need be, quantitation of the analytes.

It is a common practice to employ a battery of presumptive and confirmatory tests on the basis of their applicability in routine cases as well as their adaptability in unusual cases. Of course, the overriding criterion in the selection of the analytical methods utilized is the goal of obtaining accurate results. However, it is also reasonable that the strategy and the methods employed should be the simplest and most economical, consistent with accurate results.

5.2.1 PRESUMPTIVE OR SCREENING METHODS

The purpose of initial presumptive, or screening, tests, which are widely used for both forensic and clinical purposes, is to determine the presence or absence of a large number of drugs, not only those suspected of being present in a sample, but also those that are not specifically indicated in the case, but which may be detected frequently due to their widespread use and abuse. Presumptive methods of analysis have low detection limits, usually in the ng/mL range, are simple to perform, relatively inexpensive, and easily adaptable to automated batch analysis. One of the important benefits of presumptive testing is that due to the low detection limits of the methods used, negative results are a strong indication that the analytes *are not* present and that further analyses requiring time-consuming and expensive methods for the detection of those analytes are not warranted. By extension, positive results are an indication that one or more analytes of interest may be present and thus confirmatory analysis, of this or another type of sample, by means of a method with a different theoretical basis, is required.

Typically employed presumptive screening methods include color tests, immunoassays, TLC, GC, GC/MS (MS), and LC/MS (MS). Immunoassays, which are commonly employed as presumptive methods, generally have low specificity for individual analytes, as several members of a specific drug class are detectable with their use. For example, several, but not all, opioids and/or their metabolites may be detected by use of an immunoassay designed to detect opioids, but the specific opioids or metabolites detected cannot be identified. However, this lack of specificity of immunoassays often is advantageous since the presumptive detection of a large number of drugs—including many members of a drug class, as well as their metabolites and analogs—may be detected rapidly and inexpensively by the use of a single immunoassay. A single analysis using GC/MS (MS) or LC/MS (MS) allows for the detection of a broad spectrum of drugs, metabolites, and analogs of a specific class or of several drug classes with a degree of specificity that often permits not only detection, but also identification.

Samples used for presumptive analyses should include those in which it is likely that the analyte drugs and/or their metabolites will be present following use or abuse. Further, the samples should be amenable to analysis in a rapid and reliable manner by means of several different types of analytical methods, which may be applied to a large number of samples without the incidence of any unusual analytical problems. In antemortem cases, urine, hair, and saliva are widely used for screening purposes, urine being the most commonly employed. Of course, a wider variety of samples is available for postmortem qualitative analysis. In both antemortem and postmortem cases, blood is commonly used for quantitative confirmatory analysis because the current databases correlating blood levels of drugs and/or their analytes with physiological and toxicological effects are more extensive than for other biological samples.

It is essential that the interpretation and significance of presumptive results are understood by those who utilize them. For example, attorneys and physicians often are not familiar with the limitations of presumptive methods and as a result may assume erroneously that a report of "no drugs detected" as the result of a "drug screen" is consistent with the absence of *any* drugs.

5.2.2 NON-STA METHODS

Analyses for specific drugs that are not detectable by the battery of tests in a routine STA, especially those that are not detectable by the presumptive methods, should be conducted when the investigative evidence in a case suggests them to be necessary. For example, if a body with red lividity is found inside a car in a closed garage with an empty gas tank, an analysis of blood for the detection of carbon monoxide, an analyte that may not be a component of the analytical strategy, must be conducted. Additional cases in which specific methods should be considered in a toxicological investigation are those in which the presence of drugs, although not suggested by the facts of a specific case, may be anticipated to be encountered in a meaningful number of cases due to widespread regional use or abuse. For example, analysis for the presence of oxycodone would be warranted if the sample was collected from a subject living in a geographic area, and of the age group, in which Oxycontin® abuse has taken on near epidemic-like proportions. Although specific methods require a greater expenditure of time and labor than the methods in the STA, it is important that they are utilized when warranted by the specific circumstances of a case.

5.2.3 CONFIRMATORY METHODS

The use of a confirmatory method is essential for the identification of an analyte detected by most initial presumptive analyses. A positive result obtained by the utilization of a single presumptive method of analysis, such as immunoassay or GC/MS, regardless of the specificity of the method, must, with few exceptions, be confirmed by a second, or confirmatory, method.

The SOFT/AAFS Forensic Toxicology Laboratory Guidelines (SOFT/AAFS, 2006) state that

> *As a matter of scientific and forensic principle, the detection or initial identification of drugs and other toxins should be confirmed whenever possible by a second technique **based on a different chemical principle.** (emphasis added)*

It is important to emphasize that a confirmatory method must be based on a different principle of analysis than the initial presumptive test. For example, a positive result obtained by an enzyme-multiplied immunoassay (EMIT) should not be confirmed by means of fluorescence polarization immunoassay (FPIA), but rather by a nonimmunoassay such as GC/MS, which has been used for several years for this purpose and referred to as the "gold standard" of confirmatory methods. Recently, LC/MS/MS has been used increasingly in a confirmatory role because it offers several benefits including the detection of nonvolatile, thermal-labile, and high-molecular-weight compounds (usually without the need for derivatization). LC/MS/MS analysis also allows for the detection of dozens or hundreds of compounds, in a single sample, often at lower detection limits than possible with many other methods.

The importance of confirmatory analyses cannot be overestimated. However, an important differentiation between *confirmation* and *identification* has been made by de Zeeuw who has opined that the confirmation of presumptive screening results, as commonly conducted, is not an identification, but only an affirmation that the result of confirmatory testing "… is not against the presumption" of the screening result (457 de Zeeuw, 2004). The confirmatory methods employed generally do not determine whether there are other compounds present in the sample that meet the confirmatory criteria for a positive result (Hartstra, et al., 2000). Thus, the interpretation of the results is directed by the preconception that the analyte suggested by the screening result is the analyte detected by the confirmatory method. The reasoning might go something like this: Screening test results were consistent with the presence of drug X and the confirmatory results did not deviate from this consistency. Therefore, the drug present in the sample must be drug X. de Zeeuw argues persuasively that identification is necessary, i.e., other drugs must be excluded. Without the implementation of strict and rigorous criteria of identification, confirmation as presently conducted may result in serious errors as a result of confirmatory bias, i.e., "the tendency to look for and perceive evidence consistent with our hypotheses and to deny, dismiss or distort evidence that is not" (458 Littlefield, 2010).

5.3 SAMPLES

The selection of samples to be included in the analytical strategy depends upon the purpose of the analysis, the specific analytes being sought, the ease of analysis, and the type of information provided by the analysis of specific samples.

Since presumptive analyses are conducted for the purpose of determining which analytes **may be** present, the samples used for such analyses should be those in which a large number of drugs and/or their metabolites are likely to be present if subjects had been exposed to these drugs. Urine is the sample most commonly used for this purpose, since it is a major route of drug and metabolite excretion. Oral fluid and hair, which offer the advantages of ease of collection and detection of analytes over a longer period, respectively, are being used increasingly, especially in antemortem cases.

If the sole goal of the analysis is to determine whether specific analytes are present, qualitative confirmatory methods may be conducted using either the same samples used for the presumptive testing or other samples. If the goal is to draw additional conclusions, such as whether the drugs/metabolites detected may be associated with an adverse effect experienced by the subject, then quantitative confirmatory methods must be employed using samples that may provide the results necessary for that purpose, e.g., blood. The benefits and disadvantages of the use of various samples are discussed in Chapter 6.

5.4 ANALYTES
5.4.1 ANALYTES INCLUDED IN THE STA

In general, substances of interest to forensic toxicologists include legal and illegal drugs and their metabolites, industrial chemicals, environmental pollutants, and naturally occurring botanicals and metals. Of the vast number of known compounds[3] included in these categories of interest, only a small fraction can be detected via routine analyses, regardless of the analytical strategy employed.

---

[3]In 2011, Chemical Abstracts Service estimated that there were more than 54 million commercially available compounds (Chemical Abstracts Service, 2012).

A pivotal initial step in the development of an effective STA is the designation of the analytes to be detected, which generally include legal and illegal drugs, their metabolites, and their analogs. Licit and illicit drugs, which are used or abused, that are commonly included in an analytical strategy include ethanol and other volatile organic compounds, opioids, CNS stimulants, hallucinogens, cannabinoids, hypnotics, anxiolytics, antipsychotics, and antidepressants. Additionally, STA analyses are often designed to detect certain environmental substances, such as pesticides, cyanide, and carbon monoxide, to which persons may be exposed either accidentally or intentionally.

The selection of analytes to be included in the STA should be based on knowledge of the international, national, regional, and local patterns of use and abuse of specific drugs and chemicals. Even if the use and abuse of specific drugs at the international and national levels are not yet evident in the regional and local regions serviced by forensic toxicology laboratories, they may be harbingers of future abuse trends. A case in point is the abuse of synthetic cannabinoids, a problem recognized in Europe before federal action was taken in the United States in 2011 and 2012 to control the abuse of these drugs (Johnston et al., 2014).

In regional and local areas, data obtained from local law enforcement agencies and medical sources can be used to gain an understanding of the extent of drug use and abuse. These data include the rates at which drugs are being diverted from legal to illegal uses either by theft or by "doctor shopping," local drug abuse patterns, law enforcement reports regarding the prevalence of illegal laboratories synthesizing drugs of abuse, the availability of drugs of abuse "on the street," the number of drug abuse-related emergency room visits, and the number of prescriptions for specific drugs filled.

In the United States, geographically distinct patterns of widespread drug abuse in local regions have been exemplified by:

- the extent of phencyclidine (PCP) abuse in the metropolitan Washington, DC, area. In 1987, 44% of all emergency room mentions and 41% of all PCP-related deaths reported to the Drug Abuse Warning Network were from the DC area (Thombs, 1989); and
- the high rate of false prescriptions written for oxycodone-containing products in Maryland. In 1999, approximately 85% of all arrests in Maryland for written false prescriptions were for these products (U.S. Department of Justice, January 2001).

5.4.2 UNCOMMON ANALYTES

Although forensic toxicology laboratories generally are well equipped to detect drugs and chemicals that are commonly present in biological samples, compounds encountered less frequently by forensic toxicologists pose an additional analytical challenge. This challenge arises because the methods for the detection of such infrequently encountered drugs and chemicals may not be included as components of the routine analytical strategy, or the laboratory may not have the analytical capability to perform the methodologies required for detection and identification. Two notorious examples of substances in this category, which have been used in homicide cases, are the hormone insulin and ricin, a protein derived from the castor bean. Because insulin, ricin, and other rarely encountered substances are unlikely to be detected by routine methods, in cases in which their use is suspected, special methods outside of the routine analytical strategy have to be employed for their detection and identification. In some cases, this may necessitate that the analyses are performed by another laboratory that has the required instrumentation and/or analytical expertise.

5.4.3 THE CHANGING ANALYTE PROFILE

The drugs and chemicals of interest to and encountered by forensic toxicologists have changed during the development and practice of forensic toxicology; this can be attributed largely to societal, technological, and pharmaceutical advances. In the mid-nineteenth century, homicidal poisonings most commonly involved arsenic, opium, oxalic acid, mercuric chloride, or strychnine (Coley, 1991). In the early twentieth century, as Gettler and his coworkers were establishing the foundations of forensic toxicology in the United States, the drugs and chemicals that they encountered most frequently included ethanol, methanol, arsenic, mercury, and CO (Blum, 2010). In the mid-twentieth century, from 1942 to 1950, a survey of drugs involved in fatal poisonings in the three large metropolitan areas of Cleveland, Los Angeles, and Baltimore (Sunshine and Adelson, 1954) determined that carbon monoxide and barbiturates were responsible for approximately 70% of all such fatalities, and heavy metals were responsible for an additional 10% (ethanol was not considered in this study). In the late twentieth century, studies of drug-related deaths (Caplan et al., 1985), drug-impaired drivers (McLinden, 1987), clinical urine samples (Jones et al., 1985), and trauma victims (Rivara et al., 1989) demonstrated that although commonly encountered drugs included those that had been of concern for many years—ethanol, carbon monoxide, and barbiturates—newly available therapeutic drugs including tricyclic antidepressants, synthetic narcotics, and benzodiazepines, as well as drugs of abuse, including marihuana, cocaine, hallucinogens, and designer drugs, contributed significantly to cases of drug abuse and toxicity.

Presently, the list of analytes encountered by forensic toxicologists includes not only several that were of interest in previous decades, but also many new classes of therapeutic and abused drugs. The continually escalating variety and availability of designer or "smart" drugs of abuse, a number of which were originally synthesized for clinical and research use, but which have been diverted to abuse, present a current and consequential problem. Several of these designer drugs were not regulated under the Controlled Substance Act for prolonged periods of time after their widespread emergence in the United States.[4] In the absence of such regulation, these

---

[4]However, several of these drugs such as cannabinomimetics (Spice), cathinone derivatives (bath salts), and phenethylamines (2C drugs) were added to the Controlled Substances Act in 2012 as Schedule I drugs, either permanently or temporarily (Drug Enforcement Administration, 2013).

drugs were synthesized, distributed, and frequently easily available online as "legal highs" (Zawilska, 2011).

At present, a large number of relatively "new" abused drugs have gained popularity (Table 5.1). Among these, synthetic cannabinoids may present the greatest problem and as such are a source of major concern for forensic toxicologists. Synthetic cannabinoids, which are commonly identified as "herbal blends" and often sold under the product names K2 and Spice, are reported to bind to cannabinoid receptors and to produce effects with greater potencies than marihuana. Often these drugs are sold in mixtures containing any of a variety of synthetic cannabinoids, including CP-47,497, JWH-018 and HU-210, and related compounds (Fuller, 2011). An additional group of relatively new abused drugs—the so-called "bath salts," which are sold under a variety of names, e.g., Tranquility, Kush Blitz, and XOXO— has been shown to contain methylone and 3,4-methylenedioxypyrovalerone (MDPV)—both of which are similar in effect to MDMA (Frazee et al., 2011).

A sampling of additional "designer" drugs that forensic toxicologists may encounter include (Maurer, 2010b; Peters and Martinez-Ramirez, 2010) phenethylamine derivatives (2Cs), e.g., 4-methyl-2,5-dimethoxy-phenethylamine (2C-D); 4-substituted amphetamines, e.g., *para*-methoxyamphetamine (PMA); 2,5-dimethoxy amphetamines, e.g., 2,5-dimethoxy amphetamine (DMA); β-keto-amphetamines, e.g., mephedrone; pyrrolidinophenones, e.g., pyrrolidinopropiophenone (PPP); piperazines, e.g., benzylpiperazine (BZP); and a new class of drugs, the aminoindanes, amphetamine analogs, e.g., 5,6-methylenedioxy-2-aminoindane (Sainsbry et al., 2011). The structures of several of these abused designer drugs are presented in Table5.1. Fortunately, forensic toxicologists have risen to the challenge of identifying new drugs in biological samples and have developed methods of analysis for this purpose (Meyer and Peters, 2012; Peters and Martinez-Ramirez, 2010; Wohlfarth and Weinmann, 2010).

As history has shown, the identities of used and abused drugs, as well as the drugs of accidental exposure, are continually changing, often in parallel with both advances in synthetic organic chemistry and the rapid dissemination of information among illegal drug distributors and abusers. Although it would be difficult for forensic toxicologists to anticipate the identity of future compounds that either will be diverted from legitimate use or synthesized specifically for purposes of abuse, they must be aware of the emergence of these "new" drugs of abuse when they become components of the drug abuse counter culture. Such an awareness of the pharmaceutical climate is vital to the development of new analytical strategies and methods of analysis that are adequate for the detection, identification, and quantitation of the drugs and chemicals that forensic toxicologists are likely to encounter in their laboratories.

Given the necessity for a forensic toxicological analysis to detect both suspected as well as unsuspected drugs and chemicals in biological samples, a successful analytical strategy must incorporate several different types of samples, a variety of presumptive screening tests and special analyses, as well as the appropriate confirmatory analyses. A typical analytical strategy might include the use

Table 5.1 Designer Drugs

Drugs	Structures	Drugs	Structures
Cannabinomimetics		**Cathinones**	
CP-47,497[a]		Mephedrone[b]	
JWH-073[c]		MDPV[d]	
JWH-018[e]		Methylone[f]	
HU-210[g]			
Phenethylamines		**Piperazines**	
2C-E[h]		BZP[i]	

Continued

Table 5.1 Designer Drugs—cont'd

Drugs	Structures	Drugs	Structures
Phenethylamines		**Piperazines**	
2CI[j]		TFMPP[k]	
Bromo-Dragonfly[l]			
Aminoindanes		**Pipradols**	
MDAI[m]		D2PM[n]	
MMAI[o]		2-DPMP[p]	

[a] 5-(1,1-Dimethylheptyl)-2-[(1R,3S)-3-hydroxycyclohexyl]-phenol.
[b] 4-Methylmethcathinone.
[c] 1-Butyl-3-(1-naphthoyl)indole.
[d] 3,4-Methylenedioxypyrovalerone.
[e] 1-Pentyl-3-(1-naphthoyl)indole.
[f] 3,4-Methylenedioxy-N-methylcathinone.
[g] (6aR,10aR)-9-(hydroxymethyl)-6,6-dimethyl-3-(2-methyloctan-2-yl)-6a,7,10,10a-tetrahydrobenzo[c]chromen-1-ol.
[h] 2,5-Dimethoxy-4-ethylphenethylamine.
[i] 1-Benzylpiperazine.
[j] 2-(4-Iodo-2,5-dimethoxyphenyl)ethanamine.
[k] 1-(3-Trifluoromethyphenyl) piperazine.
[l] 1-(8-Bromobenzo[1,2-b;4,5-b′]difuran-4-yl)-2-aminopropane.
[m] 5,6-Methylendioxy-2-aminoindane.
[n] Diphenyl-2-pyrrolodinyl-methanol.
[o] 5-Methoxy-6-methyl-2-aminoindane.
[p] 2-Diphenylmethylpiperidine.

of immunoassays for the presumptive detection of several common drugs of abuse in urine, GC/MS for the detection of drugs in blood, GC for the detection of ethanol and other volatiles in blood, vitreous humor, and urine, GC for the detection of carbon monoxide, and any additional methods deemed necessary for the detection of specific or uncommon drugs as appropriate. If all of the aforementioned presumptive analyses yield negative results, then a decision would be made as to whether additional, potentially time-consuming, testing for additional drugs would be warranted.

In summary, implementation of an analytical strategy and achievement of its goals depends on

- operating budgets suitable for the goals of the strategy,
- availability and maintenance of required equipment,
- the case load of the laboratory,
- the availability of the necessary biological samples,
- the development of a validated method of analysis for the detection, identification, and quantitation of relevant drugs and/or their metabolites, and
- a laboratory staff who possesses the skills, knowledge, and competence to perform the analysis in a reliable and accurate manner.

REVIEW QUESTIONS

1. Describe the differences between the directed search and the general unknown screening (GUS) analytical strategies.
2. Define the systematic toxicological analysis (STA) method.
3. Under what conditions would non-STA methods of analysis be necessary?
4. Why is it important that multiple analytical methodologies be utilized in toxicological analyses?
5. Under what conditions would a confirmatory test not be required in the common strategy?

APPLICATION QUESTIONS

1. Discuss the major weaknesses of the general unknown screening (GUS) strategy of analysis, and explain how the systematic toxicological analysis (STA) approach overcomes or circumvents these weaknesses.
2. Discuss the major strengths of the two-stage approach to analysis employed in the common strategy. Describe the analytical methods that you might utilize in the presumptive screening stage and in the confirmatory stage of the strategy.
3. Describe the major factors that must be considered when selecting the biological sample (or samples) to be analyzed via the common strategy. How would you, as a toxicologist, proceed if the optimal biological sample type was not available for analysis?

4. Describe how you would determine which analytes to test for in a toxicological analysis. What factors would influence your decision? Why might the choice of analytes vary at different toxicology laboratories, or at different periods in time?

REFERENCES

Anders, M.W., Mannering, G.J., 1967. Application of gas chromatography to toxicology. In: Stolman, A. (Ed.), Progress in Chemical Toxicology, vol. 3. Academic Press, New York.

Blum, D., 2010. The Poisoner's Handbook. The Penguin Press, New York.

Bogusz, M., Wijsbeek, J., Franke, J.P., de Zeeuw, R.A., 1983. Applicability of capillary gas chromatography to systematic toxicological analysis: occurrence of concentration-dependent retention behavior. J. Anal. Toxicol. 7, 188–192.

Burney, I.A., 2002. Testing testimony: toxicology and the law of evidence in early nineteenth-century England. Stud. Hist. Phil. Sci. 33, 289–314.

Caplan, Y.H., Ottinger, W.E., Park, J., Smith, T.D., 1985. Drug and chemical related deaths: incidence in the state of Maryland - 1975–1980. J. Forensic Sci. 30, 1012–1021.

Chemical Abstracts Service, 2012. CAS Registry. Retrieved September 1, 2012, from: http://www.cas.org/content/chemical-substances.

Coley, N.G., 1991. Alfred Swaine Taylor, MD, FRS (1806–1880): forensic toxicologist. Med. Hist. 35, 409–427.

Curry, A.S., 1960. Outline of a systematic search for an unknown poison in viscera. In: Stewart, C.P., Stolman, A. (Eds.), Toxicology: Mechanisms and Analytical Methods, vol. 1. Academic Press, New York.

Curry, A.S., 1961. Acidic and neutral poisons (other than barbiturates). In: Stewart, C.P., Stolman, A. (Eds.), Toxicology: Mechanisms and Analytical Methods, vol. 2. Academic Press, New York.

de Zeeuw, R.A., 2004. Substance identification: the weak link in analytical toxicology. J. Chromatogr. B 811, 3–12.

Drug Enforcement Administration, May 16, 2013. Schedules of controlled substances: temporary placement of three synthetic cannabinoids into schedule I. Final order. Fed. Reg. 78 (95), 28735–28739.

Drummer, O.H., 1999. Chromatographic screening techniques in systematic toxicological analysis. J. Chromatogr. B 733, 27–45.

Drummer, O.H., 2007. Requirements for bioanalytical procedures in postmortem toxicology. Anal. Bioanal. Chem. 388, 1495–1503.

Drummer, O.H., 2010. Forensic toxicology. EXS 100, 579–603.

Drummer, O.H., Gerastamoulos, J., 2002. Postmortem drug analysis: analytical and toxicological aspects. Ther. Drug Monit. 24 (1), 199–209.

Farmilo, C.G., Genest, K., 1961. Alkaloids and related bases: identification. In: Stewart, C.P., Stolman, A. (Eds.), Toxicology: Mechanisms and Analytical Methods, vol. 2. Academic Press, New York.

Frazee, C.C., Johnson, L., Scott, D., 2011. Bath Salts: Analysis of Three Versions of New Street Drugs. Retrieved September 26, 2011 from: http://www.soft-tox.org/index.php?option=com_jdownloads&Itemid=109&view=finish&cid=131&catid=3.

Fuller, D.C., 2011. Herbal Incensed. Retrieved September 26, 2011 from: http://www.soft-tox.org/index.php?option=com_jdownloads&Itemid=109&view=finish&cid=19&catid=3.

Gergov, M., LeBeau, M., Muller, R.K., Sporkert, F., Weinmann, W., 2015. TIAFT Committee on Systematic Toxicological Analysis and Guidelines. Retrieved January 2, 2015 from: http://www.tiaft.org/tiaft-guidelines.html.

Goldbaum, L.R., Domanski, T.J., 1965. An approach to the analysis of biological specimens for basic drugs. In: Stolman, A. (Ed.), Progress in Chemical Toxicology, vol. 2. Academic Press, New York.

Goldbaum, L.R., Dominguez, A.M., 1974. Analysis of drugs in biological specimens. In: Stolman, A. (Ed.), Progress in Chemical Toxicology, vol. 5. Academic Press, New York.

Hartstra, J., Franke, J.P., de Zeeuw, R.A., 2000. How to approach substance identification in qualitative bioanalysis. J. Chromatogr. B Biomed. Sci. Appl. 739, 125—137.

Johnston, L.D., O'Malley, P.M., Miech, R.A., Bachman, J.G., Schulenberg, J.E., 2014. Monitoring the Future, National Results on Drug Use: 1975—2013: Overview, Key Findings on Adolescent Drug Use. Retrieved October 6, 2014 from: http://www.monitoringthefuture.org/pubs/monographs/mtf-overview2013.pdf.

Jones, D.W., Adams, D., Martel, P.A., Rousseau, R.J., 1985. Drug population in one thousand geographically distributed urine specimens. J. Anal. Toxicol. 9, 125—130.

Littlefield, S.O., 2010. Fudge factor. Sci. Am. 303, 18.

Maurer, H.H., 2010a. Analytical toxicology. EXS 100, 317—337.

Maurer, H.M., 2010b. Chemistry, pharmacology, and metabolism of emerging drugs of abuse. Ther. Drug Monit. 32, 544—549.

McLinden, V.J., 1987. Experiences in relation to drugs/driving offences. J. Forensic Sci. 27, 73—80.

Meyer, M.R., Peters, F.T., 2012. Analytical toxicology of emerging drugs of abuse—an update. Ther. Drug Monit. 34, 615—621.

Peters, F.T., Martinez-Ramirez, J.A., 2010. Analytical toxicology of emerging drugs of abuse. Ther. Drug Monit. 32, 532—539.

Reese, J.J., 1874. A Manual of Toxicology, Including the Consideration of the Nature, Properties, Effects, and Means of Detection of Poisons, More Especially in their Medico-Legal Relations. J.B. Lippincott & Co., Philadelphia. http://www.archive.org/stream/manualoftoxicolo00reesiala/manualoftoxicolo00reesiala_djvu.txt.

Rivara, F.P., Mueller, B.A., Fligner, C.L., Luna, G., Raisys, V.A., Copass, M., et al., 1989. Drug use in trauma victims. J. Trauma 29, 462—470.

Sainsbry, P.D., Kicman, A.T., Archer, R.P., King, L.A., Braithwaite, R.A., 2011. Aminoindanes—the next wave of "legal highs"? Drug Test. Anal. 3, 479—482.

SOFT/AAFS, 2006. Forensic Toxicology Laboratory Guidelines. Retrieved April 29, 2009 from: http://www.soft-tox.org/files/Guidelines_2006_Final.pdf/.

Stajic, M., 1981. The general unknown. In: Cravey, R.H., Baselt, R.C. (Eds.), Introduction to Forensic Toxicology. Biomedical Publications, Davis, CA.

Stolman, A., 1965. Thin layer chromatography application in toxicology. In: Stolman, A. (Ed.), Progress in Chemical Toxicology, vol. 2. Academic Press, New York.

Sunshine, I., 1977. Forensic toxicology: role of the laboratory. In: Thoma, J.J., Bondo, P.B., Sunshine, I. (Eds.), Guidelines for Analytical Toxicology Programs. CRC Press Inc., Cleveland, OH.

Sunshine, I., Adelson, L., 1954. Fatal and non-fatal poisonings: a statistical survey. J. Crim. Law Criminol. Pol. Sci. 44, 116—123.

Thombs, D.L., 1989. A review of PCP abuse trends and perceptions. Public Health Rep. 104, 325328.

U.S. Department of Justice, January 2001. Oxycontin Diversion and Abuse. http://www.justice.gov/archive/ndic/pubs/651/abuse.htm.

Van Boexlaer, J.F., 2005. Recent trends in analytical procedures in forensic toxicology. Ther. Drug Monit. 27, 752–755.

Wohlfarth, A., Weinmann, W., 2010. Bioanalysis of new designer drugs. Bioanalysis 2, 965–979.

Wu Chen, N.B., Schaffer, M.I., Lin, R., Kurland, M.L., Donoghue, E.R., Stein, R.J., 1983. The general toxicology unknown: I. the systematic approach. J. Forensic Sci. 28, 391–397.

Zawilska, J.B., 2011. "Legal highs"—new players in the old drama [Electronic version]. Curr. Drug Abuse Rev. 4 (2), 122–130.

Sample Handling

6

*… great care should be exercised not to subject the matter to any process
that would preclude the possibility of examining for any poison for which it
might afterwards become necessary to look.*
T.G. Wormley (1867)

Prior to the detection, identification, and quantitation of analytes, the important procedures of sample selection, collection, storage/preservation, and transport take place. Although these procedures have been referred to as "preanalytical" (Skoop, 2004), they should not be considered as separate entities, apart from the analysis, but rather as important analytical components, since the manner in which they are conducted often determines the validity of the analytical results. For convenience, in this and subsequent chapters, the procedures of sample selection, collection, preservation, and transmittal will be referred to, collectively, as sample handling.

The importance of sample handling in obtaining accurate analytical results cannot be overemphasized, since if it is not conducted in an appropriate and accurate manner, alterations of sample structure and analyte concentrations may result causing any subsequent analyses, no matter how sophisticated, to be comprised, leading to inaccurate interpretations and conclusions. The proper handling of samples is the foundation for the accuracy of all analyses that follow and therefore, utmost caution and care must be taken in the execution of these initial procedures of the analysis so that they do not adversely influence the accuracy of the analytical results. Any errors in these procedures may render all subsequent analyses at best suspect and at worst worthless. Not only must forensic toxicologists be trained in the correct methods of sample handling, but also since generally they are not involved in the collection, initial preservation, and transport of samples to the laboratory, they should be involved in the training of those persons who are involved in these procedures to ensure that the proper methods are employed.

Forensic toxicologists are commonly called upon to determine whether drugs and exogenous chemicals are present in several different types of sample, which possess dissimilar physical and chemical characteristics, e.g., urine differs greatly both structurally and biochemically from liver tissue, as hair differs from blood, etc. An appropriate sample-handling protocol must be utilized for each type of sample to ensure, to the extent possible, that neither the composition of the samples nor the presence or the concentration of any drugs contained therein is altered prior to

Forensic Toxicology. http://dx.doi.org/10.1016/B978-0-12-799967-8.00006-2

analysis. In addition, legal requirements, such as the maintenance of a chain of custody (COC), must be satisfied throughout the implementation of the sample-handling procedures.

The protocols employed in the various aspects of sample handling must be evaluated prior to use and determined to be consistent with minimizing the alteration of sample matrices and analyte concentrations. Generally, forensic toxicologists analyze samples obtained from humans, but occasionally they are requested to analyze samples obtained from domesticated and farm animals to determine whether there is any evidence that the animals may have been exposed to harmful substances, either intentionally or unintentionally. In addition, materials such as food, liquids, tablets, capsules, powders, and clothing obtained from the scene of a suspicious event may be submitted to forensic toxicologists for analysis. The strictures that apply to the handling of human samples apply to these samples as well.

6.1 SAMPLE SELECTION
6.1.1 CRITERIA FOR SAMPLE SELECTION

The initial, and in many regards the most important, step in the analytical process is the selection of appropriate samples. Several of the criteria that should be considered in the selection of samples are listed in Table 6.1. The most important criterion in sample selection is a clear understanding of the purpose of the analysis. For example, if the purpose of the analysis is to establish whether a subject used a drug or been exposed to a chemical, then samples suitable for presumptive or screening analyses should be selected. However, if the purpose of the analysis is to attempt more far-reaching conclusions, for example, a determination of the effects that would be consistent with the concentrations of any drugs or chemicals identified in the samples, or the estimation of the time at which the subject was exposed to the analytes, then different or additional samples must be selected. In either case, samples chosen for analysis are those for which the detection and/or quantitation of exogenous substances and/or their metabolites will provide the data necessary to achieve the specific purpose(s) of the analysis.

Table 6.1 Criteria for Sample Selection

Purpose of the analysis
Antemortem or postmortem case
Sample availability
Condition of the samples
Type of interpretation
Ease of analysis
Drug stability

Samples used for presumptive or qualitative analyses are those in which it is likely that exogenous substances and/or their metabolites will be present following intentional or unintentional use or exposure. Usually, the results obtained from the analysis of these samples are not sufficient to formulate any interpretations beyond the conclusion that the subject from whom the samples were obtained had been exposed to the analyte, either intentionally or unintentionally. It is desirable that samples selected for this purpose can be analyzed in a rapid and reliable manner by means of several different types of analytical methods that are relatively inexpensive, amenable to batch analysis preferably by automated methods, and unlikely to result in any unusual analytical problems. In short, the most preferable methods of analysis are those that can be performed in the simplest manner possible, consistent with accurate results. In both ante- and postmortem cases, urine is the sample most commonly employed for screening purposes because it meets the aforementioned criteria for the majority of the drugs of interest. However, hair, oral fluid, and sweat are being used with increasing frequency as they afford certain benefits, including decreased invasion of privacy during collection and, in the case of hair, both a longer detection period after the last use of the substance and increased drug stability compared to the other samples frequently used for this purpose. An analysis of the combined analytical results from multiple types of samples is sometime beneficial in providing a chronology of a pattern of drug use, from hours (blood or oral fluid) to days (urine) to weeks, months, or possibly centuries (hair).

Samples used for quantitative analyses are selected with the intent of correlating the analyte concentrations in these samples with the effects produced by the analytes. Such correlations may be of value in determining whether the presence of analytes at the concentrations detected may have caused or contributed to an adverse effect, e.g., an automobile accident or aggressive behavior by the subject. Blood is the sample most commonly selected for quantitative analysis because the existing database correlating blood levels with effects is more extensive than for other samples. However, in the absence of blood, it may be possible to use other samples, e.g., vitreous humor, in which the drug concentration determined may either be correlated with a corresponding blood concentration of the drug or be correlated directly with an effect. Interpretations of drug concentrations in fluids and tissues, and the factors that influence these interpretations, are the topics of Chapters 12 and 13.

The selection of antemortem samples is necessarily limited as only a small number of sample types is available from the living—blood, urine, hair, nails, and oral fluid. Even though postmortem fluids or tissues can generally be obtained in the desired quantities from relatively well-preserved bodies at autopsy, a limited number of samples are collected routinely for analysis. In "routine" cases in which either there is no evidence of drug involvement, or the suspected drug involvement involves commonly encountered drugs, the samples selected generally are those that are a component of the systematic toxicological analysis (Chapter 5), e.g., blood, urine, and vitreous humor. However, it is reasonable to assume that virtually any sample available at autopsy should be considered to be a suitable analytical sample for the detection of any analyte unless and until experience compels the contrary.

The use of the so-called alternative samples may be required when the desired samples are not available in postmortem cases due to conditions such as incineration, severe decomposition, putrefaction, or skeletonization. Alternative samples include those that are not collected routinely, such as hair, bile, muscle, kidney, lung, and finger- and toenails, as well as those, such as meconium, bone marrow, adipocere, and insect larvae, that are collected rarely and then usually under specific circumstances or for specific purposes. Apart from a lack of the desired samples, the specific circumstances of a case may require the analysis of a particular alternative sample, in order to facilitate the proper analysis or to provide additional data for the interpretation, e.g., breast milk may be collected to determine whether an infant was exposed to a drug through that route, or hair may be collected to determine the chronology of drug abuse. The criteria for the selection of alternative samples are the same as those summarized in Table 6.1 for the selection of the desired samples.

6.1.2 NUMBER OF SAMPLES

In both ante- and postmortem cases, the collection of multiple samples of the same or different types is beneficial because this practice often allows interpretations to be made that are either more difficult, or not possible, to make if the results of only a single sample type are available (Table 6.2). In antemortem cases, the collection and subsequent analysis of two breath or blood samples at different times may enable a determination to be made as to whether the subject's blood ethanol concentration is on the ascending or descending portion of the blood alcohol curve, which in turn

Table 6.2 Advantages of the Collection of Multiple Samples

Advantages of the Collection of Multiple Samples of the Same Type	Advantages of the Collection of Multiple Samples of Different Types
A difference in analytical results may indicate that postmortem redistribution has occurred and may minimize the likelihood that elevated analyte concentrations due to postmortem redistribution are accepted as indications of antemortem concentrations.	The detection of analytes in specific samples may allow a determination of the route of administration to be made.
Consistent results in two or more samples of the same type support the reliability of the analytical results.	Meaningfully inconsistent analytical results in two or more different sample types suggest the postmortem synthesis of the analyte, especially if the sample in which the lower concentration is detected is a sample generally resistant to putrefaction, e.g., vitreous humor.
In living subjects, analysis of samples, e.g., blood or breath, collected at different times, may allow an estimate of the analyte concentration, e.g., the blood alcohol concentration (BAC), at a time prior to the time of sample collection.	The ratio of analyte concentrations in two or more sample types may indicate whether drug equilibrium has been established.

may allow a more accurate estimate of a subject's blood ethanol concentration at a time of interest prior to sample collection. In postmortem cases, the collection of multiple specimens of the same sample type, most commonly blood, from different sites in the body is a common practice. The evaluation of differences in the results obtained from the multiple samples may provide an insight to the likelihood that postmortem redistribution or synthesis may have occurred. For these reasons in many postmortem forensic toxicology laboratories, the standard operating procedure in "routine" cases is the collection of blood from more than one anatomical site, commonly from the heart and a femoral vessel, as well as the collection of urine and vitreous humor. This is an excellent practice, widely employed.

6.2 SAMPLE COLLECTION

The collection of samples is the first step in sample preservation and, therefore, must be conducted with the goal of maintaining the structural integrity of the sample and the concentration of any analytes that may be present, or at a minimum, preventing meaningful changes in either so that false-positive or false-negative results are less likely to occur. For this reason, great care must be taken to ensure that, to the extent possible, the samples collected are not contaminated with other samples or any substance from the collection implements, and the physical nature of the sample is not altered in a manner that causes the concentration of any drugs present to be altered. The manner in which samples are collected must be conducted, so there is no question as to the identity of the sample collected. Generally, identification is not a problem since the sample is collected from a known anatomical location and is easily identifiable. The most common problem of sample identity arises with the collection of blood, as described in Chapter 8.

6.2.1 IMPLEMENTS USED FOR SAMPLE COLLECTION

The material composition of implements used for the collection of samples must neither alter the structural integrity of the samples, thus causing alterations in the drug concentrations, nor contaminate the content of the sample. For example, serious problems of trace metal contamination may result if metal scalpels or needles are used for collection. This problem appears to have been addressed in the early history of forensic toxicology as exemplified by the use of an ivory spatula for the collection of autopsy samples by Alfred Swaine Taylor in the nineteenth century (Rosenfeld, 1985). Since the concentrations of several metals, including nickel, chromium, zinc, manganese, and copper, may be increased as a result of the use of stainless steel scalpel blades and metal biopsy needles (Koirtyohann and Hopps, 1981; Versiek and Speecke, 1972), the use of quartz knives has been suggested as a means of preventing this type of contamination (Koirtyohann and Hopps, 1981). A problem of metal contamination led to the erroneous conclusion that nickel may have been the cause of "Legionnaire's Disease" (Chapter 13). In order to avoid the possibility of either implement contamination or sample-to-sample contamination, disposable implements and containers should be used whenever possible.

6.2.2 SAMPLE CONTAINERS

The type of containers selected for sample collection is an important decision since the composition and type of the containers may have an effect on the stability of analytes in samples that are stored in them, not only throughout the relatively short Stage II storage period, but also for the longer Stage III storage period.

Glass containers are recommended as the preferred type of container for the collection of samples, especially postmortem fluid samples (Rejent, 1981; Skoop, 2004). An important advantage of glass containers is that glass is relatively inert and, therefore, there is little likelihood of organic compounds leaching from the container walls into the sample and interfering with analytical methods, as may occur when plastic containers are used. However, the use of glass containers presents additional problems in addition to the obvious disadvantage of breakage. Trace elements may be desorbed from the glass into the sample, thus increasing the concentrations of zinc cadmium, copper, zinc, and mercury in the sample (Katz, 1984; Méranger et al., 1981; Schmitt, 1987). An additional problem with the use of glass containers for the collection of samples is that organic analytes may be adsorbed onto the glass surface. The loss of drugs due to their adsorption onto glass may be decreased by coating the glass surface with silicone compounds, an approach that has been shown to reduce, but not eliminate completely, the adsorption of many drugs, including morphine (Bhargava, 1977), buprenorphine (Hadidi and Oliver, 1998), and sufentanil (Dufresne et al., 2001).

Plastic containers, which have the benefits of being both disposable and more resistant to breakage than glass containers,[1] are used widely for the collection and subsequent storage of samples from both antemortem and postmortem subjects. Several drugs, especially those that are highly lipid soluble, such as fentanyl (Malkawi et al., 2008), can present a problem of detection, especially if the analytes are present at low concentrations (Kerrigan, 2011). The degree of analyte adsorption to plastics may be influenced by several factors including the physical characteristics of the analyte, the type of plastic used, the type of sample being stored, the temperature of storage, the pH of the sample, and the surface area of the plastic to which the sample is exposed (Jamerson et al., 2005; Roth et al., 1996; Stout et al., 2000). Because of these factors, plastic containers used for the storage of samples that may contain specific analytes must be evaluated under varying conditions as a component of method validation prior to their use. As is the case with glass containers, the analyte loss may not be extensive in absolute terms, but for drugs present at low concentrations, the relative extent of binding may be sufficient to result

---

[1]However, polystyrene containers, may crack when frozen (Flanagan et al., 2007), whereas polypropylene containers will not (Isenschmid and Hepler, 2007).

in drug concentrations decreasing below the detection limit or to values that cause a change in the interpretation of results. In spite of the potential for the adsorption of drugs onto plastics, the relative loss generally is less in samples such as solid tissues, in which the analytes have limited contact with the plastic, and gastric contents, in which relatively high drug concentrations are generally present (Isenschmid and Hepler, 2007).

The collection of serum and whole blood in blood collection tubes containing serum-separator gels has been reported to decrease the concentrations of several drugs, including lidocaine, phenobarbital, phenytoin (Dasgupta et al., 1996), amitriptyline, nortriptyline, clonazepam (Karppi et al., 2000), and methadone (Berk et al., 2006), presumably due to the binding of these drugs to the gels. Although this is generally not a problem for the storage of postmortem blood samples, as these samples are not typically collected in this type of tube, this may present a problem in clinical toxicology as these serum-separator tubes often are used for the collection of blood samples.

The selection of containers is of particular importance for the collection of samples that contain volatile analytes, such as organic solvents and carbon monoxide, or photolabile analytes. Unless proper containers are selected, volatile analytes may diffuse from a liquid sample stored in a closed container into the headspace above it, i.e., the vapor phase above the sample in a closed container. The extent of the analyte loss is proportional to the volume of the headspace and the temperature of the sample (Henry's Law) and results in erroneous analytical results. Samples thought to contain volatile compounds are most appropriately collected in containers with volumes which approximate those of the samples stored in them so that there is a minimum headspace above the sample. Since it is not known prior to analysis whether volatiles are present in samples, all fluid samples should be stored in such a manner. The transfer of volatile analytes from samples into the headspace will be decreased if the samples are refrigerated. However, if samples are removed from refrigeration and their temperatures are allowed to come to room temperature, the transfer will increase, and the analyte concentrations in the samples will decrease. In addition, each time the lid or stopper of the container is removed, the distribution equilibrium of the analyte shifts toward the vapor phase with an increasing loss of analyte. Therefore, the frequency of opening and closing storage containers should be kept to a minimum.

An additional problem posed by the collection of samples that contain volatile analytes is that these substances may diffuse through rubber stoppers of the types frequently used with test tubes. To minimize losses of volatile analytes in this manner, samples should be collected either in glass-stoppered glass tubes (Collom and Winek, 1970) or in glass containers fitted with metal foil-lined caps (Flanagan et al., 1990).

Several drugs and metabolites are known to undergo photodecomposition. In addition to the structural characteristics of analytes, important factors that influence the rate of photodecomposition include the type of sample that is stored, the composition of the container in which the sample is stored, e.g., glass, polyethylene, or polypropylene, and the wavelength of light to which the sample is exposed, e.g., sunlight or fluorescent lighting. Because lysergic acid diethylamide (LSD, also known as "acid") (Skopp et al., 2002; Webb et al., 1996) and the benzodiazepines (clonazepam, flurazepam, and nitrazepam) are known to undergo photodecomposition (Bares et al., 2004; Wad, 1986), samples thought to contain these drugs should be collected and stored in containers of opaque amber glass, opaque polyethylene, or wrapped with an aluminum foil to prevent exposure to sunlight or artificial light. Methadone demonstrates significant photodecomposition when exposed to UVB radiation; interestingly, the decomposition is greater in standard solutions than in hair, probably due to the protective effect of melanin and keratin in the hair (Favretto et al., 2014).

6.2.3 COLLECTION SITE

The body site from which the same types of samples are collected may have a profound effect on the measured analyte concentration. It should not be assumed, in the absence of data to the contrary, that drug concentrations are comparable in the same type of samples, e.g., blood, fat, and hair, collected either from different parts of the body, or from different areas of structurally heterogeneous organs, such as the brain or liver.

Because of the potential site-dependent differences in analyte concentrations, the sites from which samples are collected should be standardized, e.g., blood from the femoral vein or the right lobe of the liver, and recorded on the sample container. Unfortunately, sample collection protocols often do not specify a specific sampling site and consequently the collection sites are not identified on the containers in the toxicology report. This failure may be due simply to expedience or to the mistaken assumption that there is a homogeneous distribution of drugs within organs and tissues.

The collection of blood from fire victims should be collected from internal blood vessels or the heart because blood collected from body wounds or cavities may be contaminated with carbon monoxide and cyanide absorbed from the atmosphere at the site of the fire (Thoren et al., 2013). The extent of absorption and the resultant blood concentrations are dependent upon the concentration of these gases in the atmosphere and the duration of exposure.

Obtaining samples from semisolid organs presents potential problems because analytes may not be distributed homogeneously throughout the organ. Potential causes of heterogeneous analyte distribution within tissues and organs include an unequal blood supply to different parts of the organ and variations of structural and functional cell and tissues types in complex organs, including muscle, kidney, and brain (Koirtyohann and Hopps, 1981). Unfortunately, with the possible exception of the brain, sample collection protocols for the collection of samples from organs frequently do not specify a specific sampling site within the organ.

6.2.4 SAMPLE QUANTITY

A sufficient quantity of material must be collected so that all necessary screening tests, confirmatory analyses, and repeat analyses may be conducted. It cannot be overemphasized that a sufficient amount of each sample must be collected for all of these purposes; collecting an insufficient amount of sample is an error that often cannot be rectified at a later date.

The quantity of material required depends upon the number of analyses to be conducted and the detection limits of the analytical methods employed. Approximately 25−100 mL of blood, 50−100 g of other tissues, and all available bile, stomach contents, urine, and vitreous humor is generally sufficient for all required analyses and storage of samples in most cases (Baselt and Cravey, 1980; Butler, 1977; Rejent, 1981; SOFT/AAFS, 2006). If urine cannot be obtained at autopsy from an apparently empty bladder, the bladder should be rinsed with a small amount of water or saline to obtain any residual urine that may be present (Isenschmid and Hepler, 2007), which, due to the low detection limits of common methods of analysis, may be sufficient for the detection of a number of analytes.

6.2.5 SAMPLE LABELING

At a minimum, all samples that are collected should be labeled with a case number and/or subject name, sample type, specific site from which the sample was collected, the name and signature or initials of the collector, the date and time of collection, and the type of preservative used, if any (Molina, 2010, p. 5). The sample containers should be labeled with sample-specific accession number that allows for the identification and tracking of the sample throughout its analysis and storage. Many laboratories utilize preprinted labels that contain accession numbers and/or other identifiers. If labeling is done manually, the ink used should be waterproof and able to withstand extensive handling, exposure to chemicals and low temperatures, without being degraded to the point of illegibility.

Although not conducted routinely, DNA analysis of samples may be valuable for the identification of the subject from whom samples have been collected. DNA analysis has been used in cases of aircraft accidents, for the identification of body parts and samples (Chaturvedi et al., 1999, 2010).

6.3 SAMPLE PRESERVATION

Within the past few years, increased attention has been directed toward developing an understanding of the alterations in analyte concentrations that may result from storage conditions during storage stages II and III. It has become apparent that the improper storage of samples may constitute one of the greatest sources of errors in forensic and analytical toxicology. Because of these potential errors, forensic toxicologists and forensic pathologists should work together to establish protocols for the preservation of samples, including special precautions that may be required due to the suspected presence of storage-sensitive drugs. Common methods of sample and analyte preservation include storage at decreased temperature, addition of enzyme inhibitors, alteration of pH, and preparation of dried samples.

6.3.1 DECREASED TEMPERATURE

The method most commonly used to improve the stability of analytes in biological samples is the storage of samples at reduced temperatures: generally refrigeration for storage period II and freezing during storage period III. This strategy is often successful as most analytes exhibit greater stability in samples stored at these reduced temperatures as compared to samples stored at ambient laboratory temperatures. The temperature at which fluid and tissue samples, as well as standard solutions, are stored is extremely important because sample storage at even moderately elevated temperatures has the potential not only to accelerate the rate and extent of enzymatic or chemical degradation of the drug analytes in these samples, but also to cause alterations in the matrix of the samples.

Customarily, refrigeration is employed for the storage of samples for periods of days or weeks, i.e., Stage II storage, but is not suitable for storage periods of months or years, i.e., Stage III storage. Although refrigeration is effective for maintaining the stability of analytes during the short storage periods of Stage II, changes such as drug redistribution and degradation may occur in samples stored for prolonged periods of time at refrigeration temperature of approximately 4−5 °C. For prolonged storage periods of months or years, e.g., Stage III storage, storage at temperatures of −15°C to −20 °C or lower is more appropriate. However, storage at these decreased temperatures is not without problems of matrix alterations such as cell hemolysis, leakage of fluid from tissue, and loss of tissue homogeneity. For example, a 5 g piece of liver may be frozen in a relatively "dry" condition in a container. When the sample is thawed, it will be obvious that a meaningful amount of fluid—containing cellular contents and blood—has been released from the tissue due to the structural damage. If a 1 g portion required for analysis is collected from the sample, the drug concentration determined may be less than was present in the sample prior to freezing due to the loss of drug in the fluid released from the tissue.

The use of reduced temperatures as a means of storage, although appropriate and generally effective, is not a panacea for all of the problems of drug or sample stability—especially over the long term. Freezing may increase rather than decrease the rate of certain chemical reactions possibly as a result of increased solute concentration due to the freezing of water, pH shift, or increased catalytic action due to the formation of ice surfaces (Poulsen and Lindelov, 1981). Thus, the metabolic or chemical degradation of drugs, or the synthesis of postmortem products may continue even after the sample has been frozen.

6.3.2 INHIBITORS

Although chemical additives are employed frequently as sample and analyte preservatives, it must be reemphasized that the addition of anything to a sample must be evaluated and shown neither to alter the concentration of analytes present in the sample nor to affect the analysis of the sample. To ensure the integrity of the analytical results, two aliquots of a sample should be collected—one with and one without the preservative—so that an unexpected effect of the additive either on the analyte concentration or on the method of analysis may be identified (Flanagan et al., 2005).

A number of chemical additives have been used in order to prevent the enzymatic synthesis or metabolism of analytes. Some of these additives, including inhibitors such as sodium azide and sodium fluoride, are intended for the general inhibition of bacteria or enzymes that may metabolize or synthesize drug analytes, respectively. Although sodium azide (NaN_3) is used widely as a bacteriostatic agent in biological samples, it is effective against Gram-negative, but not Gram-positive bacteria (Snyder and Lichstein, 1940). A 2% (w/v) sodium fluoride concentration (Flanagan et al., 2005) is commonly used as a preservative to prevent the fermentation of glucose to ethanol and the enzymatic hydrolysis of esters. Physostigmine, a cholinesterase inhibitor, has also been used to increase the stability of esters such as the drug succinylcholine, a dicholine ester of succinic acid (Baldwin and Forney, 1988).

6.3.3 pH ALTERATIONS

Decreasing the pH of stored samples has been used to improve the stability of certain drugs such as esters, which are more stable under acidic conditions, since they may be hydrolyzed nonenzymatically under alkaline conditions. The increased stability of esters in acidified samples has been demonstrated in samples that have been acidified intentionally by the addition of buffers and by storage in formalin, or unintentionally as a result of postmortem events.

6.3.4 DRYING

The preservation of analytes in blood samples as dried spots (DBS), a method used widely in clinical settings (Deglon et al., 2009; Edelbroek et al., 2009; la Marca et al., 2009; Li and Tse, 2010; Wiseman et al., 2010), often provides improved analyte stability as well as having the benefits of ease of storage and transport. Although the detection of drugs in dried bloodstains was suggested decades ago as a means of differentiating bloodstains from suspects and victims of a crime (Curry, 1965; Kind, 1961), it was several years before the detection of drugs in dried bloodstains found at the scene of an incident was reported (Shaler et al., 1978; Smith, 1985). Since then, the use of DBS in forensic toxicology as a means of preservation has been employed to a limited (Chace et al., 2001; Elian, 1999), but increasing extent for the collection and storage of blood samples of 100 µL or less for the detection of subnanogram quantities of several drugs of forensic interest such as opioids, cocaine and benzoylecgonine, benzodiazepines, and amphetamines (Chace and Lappas, 2014). Several therapeutic and abused drugs have greater stability in dried samples of urine (DuBey and Caplan, 1996) and blood (Chace and Lappas, 2014; Demirev, 2013), than in fluid samples. In addition to improved stability, an added benefit of dried stains is that they are more convenient to store and transmit than are fluid samples.

6.4 SAMPLE TRANSPORT

Samples must be transmitted to the laboratory in a manner that preserves both their legal and scientific integrity. Each sample must be packaged individually, stored at a reduced temperature prior to transport (Jones, 2008; Rejent, 1981), protected from light and transmitted to the forensic toxicology laboratory as rapidly as possible. If samples must be sent to a distant laboratory, the submitting agency should follow the packing and shipping directions of the receiving laboratory, including the use of appropriate preservation methods, e.g., packing samples in dry ice or altering their pH by the use of buffers. The Armed Forces Institute of Pathology recommends that frozen samples that have to be mailed should be packed with an amount of dry ice equal to approximately three times the weight of the sample and that samples should not be sent by Registered, Certified, Air Freight, or "Return receipt requested" as these may delay receipt of the samples at the laboratory, but rather by FedEx®, U.S. Express/Priority Mail, or U.S. Second-Day Mail (Armed Forces Institute of Pathology, January 2008).

A record must be maintained of the movement of samples from the time of their collection until the time of their disposal. This record is the COC—a legal requirement, the purpose of which is to establish the authentication of the identity of the person from whom the sample was obtained, the identification of those persons who had possession of the sample, the identification of the location of sample storage, and the verification that the storage location was secure. By the maintenance of a COC it is anticipated that the likelihood of sample tampering by persons unauthorized to be in possession of the sample will be minimized and hopefully eliminated. The COC must include signatures of the person(s) from whom a sample has been received and the person(s) who receives it, the date on which the transfer of the sample was made from one person to the next, and the change in the location of the sample. In order to achieve this, it has been recommended that only specifically authorized personnel should have access to the laboratory, that receipt of the sample is verified by the signature of the person receiving it, that the date of the receipt is recorded, and that the transfer of the samples or aliquots within the laboratory for purposes of analysis or storage should be documented in the same manner (SOFT/AAFS, 2006). Many laboratories, mainly commercial laboratories, upon subpoena, will provide the so-called "litigation packet" that contains not only the essential documents pertaining to the analyses conducted, but also the COC documents from the time of sample collection, to receipt in the laboratory, through the analysis, storage, and ultimate disposal of the sample.

Although many attorneys may not be knowledgeable about the principles, concepts, and the methods of forensic and analytical toxicology, they are acutely aware of the COC requirements and will challenge the admissibility of evidence at the slightest hint of a broken chain. Many interpretations, and the analytical results on which they are based, have been excluded at the trial due to a break in the COC. Although forensic toxicology laboratories are aware of and usually careful about maintaining the COC, nonforensic laboratories, e.g., hospital laboratories, frequently are less careful and/or make no attempt to establish and maintain a COC, with the resultant consequence that the analytical results obtained from the samples are excluded from introduction as evidence at trial. The importance of maintaining the COC cannot be overemphasized as a break in the chain may render the analytical results inadmissible and negate any significance that may have been attached to them.

6.5 SAMPLE ACQUISITION

Following their transport, samples are acquired on the record upon arrival at forensic toxicology laboratories. The acquisition of samples by the laboratory must be conducted in an appropriate manner, because, if it is not, all subsequent analyses and interpretations will be invalidated. There are two important sources of potential errors in the process of sample acquisition—sample processing and bias.

Errors may occur at any of the steps in sample processing, such as inaccurate labeling, mistaken identity of samples, or failure to maintain a COC. The use of computer labeling and monitoring by means of accession numbers minimize certain of these errors to a meaningful extent. However, in a large laboratory that receives hundreds or even thousands of samples each day, a processing accuracy rate of even 99.9% will result in errors being made in dozens of samples.

In its landmark report *Strengthening Forensic Science in the United States: A Path Forward*, the National Research Council has recommended that further research is required to identify the extent of bias in forensic laboratories and to implement "… standard operating procedures (that will lay the foundation for model protocols) to minimize, to the greatest extent reasonably possible, potential bias and sources of human error in forensic practice" (National Research Council, 2009, p. 24). Bias may develop if the person who receives the samples is given information not required for the analysis of the samples, and this same individual subsequently analyzes the samples. The type of bias that may develop in such a situation is known as contextual bias, or context effect, and has been defined as the use of "… existing information or consistency to reinforce a position" (Budowle et al., 2009). Since forensic scientists are human, they are susceptible to a failure of objectivity caused by contextual bias that cannot be eliminated by the use of controls and blanks.

At first glance, it may appear that errors caused by contextual bias occur most frequently in the forensic sciences in which identifications are made as a result of "matches" based on human judgment and experience, e.g., fingerprint and firearm comparisons. However, a similar situation exists in forensic toxicology because analyte identifications commonly are made by means of comparisons, or "matches," of data, such as gas chromatography retention times and mass spectrometer-specific ion ratios, obtained from unknown samples with those of standard or control samples. In cases in which nonanalytical information has been given to the forensic toxicologists conducting the analyses or reviewing the results, contextual bias may influence them to conclude erroneously that the analytical data are consistent with identification criteria to identify the analyte (Of Interest 6.1).

OF INTEREST 6.1 CONTEXTUAL BIAS

An example of contextual bias is the case of a forensic toxicologist who received a blood sample from a police officer who informed him that the sample had been obtained from a subject who had been apprehended on several occasions for driving under the influence of various drugs and "… this time as a result of his drugged driving, he killed someone." In this case, although the toxicologist who received the sample and the specific case information did not perform the analysis, he reviewed the results of a gas chromatography-mass spectrometry (GC/MS) analysis, which did not meet the criteria for a positive identification of amphetamine. However, the toxicologist concluded that the sample was positive for amphetamine because the GC/MS results were "… close enough" to the required criteria and were consistent with the history of the subject.

This seems a clear case of contextual bias since the prior knowledge obtained from the police officer likely influenced the toxicologist's interpretation of the analytical results.

Because of the potential effects of contextual bias, forensic toxicology laboratories should establish protocols by which samples are received by someone other than the forensic toxicologists who will conduct any of the subsequent analyses. In this manner, the toxicologists are shielded from information such as the identity of the person from whom the samples were obtained and any of the circumstances of the case under investigation that may influence their impartiality. An approach to this problem is the use of a case manager (Thompson et al., 2011). A staff toxicologist can be assigned the role of the case manager. The case manager will receive samples delivered by autopsy technicians, police officers, etc., will be informed of the facts of the case and will act as a bridge between the acquisition of the samples with the associated case information and the analyst conducting the analyses. The case manager can discuss the case with the chief toxicologist, medical examiner, police, and others who may be involved and possess relevant information about the case. On the basis of the sample types and the information received, the case manager will direct the analytical protocol to be followed for the case by determining the analyses that should be conducted, including those routinely performed by the laboratory and any others that are specifically appropriate for the case at hand, but not routinely performed. By the use of a case manager in this manner, forensic toxicologists who conduct the analyses are not informed of the specific nature of the case and are not provided any information other than that required to conduct the analyses that are assigned by the case manager.

REVIEW QUESTIONS

1. The term "sample handling" encompasses several procedures—list and define each of the procedures.
2. Describe the criteria that should be utilized in the selection of samples to collect in antemortem and postmortem cases.
3. Describe the information that should be included on a sample label.
4. Define contextual bias, in the context of a forensic toxicology laboratory.

5. Discuss the advantages and disadvantages of utilizing glass containers or plastic containers for sample storage. What are some factors that must be considered when using each type of container?

APPLICATION QUESTIONS

1. Discuss the potential issues associated with the collection of only a single sample, e.g., blood, from a single location, in a postmortem analysis. Describe the ways in which you would alter the sample collection protocol to avoid these potential issues.

2. Discuss three methods of sample preservation that are commonly utilized to ensure, to the extent possible, that neither the presence nor concentration of any drugs in a sample is altered during storage period II or storage period III. Are certain preservation methods more appropriate for use during short-term or long-term storage, why?

3. Discuss the value of utilizing a case manager in a forensic toxicology laboratory. Are there disadvantages associated with utilizing a case manager? In your opinion, do the advantages outweigh the disadvantages, why or why not?

4. Discuss the ways in which you, as a forensic toxicologist, would help to maintain the chain of custody (COC) of a sample. What legal and or professional obligations do you have when interacting with a sample?
In your opinion, what are the major reasons why a COC might be broken?

REFERENCES

Armed Forces Institute of Pathology, January 2008. Guidelines for the Collection and Shipment of Specimens for Toxicological Analysis. Retrieved August 22, 2009 from: http://www.afip.org/consultation/AFMES/operations/forms/toxguidelines.pdf.

Baldwin, K.A., Forney Jr., R., 1988. The influence of storage temperature and chemical preservation on the stability of succinylcholine in canine tissue. J. For. Sci. 33 (2), 462–469.

Bares, I.F., Pehourcq, F., Jarry, C., 2004. Development of a rapid RP-HPLC method for the determination of clonazepam in human plasma. J. Pharm. Biomed. Anal. 36 (4), 865–869.

Baselt, R.C., Cravey, R.H., 1980. Forensic toxicology. In: Doull, J., Klaassen, C.D., Amdur, M.O. (Eds.), Toxicology: The Basic Science of Poisons, second ed. Macmillan Publishing Company, New York.

Berk, S., Litwin, A.H., Du, Y., Cruikshank, G., Gourevitch, M.N., Arnsten, J.H., 2006. False reduction in serum methadone concentrations by BD Vacutainer serum separator tubes (SSTTM). Clin. Chem. 52, 1972–1973.

Bhargava, H.N., 1977. Improved recovery of morphine from biological tissues using siliconized glassware. J. Pharm. Sci. 66, 1044–1045.

Budowle, B., Bottrell, M.C., Bunch, S.G., Fram, R., Harrison, D., Meagher, S., Oien, C.T., Peterson, P.E., Seiger, D.P., Smith, M.B., Smrz, M.A., Soltis, G.L., Stacey, R.B., 2009. A perspective on errors, bias and interpretation in the forensic sciences and direction for continuing advancement. J. Forensic Sci. 54, 798–809.

Butler, T.J., 1977. The specimen. In: Thoma, J.J. (Ed.), Guidelines for Analytical Toxicology Programs, vol. 1. CRC Press, Cleveland.

Chace, D.H., DiPerna, J.C., Mitchell, B.L., Sgroi, B., Hofman, L.F., Naylor, E.W., 2001. Electrospray tandem mass spectrometry for analysis of acylcarnitines in dried postmortem blood specimens collected at autopsy from infants with unexplained cause of death. Clin. Chem. 47 (7), 1166—1182.

Chace, D.H., Lappas, N.T., 2014. The use of dried blood spots and stains in forensic science. In: Li, W., Lee, M. (Eds.), Dried Blood Spots: Applications and Techniques. John Wiley & Sons, Hoboken, New Jersey.

Chaturvedi, A.K., Craft, K.J., Kupfer, D.M., Burian, D., Canfield, D.V., 2010. Resolution of aviation forensic toxicology findings with the aid of DNA profiling. [Electronic version]. Forensic Sci. Int. 206 (1—3), 81—86.

Chaturvedi, A.K., Vu, N.T., Ritter, R.M., Canfield, D.V., 1999. DNA typing as a strategy for resolving issues relevant to forensic toxicology. [Electronic version]. J. Forensic Sci. 44 (1), 189—192.

Collom, W.D., Winek, C.L., 1970. Detection of glue constituents in fatalities due to glue sniffing. Clin. Tox. 3, 125—130.

Curry, A.S., 1965. Science against crime. Int. Sci. Tech. 47, 39—48.

Dasgupta, A., Blackwell, W., Bard, D., 1996. Stability of therapeutic drug measurement in specimens collected in VACUTAINER plastic blood-collection tubes. Ther. Drug Monit. 18, 306—309.

Deglon, J., Thomas, A., Cataldo, A., Mangin, P., Staub, C., 2009. On-line desorption of dried blood spot: a novel approach for the direct LC/MS analysis of micro-whole blood samples. J. Pharm. Biomed. Anal. 49 (4), 1034—1039.

Demirev, P.A., 2013. Dried blood spots: analysis and applications. Anal. Chem. 85, 779—789.

DuBey, I.S., Caplan, Y.H., 1996. The storage of forensic urine drug specimens as dry stains: recovery and stability. [Electronic version]. J. Forensic Sci. 41 (5), 845—850.

Dufresne, C., Favetta, P., Paradis, C., Boulieu, R., 2001. Stability of sufentanil in human plasma samples. [Electronic version]. Ther. Drug Monit. 23 (5), 550—552.

Edelbroek, P.M., van der Heijden, J., Stolk, L.M., 2009. Dried blood spot methods in therapeutic drug monitoring: methods, assays, and pitfalls. Ther. Drug Monit. 31 (3), 327—336.

Elian, A.A., 1999. Detection of low levels of flunitrazepam and its metabolites in blood and bloodstains. Forensic Sci. Int. 101 (2), 107—111.

Favretto, D., Tucci, M., Monaldi, A., Ferrara, S.D., Miolo, G., 2014. A study on photodegradation of methadone, EDDP, and other drugs of abuse in hair exposed to controlled UVB radiation. Drug Test. Anal. 6 (Suppl. 1), 78—84.

Flanagan, R.J., Ruprah, M., Meredith, T.J., Ramsey, J.D., 1990. An introduction to the clinical toxicology of volatile substances. Drug Saf. 5, 359—383.

Flanagan, R.J., Connally, G., Evans, J.M., 2005. Guidelines for sample collection postmortem. Toxicol. Rev. 24, 63—71.

Flanagan, R.J., Taylor, A., Watson, I.D., Whelton, R., 2007. Fundamentals of Analytical Toxicology. John Wiley & Sons, Hoboken, NJ.

Hadidi, K.A., Oliver, J.S., 1998. Stability of morphine and buprenorphine in whole blood. [Electronic version]. Int. J. Leg. Med. 111 (3), 165—167.

Isenschmid, D.S., Hepler, B.R., 2007. Specimen selection, collection, preservation and security. In: Karch, S.B. (Ed.), Postmortem Toxicology of Abused Drugs.

Jamerson, M.H., McCue, J.J., Klette, K.L., 2005. Urine pH, container composition, and exposure time influence adsorptive loss of 11-nor-delta9-tetrahydrocannabinol-9-carboxylic acid. [Electronic version]. J. Anal. Toxicol. 29 (7), 627–631.

Jones, G.R., 2008. Postmortem toxicology. In: Jickells, S., Negrusz, A. (Eds.), Clarke's Analyical Forensic Toxioclogy. Pharmaceutical Press, Chicago.

Karppi, J., Akerman, K.K., Parviainen, M., 2000. Suitability of collection tubes with separator gels for collecting and storing blood samples for therapeutic drug monitoring. Clin. Chem. Lab. Med. 38, 313–320.

Katz, S.A., 1984. Collection and preparation of biological tissues and fluids. Am. Biotechnol. Lab 2, 24–30.

Kerrigan, S., 2011. Sampling, storage and stability. In: Moffat, A.C., Osselton, M.D., Widdop, B., Watts, J. (Eds.), Clarke's Analysis of Drugs and Poisons, fourth ed. Pharmaceutical Press, Chicago.

Kind, S.S., 1961. The individuality of human bloodstaining. J. Forensic Sci. Soc. 2, 75.

Koirtyohann, S.R., Hopps, H.C., 1981. Sample selection, collection, preservation, and storage for a data bank on trace elements in human tissue. Fed. Proc. 40, 2143–2146.

la Marca, G., Malvagia, S., Filippi, L., Luceri, F., Moneti, G., Guerrini, R., 2009. A new rapid micromethod for the assay of phenobarbital from dried blood spots by LC-tandem mass spectrometry. Epilepsia 50 (12), 2658–2662.

Li, W., Tse, F.L., 2010. Dried blood spot sampling in combination with LC-MS/MS for quantitative analysis of small molecules. BMC 24 (1), 49–65.

Malkawi, A.H., Al-Ghananeem, A.M., Crooks, P.A., 2008. Development of a GC-MS assay for the determination of fentanyl pharmacokinetics in rabbit plasma after sublingual spray delivery. AAPS J. 10, 261–267.

Méranger, J.C., Hollebone, B.R., Blanchette, G.A., 1981. The effects of storage times, temperatures and container types on the accuracy of atomic-absorption determinations of Cd, Cu, Hg, Pb and Zn in whole heparinized blood. J. Analyt. Tox. 5 (1), 33–41.

Molina, D.K., 2010. Handbook of Forensic Toxicology for Medical Examiners. CRC Press, New York.

National Research Council, 2009. Strengthening Forensic Sciences in the United States. National Academy Press, Washington, D.C.

Poulsen, K.P., Lindelov, F., 1981. Acceleration of chemical reactions due to freezing. In: Rockland, L.B., Stewart, G.F. (Eds.), Water Activity: Influences on Food Quality. Academic Press, New York.

Rejent, T.A., 1981. Collection and storage of evidence. In: Cravey, R.H., Baselt, R.C. (Eds.), Introduction to Forensic Toxicology. Biomedical Publications, Davis, CA.

Rosenfeld, L., 1985. Alfred swaine taylor (1806–1880), pioneer toxicologist—and a slight case of murder. Clin. Chem. 31, 1235–1236.

Roth, K.D., Siegel, N.A., Johnson Jr., R.W., Litauszki, L., Salvati Jr., L., Harrington, C.A., et al., 1996. Investigation of the effects of solution composition and container material type on the loss of 11-nor-delta 9-THC-9-carboxylic acid. [Electronic version]. J. Anal. Toxicol. 20 (5), 291–300.

Schmitt, Y., 1987. Influence of preanalytical factors on the atomic absorption spectrometry determination of trace elements in biological samples. J. Trace Elem. Electrolytes Health Dis. 1, 107–114.

Shaler, R.C., Smith, F.P., Mortimer, C.E., 1978. Detection of drugs in a bloodstain. I: Diphenylhydantoin. J. Forensic Sci. 23, 701–706.

Skoop, G., 2004. Preanalytic aspects in postmortem toxicology. Forensic Sci. Int. 142, 75–100.

Skopp, G., Potsch, L., Mattern, R., Aderjan, R., 2002. Short-term stability of lysergic acid diethylamide (LSD), N-desmethyl-LSD, and 2-oxo-3-hydroxy-LSD in urine, assessed by liquid chromatography-tandem mass spectrometry. [Electronic version]. Clin. Chem. 48 (9), 1615–1618.

Smith, F.P., 1985. The detection of drugs in bloodstains. In: Lee, H.C., Gaensslen, R.E. (Eds.), Advances in Forensic Sciences. Biomedical Publications, Foster City, CA, p. 238.

Snyder, M.L., Lichstein, H.C., 1940. Sodium azide as an inhibiting substance for gram-negative bacteria. J. Infect. Dis. 67, 113–115.

SOFT/AAFS, 2006. Forensic Toxicology Laboratory Guidelines. Retrieved November 3, 2012 from: http://www.soft-tox.org/files/Guidelines_2006_Final.pdf.

Stout, P.R., Horn, C.K., Lesser, D.R., 2000. Loss of THCCOOH from urine specimens stored in polypropylene and polyethylene containers at different temperatures. J. Anal. Toxicol. 24 (7), 567–571.

Thompson, W.C., et al., 2011. Commentary on Thornton, J. L. (letter to the editor - a rejection of "working blind" as a cure for contextual bias). J. For. Sci. 55 (6), 1663.

Thoren, T.M., Thompson, K.S., Cardona, P.S., Chaturvedi, A.K., Canfield, D.V., 2013. In vitro absorption of atmospheric carbon monoxide and hydrogen cyanide in undisturbed pooled blood. J. Anal. Tox. 39 (4), 203–207.

Versiek, J.M.J., Speecke, A.B.H., 1972. Contamination induced by collection of liver biopsies and human blood, as cited in Koirtyohann, S.R., Hopps, H.C., 1981. Sample selection, collection, preservation, and storage for a data bank on trace elements in human tissue, Fed. Proc. 40, 2143–2146.

Wad, N., 1986. Degradation of clonazepam in serum by light confirmed by means of a high performance liquid chromatographic method. [Electronic version]. Ther. Drug Monit. 8 (3), 358–360.

Webb, K.S., Baker, P.B., Cassells, N.P., Francis, J.M., Johnston, D.E., Lancaster, S.L., et al., 1996. The analysis of lysergide (LSD): the development of novel enzyme immunoassay and immunoaffinity extraction procedures together with an HPLC-MS confirmation procedure. [Electronic version]. J. Forensic Sci. 41 (6), 938–946.

Wiseman, J.M., Evans, C.A., Bowen, C.L., Kennedy, J.H., 2010. Direct analysis of dried blood spots utilizing desorption electrospray ionization (DESI) mass spectrometry. Analyst 135 (4), 720–725.

Wormley, T.G., 1867. Micro-Chemistry of Poisons Including their Physiological, Pathological, and Legal Relations, Adapted to the Use of the Medical Jurist, Physician, and General Chemist. Baillier Brothers, New York, p. 22.

Storage Stability of Analytes

7

In regard to the effects of chemical changes and decomposition in removing poison beyond the reach of analysis, it may be remarked that some of the organic poisons, especially when of a volatile nature, may undergo a change … in the dead body after very short periods.
T.G. Wormley (1867)

It cannot be doubted that during the putrefactive changes which occur after death, some poisons may be altered, and even entirely disappear.
John James Reese (1874)

In the ideal universe, sample matrices would remain unchanged during storage, the concentrations of the drugs present in samples would remain constant, and postmortem products would not be produced. Unfortunately, in the real world of forensic toxicologists, all samples are stored for varying periods of time under widely differing and often extreme conditions. For example, a body may not be discovered immediately after death and as a result, samples may be subjected to extremes of temperature and humidity prior to their collection, causing the alteration in concentration, or loss of analytes present in the samples at the time of death. Following their collection, the improper storage of samples, for even relatively short periods prior to analysis, can also cause alterations of analyte concentrations.

It is apparent from the works of Wormley and Reese that forensic toxicologists have long been both aware of and concerned about the problem of analyte stability in stored samples. Within the past few years, as a result of the great deal of attention directed toward developing an understanding of the alterations in analyte concentrations that may occur during the storage of samples, it has become apparent that the inappropriate storage of samples is an important source of errors in forensic and analytical toxicology. Therefore, forensic toxicologists must be aware of the potential for these problems and take appropriate precautions in order to prevent them.

For purposes of this discussion, the storage periods to which a sample may be subjected are referred to as storage periods I, II, and III. As described in Chapter 3, storage period I occurs between the event of interest, e.g., the death of an individual or an automobile accident, and the collection of samples, during which time the analytes are stored in situ; storage period II is the time interval between the

Forensic Toxicology. http://dx.doi.org/10.1016/B978-0-12-799967-8.00007-4

collection of samples and their initial analysis; and storage period III is the storage period that begins when the initial analysis of the samples has been completed and extends until to the time that the samples are discarded.

Numerous cellular activities can continue throughout one or more of these storage periods and as a result analyte concentrations in stored samples may be:

- considered to be unchanged if the alteration in the concentration either is not statistically significant or is insufficient to cause the interpretation of the concentration to be altered from a prestorage interpretation;
- decreased due to chemical degradation, endogenous, or exogenous enzymatic activity, or the type of storage container used;
- increased due to de novo synthesis or conversion of metabolites to parent compounds and vice versa.

In antemortem samples, normal physiological and biochemical activities continue, generally at normal rates and to normal extents during storage period I until samples are collected. Although postmortem cells are moribund during storage period I, they are not yet completely quiescent and may not be dead; within these samples, there still persist "normal" cellular physiological and biochemical activities albeit at decreasing rates and to decreasing extents. Also, importantly, events that do not occur in antemortem cells may occur in postmortem cells as a result of autolysis and putrefaction that can occur during this period. Samples that move from storage period II to storage period III may not be uniform in their morphology and composition; nonetheless, the methods used to minimize alterations in analyte concentrations are similar if not identical for samples during both periods.

The stability of analytes following storage in the three storage periods depends on a number of factors:

- *The initial analyte concentration*: The greater the initial analyte concentration prior at storage, the more likely it is that the analyte will be detected at the end of the storage period.
- *The specificity and the sensitivity of the analytical method*: The method used for the detection of analytes must be able to differentiate among the analyte, its metabolites—which are frequently produced, and other substances that might be produced during storage. In addition, the lower the detection limits of the analytical methods used, the longer analytes will be detected and the greater the reported stability.
- *The type of samples in which analytes have been stored*: The enzyme types and cofactor concentrations present in samples of varying types, e.g., vitreous humor compared to liver, can influence sample stability. Also, the stability of analytes in postmortem samples may differ from that in antemortem samples due to the greater likelihood of microbial activity in the former,
- *The length of the storage period*: Storage periods of greater lengths of time would be expected to result in a greater alteration of analyte concentrations than would storage periods of shorter lengths of time.

- *The use of preservatives*: The use of preservatives such as enzyme inhibitors and pH buffers generally are effective in stabilizing analyte concentrations during storage periods II and III.
- *The conditions of storage*: During storage period I, temperature, moisture, and postmortem pH changes during autolysis and putrefaction, all have the potential to affect both the rate and extent of endogenous and exogenous (microorganisms) chemical and enzymatic reactions, resulting in increased or decreased analyte concentrations. During storage periods II and III, temperature, light, decomposition, storage in formaldehyde or in embalmed bodies can have an effect on analyte stability. Because the conditions that exist during storage periods greatly influence the stability of analytes, it is essential that the effects of these conditions on specific analytes are determined. Although forensic toxicologists cannot alter the storage conditions of storage period I, they must be aware of the changes that can occur in order to make the appropriate interpretations of measured analyte concentrations. However, procedures can and must be implemented during storage periods II and III to prevent or minimize any alterations of analyte concentrations that may occur during these periods.

7.1 STABILITY STUDIES

Stability studies are an evaluation of the stability of analytes under a specific set of factors as described above. Therefore, in such studies, all samples should be prepared in the same manner, stored at the same volume or weight in containers of the same type, stored under identical conditions of temperature, humidity, and light, sampled in the same manner and analyzed by the same method using instruments whose performance is unaltered over the course of the study and preferably using reagents from the same manufacturer's lots. The method of analysis used to determine the drug concentration in the stored samples must be able to differentiate between the analyte drug and any metabolic, degradative, synthesized, or putrefactive compounds produced during the storage period so that the loss or gain of analytes may be detected and not affected by the nonspecific detection of any storage products. Since analyte stability is determined under specific conditions, the results cannot be assumed to hold for other sample types or storage conditions.

Stability studies may be conducted using several different types of samples: case samples, experimental samples obtained from drug-treated human volunteers or experimental animals, or fortified ("spiked") samples prepared by the addition of a known quantity of analyte to a selected sample.

7.1.1 CASE SAMPLES

Both antemortem and postmortem case samples, which may be used in stability studies, have the advantage of being "authentic" samples that mirror the types of samples that forensic toxicologists will encounter. A disadvantage of the use of case samples is that the samples must be taken and used "as is," with no knowledge of the presence of other drugs and metabolites, existing pathologies or abnormalities of drug metabolism. In the case of postmortem case samples, the degree of decomposition and presence of postmortem putrefactive products may influence the stability of analytes. These problems are compounded if samples of sufficient volume or weight cannot be obtained from a single subject, necessitating mixing of samples from several subjects, thereby increasing the likelihood of the presence of unidentified and potentially interring substances.

7.1.2 EXPERIMENTAL SAMPLES

The use of samples obtained from drug-treated human volunteers or experimental animals eliminates many of the problems encountered with the use of case samples. Blood, urine, and hair obtained from human volunteers, and organs such as liver, brain, and kidney obtained from experimental animals, may offer several advantages. The samples would contain only the drug of interest and its metabolites and could be stored under a variety of conditions immediately upon collection. The absence of unknown exogenous substances other than the administered substance and its metabolites would eliminate the possibility of interactions, such as metabolic interactions, that might affect stability.

7.1.3 FORTIFIED SAMPLES

The use of samples fortified ("spiked") with analytes enables the greatest level of organization and control of all aspects of sample preparation and storage. The samples to be fortified should be prepared using a pool of material obtained from several test subjects so that any unusual characteristics of a few samples do not unduly influence the "normal" nature of the pool. All samples used must be analyzed to ensure that they are drug-free and that the concentrations of endogenous substances such as hemoglobin, albumin, and erythrocytes are within normal ranges, as abnormalities in the concentrations of these and other endogenous substances may alter the normal patterns of drug binding and distribution within the samples. The preparation of liquid samples such as blood or urine generally is effectively achieved by adding the appropriate volume of an alcoholic solution of the drug to a volumetric flask, evaporating the alcohol and then mixing and diluting the drug residue with the required volume of sample. However, when nonliquid samples are used, e.g., liver, brain, or muscle, the samples are homogenized. The volume and type of homogenizing fluid used may influence the stability of the drug and so should be chosen carefully—water, saline, or buffers usually are effective and unreactive solvents. A drawback to the use of homogenates is that the resultant fortified homogenate is at best a diluted approximation of the actual tissue, in which the disruption of the normal tissue matrix may not reflect the "normal" stability of the drug in intact tissue. The distribution of the drug and the availability of metabolic enzymes and substances normally sequestered within the cells undoubtedly will be different in the disrupted tissue than in the intact tissue. Also, samples used to prepare these pooled samples usually are less likely to have undergone any decomposition, so that the effect of microbial action is minimized or eliminated.

7.1.4 INTERPRETATION OF STABILITY STUDIES

The results of stability studies may be interpreted in two manners. The drug concentration after storage may be compared to the original concentration in order to determine whether (1) there has been a predefined or statistically significant change in concentration or (2) the change in the analyte concentration following storage differs sufficiently from that of the original analysis to cause a change in the interpretation of the analytical results.

Neither a large predefined, e.g., ±20%, nor a statistically significant change in concentration may be appropriate as a standard since neither may be consistent with a toxicologically significant change, i.e., the changes may not be sufficiently large to alter the initial interpretation of analyte concentrations. For many drugs, concentration ranges that are consistent with therapeutic, toxic, and lethal effects are broad, often an order of magnitude or greater. Because of this, although there may be a statistically significant alteration of the analyte concentration as a result of storage, it may not be sufficiently great as to change the initial interpretation, e.g., drug concentrations prior to and following storage both may be in the toxic concentration range even though the difference between the two concentrations is statistically significant. Therefore, a more meaningful measure of stability is whether any change in analyte concentrations results in an alteration of the interpretation of the analytical results. For example, a decrease in the prestorage concentration from a concentration consistent with toxicity to a poststorage concentration consistent with therapeutic use is meaningful and can have far reaching consequences.

7.2 STORAGE PERIODS
7.2.1 STORAGE PERIOD I

The length of storage period I may vary from hours to centuries and the storage conditions may vary from hot and dry to cold and wet. Therefore, during this storage period, samples and the analytes they contain may be exposed to mild conditions for short periods, as is the case of samples collected from living persons, or to extreme conditions for very long periods, which can be the case of postmortem samples. In the former, it is likely that little change will occur in sample matrices or in analyte concentrations because of the types of samples that are collected and because the samples can be stored appropriately soon after their collection. However, the longer duration of storage period I in postmortem cases can result in extensive alterations of both sample matrices and analyte concentrations.

It is common for postmortem samples to be of poor quality due to the several events that may be related to the cause of death, e.g., trauma, or that occur following death, e.g., decomposition. Of the two, postmortem decomposition likely has the greater potential to affect analyte stability. Postmortem decomposition, which begins minutes after death (Vass et al., 2002), is a complex process consisting of autolysis (self-digestion), the process by which cells are dissolved by intracellular enzymes, putrefaction, the process by which the soft tissues of the body are converted to gases, liquids, and small molecules by microorganisms, and often insect activity and animal predation (Levy and Harcke, 2010; Vass et al., 2002).

Shortly after death, during autolysis, the activity of intracellular enzymes causes a decrease in pH, whereas as putrefaction develops there is an increase in pH due to the enzymatic action of microbial enzymes on lipids, carbohydrates, and proteins (Skoop, 2004). Also, dehydration is likely to occur throughout the process of decomposition. During extensive decomposition, there is widespread autolysis and putrefaction of semisolid tissues to the extent that bone and the keratinous samples, nails, and hair, often are the only acceptable samples available for toxicological analysis.

Although the decomposition of soft tissues and fluids during storage period I may be extensive, many analytes demonstrate resistance to the degradative effects of autolysis and/or putrefaction and may be detected in these samples. Examples of drugs that remain detectable in case samples after a prolonged storage period I are presented in Table 7.1. A number of these drugs are stable for years, not only due to their chemical structures, but also due to the manner in which the body was stored. For example, under ideal storage conditions of low humidity and moderate temperatures, organic molecules may persist in hair for prolonged periods of time (Kintz, 2004), possibly for centuries (Balabanova et al., 1992; Musshoff et al., 2009; Springfield et al., 1993; Wilson et al., 2013). However, the stability of drugs and metabolites in hair is diminished if the hair has been treated with bleach, oxidizing dyes, and components of permanent wave products (Gallardo and Queiroz, 2008; Kintz et al., 2008).

Several drugs have been shown to be stable in experimental studies of fortified liver macerates (Table 7.2). Drugs that possess oxygen bonded to nitrogen, e.g., nitro groups, N-oxides, and oximes, sulfur bonded to carbon or phosphorus, e.g., $C{=}S$, $P{=}S$, or amino and phenolic hydroxyl groups on an aryl ring demonstrate the greatest instability (Stevens, 1984). This structural effect on drug stability is exemplified by the difference in the stability of benzodiazepines. As the data in Tables 7.1 and 7.2 demonstrate, benzodiazepines without a nitro group, e.g., diazepam, flurazepam, and lorazepam, are stable in liver macerates for as long as 77 days; nitrazepam, a nitro-containing benzodiazepine, is stable in liver macerates for only 12 days (Stevens, 1984). Furthermore, the nonnitro-containing benzodiazepines, diazepam, flurazepam, and triazolam, are detected in samples obtained from bodies that have been buried for several years. The instability of nitrobenzodiazepines has been attributed to their metabolism by bacteria (Robertson and Drummer, 1995).

Table 7.1 Case Sample Analytes Detected Following Storage Period I

Drug	Sample	Storage Conditions	Storage Duration (years)	Comments	References
Amitriptyline	Bone marrow	Environmental exposure	2–3	Skeletonized body	Noguchi et al. (1978)
Amitriptyline	Liver and hair	Buried	2–3	Well-preserved body	Gaillard et al. (2011)
Amphetamine and methamphetamine	Bone marrow	Buried	5	Denatured fatty material	Kojima et al. (1986)
Cocaine and benzoylecgonine	Hair	Buried	~1000	Mummified body	Springfield et al. (1993)
Diazepam	Stomach contents and liver	Buried	4.5		Karger et al. (2004)
Diazepam	Not given	Buried	4.8–7.5		Grellner and Glenewinkel (1997)
Ethyl glucuronide and ethyl sulfate	Liver, kidney, and blood clot	Entombment	27	Mummified body	Politi (2008)
Flurazepam	Not given	Buried	5.5		Grellner and Glenewinkel (1997)
Phenobarbital	Liver, heart, muscle, and skin	Environmental exposure	10	Mummified body	Giusiani et al. (2012)
Triazolam	Bone marrow and mummified muscle	Buried	4	Skeletonized body	Kudo et al. (1997)

Table 7.2 Stable Drugs in Fortified Liver Macerates[1]

Drugs	Storage Conditions	Storage Period (days)
Amitriptyline	Open to the external environment	22–77
Imipramine	Open to the external environment	22
Diazepam	Open to the external environment	22–77
Flurazepam	Open to the external environment	22–77
Lorazepam	Open to the external environment	22–77
Morphine	Open to the external environment	28–29
Meperidine	Open to the external environment	28

The samples were contaminated with blowfly borne bacteria.
[1] *Unless otherwise noted, the macerates were made using human liver.*
From Stevens (1984).

7.2.2 STORAGE PERIODS II AND III

Several of the same conditions and events that influence stability during storage period I can influence stability during storage periods II and III. Importantly, forensic toxicologists can take steps to minimize or eliminate these factors following the collection of samples. These strategies include the use of storage containers of appropriate size and composition, enzyme inhibitors and pH buffers, the protection of samples from light exposure, and storage at reduced temperatures.

Although preservation protocols employed during storage period II should be applied as soon as possible after sample collection, it may be necessary to change some aspects of storage, e.g., the type of storage container, if samples determined to contain specific drugs or chemicals must be placed into long term storage period III in order to preserve evidence.

Frequently, data obtained from drug stability studies differ among laboratories, largely due to differences in the experimental designs of these studies, which include extensive variations among the storage conditions. Because of these variations, it is not feasible to generate an exhaustive database of the stability of every drug in every storage condition. Therefore, presented below is an overview of the general stability trends of several analytes of significance in forensic toxicology.

7.3 ETHANOL

The interpretation of ethanol concentrations determined in various sample types is undoubtedly the most common interpretation made by forensic toxicologists. Therefore, the knowledge of the stability of ethanol in stored samples is of utmost importance in forensic toxicology because the interpretations of ethanol concentrations have an impact on many cases. This importance is illustrated by the voluminous literature pertaining to the effects of storage on the stability of ethanol.

Ethanol concentrations in stored samples can be increased by microbial synthesis or decreased by oxidation, volatilization, and microbial metabolism.

7.3.1 **STORAGE PERIOD I**

It has been known for decades that the synthesis of ethanol can occur during storage period I due to the action of numerous microorganisms (Anderson, 2015). Several factors influence the quantity of ethanol that will be produced during this postmortem interval (Collom, 1975). They include:

- the duration of storage period I;
- the environmental temperature during storage period I;
- the type of microorganisms that colonize the cadaver;
- the cause of death.

Longer durations and elevated temperatures in storage period I will likely cause an increased amount of ethanol to be formed as these conditions favor the growth of microorganisms. Examples of the numerous microorganisms that can synthesize ethanol from glucose include the following genera of yeasts, e.g. *Candida*; bacteria, e.g., *Aerobacter, Clostridium, Lactobacilli,* and *Streptococcus*; and molds, e.g., *Aspergillus* and *Fusarium*, that can be found in or on cadavers; in addition, several microorganisms can use other sugars as well as amino acids and fatty acids for the synthesis of ethanol (Corry, 1978). Traumatic damage to the internal organs, especially of the gastrointestinal tract, a major source of microorganisms in the body, increases the distribution of these microorganisms to other parts of the body, resulting in a more rapid and extensive colonization of the cadaver and greater ethanol synthesis than would be expected in an intact body (Collom, 1975; Wagner et al., 2015).

The influence that the conditions of storage period I have on the production of ethanol is seen in studies in which the occurrence of postmortem synthesis of ethanol ranged widely from 12% to 100% in a study of more than 800 postmortem cases (O'Neal and Poklis, 1996).

7.3.2 **STORAGE PERIODS II AND III**

The three mechanisms by which ethanol concentrations can decrease in blood samples during storage periods I and II are evaporation, oxidation, and microbial action (Brown et al., 1973; Anderson, 2015).

The loss of ethanol from blood and urine due to evaporation/volatilization appears to be caused by the failure to close and seal storage containers tightly (Brown et al., 1973; Olsen and Hearn, 2003; Sreerama and Hardin, 2003).

Ethanol in stored blood samples may be oxidized to acetaldehyde by an enzymatic reaction that requires the presence of oxyhemoglobin (Brown et al., 1973). This oxidation reaction does not occur in either serum or plasma, as they do not contain hemoglobin (Brown et al., 1973; Chen et al., 1994). The oxidation is inhibited by sodium azide, but not by fluoride. The extent of oxidation by this mechanism is increased in samples stored in containers with large headspace volumes of air (Brown et al., 1973; Olsen and Hearn, 2003).

Microorganisms may either increase or decrease ethanol concentrations in stored samples. Numerous microbes, including those mentioned above, can synthesize ethanol and therefore increase its concentration in stored samples. The microorganisms may be present in the samples due to storage period I decomposition or due to contamination and improper storage during storage periods I and II. A smaller number of microorganisms utilize ethanol as a metabolic substrate and can decrease ethanol concentrations in stored samples. *Serratia marcescens* and *Pseudomonas* sp. caused ethanol concentrations in unpreserved blood samples to decrease after several days of storage at 4 °C and preserved with 1% NaF; preservation with 2% NaF at 4 °C is effective in stabilizing the concentrations (Dick and Stone, 1987). The widely accepted method for the inhibition of microbial action is the storage of samples containing 1−2% (w/v) sodium fluoride at approximately 4 °C or −20 °C (Amick and Habben, 1997; Jones et al., 1999; Kaye and Dammin, 1945; Lough and Fehn, 1993; Sulkowski et al., 1995).

Generally, the optimal stability of ethanol is attained in samples to which sodium fluoride and/or sodium azide have been added and that are stored at decreased temperatures in containers with minimal headspace volume.

7.4 OPIOIDS

Morphine and its metabolites, morphine-3-glucuronide and morphine-6-glucuronide, stored in either spiked plasma and blood or postmortem blood with no added preservatives at −20 °C and shielded from light, are stable for the duration of the experimental storage periods of 181 and 124 days, respectively (Skopp et al., 2001). Morphine and codeine are stable in spiked and autopsy blood samples with added fluorides stored at −20 °C for as long as 8 and 9 years, respectively (Hoiseth et al., 2014). Plasma samples containing several opioids, including buprenorphine, codeine, fentanyl, hydromorphone, methadone, morphine, oxycodone, and the metabolites morphine, glucuronide, and norfentanyl, can undergo several freeze (−18 °C)/ thaw cycles over the experimental storage period of 84 days with none of the analyte concentrations varying more than 10% over this period (Musshoff et al., 2006).

Exception to the generally acceptable stability of opioids in stored blood and plasma are the esters, heroin, and 6-monoacetylmorphine (6MAM). Heroin stability in stored rat samples has been determined to be greater in brain homogenates than in plasma and greater in plasma than in whole blood, presumably due to lesser esterase activity in brain and plasma than in whole blood (Jones et al., 2013). The stability of heroin is improved when all samples are stored with added NaF and frozen. The greater instability of 6MAM than morphine and codeine in blood samples stored at −20 °C for several months or years is meaningful as its detection in samples is a confirmation of heroin use (Papoutsis et al., 2014; Hoiseth et al., 2014).

The influence of sample types on analyte stability is exemplified by 6MAM, the half-life of which is increased more than threefold, when blood is stored as a dried stain rather than as a fluid (Boy et al., 2008), and which although generally not stable when stored in biological samples, is stable for 1 year when stored in nonbiological standard solutions (Karinen et al., 2011). In a small study of hairs obtained at autopsy, dihydrocodeine, morphine, and 6MAM were found to undergo decomposition when stored in water or soil for 1–6 and 6 months, respectively (Potsch et al., 1995). A dramatic decrease occurred in the concentration of dihydrocodeine and the other drugs, which was positive initially, was negative after storage. The decreased drug concentrations were associated with microscopic changes in the structure of the hair.

The stability of morphine, codeine, and 6MAM in blood is improved by the addition of NaF and storage in siliconized glass (Bhargava, 1977) rather than in polypropylene or polystyrene tubes (Papoutsis et al., 2014). The concentrations of morphine and codeine in urine samples stored at $-20\,°C$ for 1 year have been found to not decrease below the detection limits of 14 and 15 ng/mL, respectively (Dugan et al., 1994).

It can be concluded from the results of several studies investigating the stability of opioids that the alterations in the concentrations of most opioids in blood and urine, when stored for months or years at temperatures of approximately $-20\,°C$ or lower, are minimal and consistent with acceptable stability.

7.5 COCAINE

Because cocaine is an ester, its stability in biological samples is generally poor unless appropriate precautions are taken. Cocaine can be degraded, either in vivo or in vitro, by two major mechanisms, chemical and enzymatic hydrolysis. Chemical hydrolysis occurs at alkaline pH, whereas enzymatic hydrolysis is the result of esterase activity. The products of chemical and enzymatic hydrolysis are benzoylecgonine (BE) and ecgonine methyl ester (EME), respectively.

Cocaine is stable for several months in blood samples stored at $4\,°C$ or lower, if the pH has been adjusted to a value of less than 7 and to which NaF and/or a cholinesterase inhibitor has been added (Baselt et al., 1993; Isenschmid et al., 1989; Moody et al., 1999). In unpreserved urine samples stored at $-20\,°C$ for 1 year, the concentration of cocaine decreases in approximately 20% of the samples, with an average decrease of 37% (Dugan et al., 1994). The cocaine concentration has been stabilized for 3 weeks in urine samples with pH adjusted to 5 stored at $4\,°C$, in the absence or presence of NaF (Baselt, 1983); these results demonstrate the importance of the pH on the stability of cocaine in urine. The use of sodium azide should not be used as a preservative for esters, including cocaine, because it can increase the rate of cocaine hydrolysis in urine samples, possibly as the result of an attack by the azide anion on the carbonyl carbon of the ester bond (Zaitsu et al., 2008).

The concentration of BE stored in unpreserved urine samples,

- at -16 or $-18\,°C$, is stable for up to 45 days (Paul et al., 1993);
- at $-15\,°C$ for 1–8 months, decreases an average of 19%, with a wide distribution of concentration changes (Romberg and Past, 1994); and

- at $-20\,°C$ for 1 year, increases an average of 10% with a wide distribution of concentration changes; the concentrations do not decrease sufficiently to alter the original detection of BE (Dugan et al., 1994).

The importance of pH on the stability of cocaine cannot be overemphasized. Not only does pH influence the stability of cocaine in biological samples, but also in storage fluids such as formalin. The concentration of cocaine is essentially unchanged after 30 days of storage in formalin buffered to a pH of 3.5, whereas in formalin buffered to a pH of 7.4, approximately 80% of the cocaine is degraded over the same period (Viel et al., 2009).

7.6 CANNABINOIDS

Delta-9-tetrahydrocannabinol (Δ9THC) and its metabolites, 11-nor-9-carboxy delta-9-tetrahydrocannabinol (THC COOH) and 11-hydroxy delta-9-tetrahydrocannabinol (11-OH THC), stored in blood at 4 and $-10\,°C$ have been shown to be stable for as long as 4 and 6 months, respectively, whereas, when stored in plasma, they all are stable for as long as 6 months at both 4 and $-10\,°C$ (Johnson et al., 1984). There is a marked decrease in the concentration of Δ9THC in femoral blood autopsy samples, preserved with potassium fluoride at a final concentration of approximately 1% and stored at $-20\,°C$ for 12 months. However, the magnitude of the changes is not sufficiently great so as to alter the interpretation of the results (Holmgren et al., 2004). Δ9THC and THC COOH can be detected for 7 days, the longest interval studied, when stored in dried blood stains at $2-8\,°C$ (Thomas et al., 2012).

When stored in urine, the losses of THC COOH

- are average 11% (range of 0–34%) when stored in polypropylene tubes for 45 days at -16 to $-18\,°C$ (Paul et al., 1993), but average 24% (range of $+30$ to -80%) when stored at $-15\,°C$ for longer periods ranging from 1 to 10 months (Romberg and Past, 1994);
- are greater when urine samples are stored in high-density polyethylene, polypropylene, and polystyrene than when they are stored in glass containers (Roth et al., 1996). The losses due to binding to the container material range from approximately 1 ng/cm^2 in glass to 3.5–5 ng/cm^2 in the plastics. The binding reaches equilibrium in 1–2 h and does not increase after that;
- are greater in urine samples stored in polyethylene or polypropylene containers at $4\,°C$ ($<20\%$) than at $25\,°C$ ($<5\%$) (Stout et al., 2000). The greater loss at the lower temperature may be the consequence of decreased solubility of THC COOH at $4\,°C$, resulting in greater binding of the analyte to the plastics (Paul et al., 1993; Stout et al., 2000);
- are decreased by the addition of a surfactant (Welsh et al., 2009).

The loss of THC COOH in oral fluid stored in the dark for 14 days at room temperature is approximately half as great as in oral fluid exposed to fluorescent lighting

(Moore et al., 2006). THC COOH-glucuronide in plasma and urine is stable for 10 days, the maximum storage period studied, when stored in glass vials at $-20\,^{\circ}$C (Skopp and Potsch, 2002).

Although the type of the container, the sample type, and the storage temperature can influence the stability of Δ9THC, THC COOH, and 11-OH THC, the extent of the concentration changes any of these analytes generally is not meaningful, especially if samples are stored in glass containers, at $-20\,^{\circ}$C with an added preservative such as NaF.

7.7 LYSERGIC ACID DIETHYLAMIDE

Lysergic acid diethylamide (LSD) and two of its major metabolites, *N*-desmethyllysergic acid diethylamide (nor-LSD) and 2-oxo-3-hydroxy lysergic acid diethylamide (O-H-LSD), undergo decomposition when exposed to light. The decomposition of LSD in urine is more rapid when the urine is exposed to natural light than when exposed to fluorescent lighting (Webb et al., 1996; Skopp et al., 2002). The loss of O-H-LSD in urine samples has been reported to be greater when the pH of the samples is adjusted to 8 than when at acidic conditions (Li et al., 1998; Klette et al., 2002).

REVIEW QUESTIONS

1. Describe the problem of analyte stability, from the perspective of a forensic toxicologist.
2. Describe three cellular activities that might alter analyte concentration during storage period I and/or II.
3. Describe three environmental factors that might influence analyte concentration during storage periods I, II, and/or III.
4. The results of stability studies may be interpreted in two manners—what are the two main strategies of interpretation?
5. The stability of cocaine in various samples is significantly influenced by pH, why?

APPLICATION QUESTIONS

1. Discuss the major factors that influence the stability of analytes during storage periods I, II, and III.
2. Discuss the purpose of a stability study. What factors or conditions must be controlled for in the experimental design of a stability study? Describe the differences and similarities between case samples, experimental samples, and fortified samples.

3. Describe the three major mechanisms by which ethanol concentrations in stored samples may be altered during the storage period(s).
4. Opioids are generally fairly stable in stored blood and plasma. What chemical and/or physical properties of the chemicals might contribute to this stability? Are there any conditions under which opioid stability in blood is decreased, and if so, can you suggest a sample storage and/or preservation strategy that would minimize the decrease in stability?

REFERENCES

Amick, G.D., Habben, K.H., 1997. Inhibition of ethanol production by *Saccharomyces cerevisiae* in human blood by sodium fluoride. J. Forensic Sci. 42 (4), 690–692.

Anderson, W.H., 2015. Collection and storage of specimens for alcohol analysis. In: Caplan, Y.H., Goldberger, B.A. (Eds.), Garriott's Medicolegal Aspects of Alcohol, sixth ed. Lawyers & Judges Publishing Company, Inc., Tucson, AZ.

Balabanova, S., Parsche, F., Pirsig, W., 1992. First identification of drugs in Egyptian mummies. Naturwissenschafen 79, 358.

Baselt, R.C., 1983. Stability of cocaine in biological fluids. [Electronic version]. J. Chromatogr. 268 (3), 502–505.

Baselt, R.C., Yoshikawa, D., Chang, J., Li, J., 1993. Improved long-term stability of blood cocaine in evacuated collection tubes. J. Forensic Sci. 38 (4), 935–937.

Bhargava, H.N., 1977. Improved recovery of morphine from biological tissues using siliconized glassware. J. Pharmaceut. Sci. 66, 1044–1045.

Boy, R.G., Henseler, J., Mattern, R., Skopp, G., 2008. Determination of morphine and 6-acetylmorphine in blood with use of dried blood spots. Ther. Drug. Monit. 30, 733–739.

Brown, G.A., Neylan, D., Reynolds, W.J., Smalldon, K.W., 1973. The stability of ethanol in stored blood. I. Important variables and interpretation of results. [Electronic version]. Anal. Chim. Acta 66 (2), 271–283.

Chen, H.M., Lin, W.W., Ferguson, K.H., Scott, B.K., Peterson, C.M., 1994. Studies of the oxidation of ethanol to acetaldehyde by oxyhemoglobin using fluorigenic high-performance liquid chromatography. [Electronic version]. Alcohol. Clin. Exp. Res. 18 (5), 1202–1206.

Collom, W.D., 1975. Postmortem synthesis of ethanol. In: Winek, C.L. (Ed.), Toxicology Annual, 1974. Marcel Dekker, New York.

Corry, J.E., 1978. A review. Possible sources of ethanol ante- and post-mortem: Its relationship to the biochemistry and microbiology of decomposition. [Electronic version]. J. Appl. Bacteriol. 44 (1), 1–56.

Dick, G.L., Stone, H.M., 1987. Alcohol loss arising from microbial contamination of drivers' blood specimens. [Electronic version]. Forensic Sci. Int. 34 (1–2), 17–27.

Dugan, S., Bogema, S., Schwartz, R.W., Lappas, N.T., 1994. Stability of drugs of abuse in urine samples stored at −20 °C. [Electronic version]. J. Anal. Toxicol. 18 (7), 391–396.

Gaillard, Y., Breuil, R., Doche, C., Romeuf, L., Lemeur, C., Prevosto, J.M., et al., 2011. Detection of amitriptyline, nortriptyline and bromazepam in liver, CSF and hair in the homicidal poisoning of a one-month-old girl autopsied 8 months after death. For. Sci. Int. 207 (1–3), 16–18.

Gallardo, E., Queiroz, J.A., 2008. The role of alternative specimens in toxicological analysis. Biomed. Chromatogr. 22 (8), 795–821.

Giusiani, M., Chericoni, S., Domenici, R., 2012. Identification and quantification of phenobarbital in a mummified body 10 years after death. J. For. Sci. 57 (5), 1384−1387.

Grellner, W., Glenewinkel, F., 1997. Exhumations: synopsis of morphological and toxicological findings in relation to the postmortem interval. Survey on a 20-year period and review of the literature. For. Sci. Int. 90 (1−2), 139−159.

Hoiseth, G., Fjeld, B., Burns, M.L., Strand, D.H., Vindenes, V., 2014. Long-term stability of morphine, codeine, and 6-acetylmorphine in real-life whole blood samples, stored at −20 °C. For. Sci. Int. 239, 6−10.

Holmgren, P., Druid, H., Holmgren, A., Ahlner, J., 2004. Stability of drugs in stored postmortem femoral blood and vitreous humor. J. Forensic Sci. 49, 1−6.

Isenschmid, D.S., Levine, B.S., Caplan, Y.H., 1989. A comprehensive study of the stability of cocaine and its metabolites. [Electronic version]. J. Anal. Toxicol. 13 (5), 250−256.

Johnson, J.R., Jennison, T.A., Peat, M.A., Foltz, R.L., 1984. Stability of delta 9-tetrahydrocannabinol (THC), 11-hydroxy-THC, and 11-nor-9-carboxy-THC in blood and plasma. [Electronic version]. J. Anal. Toxicol. 8 (5), 202−204.

Jones, A.W., Hylen, L., Svensson, E., Helander, A., 1999. Storage of specimens at 4 °C or addition of sodium fluoride (1%) prevents formation of ethanol in urine inoculated with *Candida albicans*. [Electronic version]. J. Anal. Toxicol. 23 (5), 333−336.

Jones, J.M., Raleigh, M.D., Pentel, P.R., Harmon, T.M., Keyler, D.E., Remmel, R.P., et al., 2013. Stability of heroin, 6-monoacetylmorphine, and morphine in biological samples and validation of an LC-MS assay for delayed analyses of pharmacokinetic samples in rats. [Electronic version]. J. Pharm. Biomed. Anal. 74, 291−297.

Karger, B., Lorin de la Grandmaison, G., Bajanowski, T., Brinkmann, B., 2004. Analysis of 155 consecutive forensic exhumations with emphasis on undetected homicides. Int. J. Legal Med. 118 (2), 90−94.

Karinen, R., Oiestad, E.L., Andresen, W., Smith-Kielland, A., Christophersen, A., 2011. Comparison of the stability of stock solutions of drugs of abuse and other drugs stored in a freezer, refrigerator, and at ambient temperature for up to one year. [Electronic version]. J. Anal. Toxicol. 35 (8), 583−590.

Kaye, S., Dammin, G.J., 1945. Stability of the blood alcohol: an agent to maintain the alcohol concentration in drawn blood. Military Surg. 96, 93−95.

Kintz, P., 2004. Value of hair analysis in postmortem toxicology. Forensic Sci. Int. 142 (2−3), 127−134.

Kintz, P., Spiehler, V., Negrusz, A., 2008. Alternative specimens. In: Jickells, S., Negrusz, A. (Eds.), Clarke's Analytical Toxicology. Pharmaceutical Press, Chicago.

Klette, K.L., Horn, C.K., Stout, P.R., Anderson, C.J., 2002. LC-MS analysis of human urine specimens for 2-oxo-3-hydroxy LSD: method validation for potential interferants and stability study of 2-oxo-3-hydroxy LSD under various storage conditions. J. Anal. Toxicol. 26 (4), 193−200.

Kojima, T., Okamoto, I., Miyazaki, T., Chikasue, F., Yashiki, M., Nakamura, K., 1986. Detection of methamphetamine and amphetamine in a skeletonized body buried for 5 years. For. Sci. Int. 31 (2), 93−102.

Kudo, K., Sugie, H., Syoui, N., Kurihara, K., Jitsufuchi, N., Imamura, T., et al., 1997. Detection of triazolam in skeletal remains buried for 4 years. Int. J. Legal Med. 110 (5), 281−283.

Levy, A.D., Harcke, H.T., 2010. Essentials of Forensic Imaging. CRC Press, Boca Raton, FL.

Lough, P.S., Fehn, R., 1993. Efficacy of 1% sodium fluoride as a preservative in urine samples containing glucose and *Candida albicans*. J. Forensic Sci. 38 (2), 266−271.

Li, Z., McNally, A.J., Wang, H., Salamone, S.J., 1998. Stability study of LSD under various storage conditions. [Electronic version]. J. Anal. Toxicol. 22 (6), 520−525.

Moody, D.E., Monti, K.M., Spanbauer, A.C., 1999. Long-term stability of abused drugs and antiabuse chemotherapeutical agents stored at −20 °C. J. Anal. Toxicol. 23 (6), 535−540.

Moore, C., Vincent, M., Rana, S., Coulter, C., Agrawal, A., Soares, J., 2006. Stability of delta(9)-tetrahydrocannabinol (THC) in oral fluid using the Quantisal collection device. [Electronic version]. Forensic Sci. Int. 164 (2−3), 126−130.

Musshoff, F., Trafkowski, J., Kuepper, U., Madea, B., 2006. An automated and fully validated LC-MS/MS procedure for the simultaneous determination of 11 opioids used in palliative care, with 5 of their metabolites. [Electronic version]. J. Mass Spectrom. 41 (5), 633−640.

Musshoff, F., Rosendahl, W., Madea, B., 2009. Determination of nicotine in hair samples of pre-Columbian mummies. Forensic Sci. Int. 185, 84−88.

Noguchi, T.T., Nakamura, G.R., Griesemer, E.C., 1978. Drug analyses of skeletonizing remains. J. For. Sci. 23, 490−492.

Olsen, T., Hearn, W.L., 2003. Stability of ethanol in postmortem blood and vitreous humor in long-term refrigerated storage. J. Anal. Toxicol. 27 (7), 517−519.

O'Neal, C.L., Poklis, A., 1996. Postmortem production of ethanol and factors that influence interpretation: a critical review. Am. J. Forensic Med. Pathol. 17 (1), 8−20.

Papoutsis, I., Nikolaou, P., Pistos, C., Dona, A., Stefanidou, M., Spiliopoulou, C., et al., 2014. Stability of morphine, codeine, and 6-acetylmorphine in blood at different sampling and storage conditions. J. For. Sci. 59 (2), 550−554.

Paul, B.D., McKinley, R.M., Walsh, J.K., Jamir, T.S., Past, M.R., 1993. Effect of freezing on the concentration of drugs of abuse. J. Anal. Toxicol. 17, 378−380.

Politi, L., Morini, L., Mari, F., Groppi, A., Bertol, E., 2008. Ethyl glucuronide and ethyl sulfate in autopsy samples 27 years after death. Int. J. Legal Med. 122 (6), 507−509.

Potsch, L., Skopp, G., Becker, J., 1995. Ultrastructural alterations and environmental exposure influence the opiate concentrations in hair of drug addicts. Int. J. Legal Med. 107 (6), 301−305.

Reese, J.J., 1874. A Manual of Toxicology, Including the Consideration of the Nature, Properties, Effects, and Means of Detection of Poisons, More Especially in Their Medico-legal Relations. J.B. Lippincott & Co., Philadelphia, p. 72. http://www.archive.org/stream/manualoftoxicolo00reesiala/manualoftoxicolo00reesiala_djvu.txt.

Robertson, M.D., Drummer, O.H., 1995. Postmortem drug metabolism by bacteria. J. For. Sci. 40 (3), 382−386.

Romberg, R.W., Past, M.R., 1994. Reanalysis of forensic urine specimens containing benzoylecgonine and THC-COOH. J. Forensic Sci. 39 (2), 479−485.

Roth, K.D., Siegel, N.A., Johnson Jr., R.W., Litauszki, L., Salvati Jr., L., Harrington, C.A., et al., 1996. Investigation of the effects of solution composition and container material type on the loss of 11-nor-delta 9-THC-9-carboxylic acid. [Electronic version]. J. Anal. Toxicol. 20 (5), 291−300.

Skoop, G., 2004. Preanalytic aspects in postmortem toxicology. For. Sci. Int. 142, 75−100.

Skopp, G., Potsch, L., 2002. Stability of 11-nor-delta (9)-carboxy-tetrahydrocannabinol glucuronide in plasma and urine assessed by liquid chromatography-tandem mass spectrometry. [Electronic version]. Clin. Chem. 48 (2), 301−306.

Skopp, G., Potsch, L., Klingmann, A., Mattern, R., 2001. Stability of morphine, morphine-3-glucuronide, and morphine-6-glucuronide in fresh blood and plasma and postmortem blood samples. J. Anal. Toxicol. 25 (1), 2−7.

Skopp, G., Potsch, L., Mattern, R., Aderjan, R., 2002. Short-term stability of lysergic acid diethylamide (LSD), N-desmethyl-LSD, and 2-oxo-3-hydroxy-LSD in urine, assessed by liquid chromatography-tandem mass spectrometry. Clin. Chem. 48 (9), 1615−1618.

Springfield, A.C., Cartmell, L.W., Aufderheide, A.C., Buikstra, J., Ho, J., 1993. Cocaine and metabolites in the hair of ancient Peruvian coca leaf chewers. Forensic Sci. Int. 63, 269−275.

Sreerama, L., Hardin, G.G., 2003. Improper sealing caused by the Styrofoam integrity seals in leak-proof plastic bottles lead to significant loss of ethanol in frozen evidentiary urine samples. [Electronic version]. J. Forensic Sci. 48 (3), 672−676.

Stevens, H.M., 1984. The stability of some drugs and poisons in putrefying human liver tissues. J. For. Sci. Soc. 24, 577−589.

Stout, P.R., Horn, C.K., Lesser, D.R., 2000. Loss of THCCOOH from urine specimens stored in polypropylene and polyethylene containers at different temperatures. [Electronic version]. J. Anal. Toxicol. 24 (7), 567−571.

Sulkowski, H.A., Wu, A.H., McCarter, Y.S., 1995. In-vitro production of ethanol in urine by fermentation. [Electronic version]. J. Forensic Sci. 40 (6), 990−993.

Thomas, A., Geyer, H., Schanzer, W., Crone, C., Kellmann, M., Moehring, T., et al., 2012. Sensitive determination of prohibited drugs in dried blood spots (DBS) for doping controls by means of a benchtop quadrupole/Orbitrap mass spectrometer. [Electronic version]. Anal. Bioanal. Chem. 403 (5), 1279−1289.

Vass, A.A., Barshick, S.A., Sega, G., Caton, J., Skeen, J.T., Love, J.C., et al., 2002. Decomposition chemistry of human remains: A new methodology for determining the postmortem interval. J. For. Sci. 47 (3), 542−553.

Viel, G., Nalesso, A., Cecchetto, G., Montisci, M., Ferrara, S.D., 2009. Stability of cocaine in formalin solution and fixed tissues. [Electronic version]. Forensic Sci. Int. 193 (1−3), 79−83.

Wagner, J.R., Caplan, Y.H., Goldberger, B.A., 2015. Blood, urine and other fluid and tissue specimens for alcohol analysis. In: Caplan, Y.H., Goldberger, B.A. (Eds.), Garriott's Medicolegal Aspects of Alcohol, sixth ed. Lawyers and Judges Publishing Co., Inc., Tucson, AZ.

Webb, K.S., Baker, P.B., Cassells, N.P., Francis, J.M., Johnston, D.E., Lancaster, S.L., et al., 1996. The analysis of lysergide (LSD): The development of novel enzyme immunoassay and immunoaffinity extraction procedures together with an HPLC-MS confirmation procedure. J. For. Sci. 41 (6), 938−946.

Welsh, E.R., Snyder, J.J., Klette, K.L., 2009. Stabilization of urinary THC solutions with a simple non-ionic surfactant. [Electronic version]. J. Anal. Toxicol. 33 (1), 51−55.

Wilson, A.S., Brown, E.L., Villa, C., Lynnerup, N., Healey, A., Ceruti, M.C., et al., 2013. Archaeological, radiological, and biological evidence offer insight into Inca child sacrifice. Proc. Natl. Acad. Sci. U.S.A. 110 (33), 13322−13327.

Wormley, T.G., 1867. Micro-chemistry of poisons, including their physiological, pathological, and legal relations, adapted to the use of the medical jurist, physician, and general chemist. Baillier Brothers, New York, p. 29. https://play.google.com/books/reader?id=Vgg1AQAAMAAJ&printsec=frontcover&output=reader&authuser=0&hl=en.

Zaitsu, K., Miki, A., Katagi, M., Tsuchihashi, H., 2008. Long-term stability of various drugs and metabolites in urine, and preventive measures against their decomposition with special attention to filtration sterilization. Forensic Sci. Int. 174, 189−196.

Analytical Samples

Since the time of Orfila, the advance in chemical analysis has further extended the list of poisonous substances that have been detected in the blood, the secretions, and the tissues and organs of the body.
John James Reese (1874)

The proper selection, collection and submission of specimens for toxicological analyses is of paramount importance if analytical results are to be their subsequent interpretation is to be scientifically sound and therefore useful in the adjudication of forensic cases.
SOFT/AAFS Forensic Toxicology Laboratory Guidelines (2006)

In this chapter, the characteristics, handling, and uses of specific samples chosen for analysis are discussed. The general considerations for the proper handling of samples presented in Chapter 6 generally hold for the samples discussed in this chapter and will not be repeated here.

Antemortem samples used for toxicological analysis usually are restricted to blood, urine, oral fluid, and hair, whereas for postmortem analyses, although virtually any sample may be available at autopsy, the samples most commonly used are blood, urine, and vitreous humor. In postmortem cases, when the commonly used or preferred samples are not available or when specific samples will provide data not obtainable from other samples, then a wide assortment of uncommonly or rarely used samples (so-called alternative samples) may be selected for analysis.

Although no sample selected for analysis by forensic toxicologists is "ideal," possessing all of the characteristics summarized in Table 6.1, each type of sample has benefits and disadvantages associated with its use (Table 8.1).

8.1 BLOOD

Interpretations that are based upon the analytical results obtained from blood samples are greater than for other samples and therefore blood is arguably the most important analytical sample used in forensic toxicology. Interestingly, in spite of the normal compositional differences among plasma, serum, and whole blood and the differences between whole blood collected in a clinical setting under sterile conditions

Forensic Toxicology. http://dx.doi.org/10.1016/B978-0-12-799967-8.00008-6

Table 8.1 Advantages and Disadvantages of Common Analytical Samples

Sample	Advantages	Disadvantages
Blood	• Large database for correlation with effects • Several collection sites • Numerous methods of analysis	• Drug concentrations are subject to postmortem alterations in concentration • Site of collection may influence drug concentrations • Wide variation in interpersonal correlation of drug concentrations with effects • Postmortem samples are often hemolyzed or clotted • Possible unequal drug distribution between plasma and whole blood
Urine	• Many drugs and metabolites are detectable in relatively high concentrations • Detection period longer for most drugs than in blood • Ease of analysis often by direct methods, e.g., immunoassays	• Correlation of drug concentrations with blood concentrations or effects usually not possible • Frequently not available in postmortem cases • Collection presents privacy issues
Oral fluid	• Easily collected without invasion of privacy • May be analyzed with little, if any, preparation	• Drugs are detected for shorter periods than urine or hair • Drug concentration may depend on the manner of collection
Liver	• Many drugs and metabolites are present in relatively high concentrations	• Generally poor correlation with drug effects • Sample preparation may be extensive
Brain	• The target organ of many drugs of interest • Potentially difficult analysis	• Generally poor correlation with drug effects • Sample preparation may be extensive • Unequal distribution of drugs
Vitreous humor	• Less likely than many other samples to decompose or putrefy • Ease of analysis • Provides a measure of the free blood concentration of many drugs	• Correlation of drug concentration with blood concentration only after establishment of equilibrium
Hair	• May provides long-term "history" of drug use • Collection does not present privacy issues	• Problems differentiating between exterior and interior drug concentrations present analytical and interpretative difficulties

and the "whole blood" collected at autopsy, which usually is hemolyzed or clotted to varying extents, the word "blood" often is used indiscriminately. Autopsy reports, hospital laboratory reports, and state statutes[1] generally refer to "blood" without distinction or description of samples that are quite dissimilar in composition.

The use of blood for screening purposes has become more widespread with the advent of advanced methods of analysis such as LC/MS/MS, which facilitate the detection of dozens of analytes and their metabolites by means of a single analysis. A disadvantage of using blood as a screening sample is that it may require preparation such as extractions, whereas other samples, such as urine, may not require any such preparation. Also, many analytes, such as tetrahydrocannabinol (Δ9THC), cocaine, and their metabolites are detectable for shorter periods of time in blood than in either urine or hair. For these reasons, urine or hair often is a better choice for screening purposes than is blood.

The overwhelming advantage of blood as an analytical sample is that the quantitative results obtained from its analysis may be used as the basis of interpretations not possible with the analysis of most other samples. This is due to the extensive database in existence in which drug concentrations in blood obtained from both ante- and postmortem subjects are correlated with effects consistent with those concentrations. Generally, the effects in these databases are categorized as either therapeutic, toxic, or lethal. A second advantage of utilizing blood as an analytical sample is that the detection of analytes and their metabolites in blood may allow for the determination of whether drug use by the subject was chronic or acute, the route of administration, and/or whether postmortem redistribution has occurred. The interpretations of blood analyte concentrations and the factors that influence them are discussed in Chapters 12 and 13.

Of considerable importance in the collection of blood samples, particularly postmortem samples, is the site from which the blood is obtained, as drug concentrations often differ markedly in blood sample collected from different sites. This heterogeneous distribution of analytes in blood samples collected from different sites may be due to either the lack of distribution equilibrium prior to death or to postmortem redistribution. Recognition of the importance of site-dependent variability of drug concentrations in blood has resulted in the standard procedure commonly followed in postmortem cases of collecting blood from more than one site, such as a peripheral samples from the femoral vein, and central samples from both the left and right sides of the heart. Of these samples, it is widely held that blood collected from a peripheral site is a more reliable indicator of antemortem concentrations than blood collected from the heart; the latter is considered to be appropriate only for initial qualitative screening purposes (Drummer, 2001; Forrest, 1993; Skopp and Potsch, 1997).

If blood is to be collected from peripheral blood vessels, the vessels should be isolated by ligature from more central vessels prior to collection so that the blood

---

[1] For example, it is not clear that the Maryland state statutes regarding the determination of blood alcohol concentrations differentiate among the various types of "blood."

sample collected is not comingled with blood from larger contiguous and more centrally located proximal vessels (Jones and Pounder, 1987; Jones, 2011; Prouty and Anderson, 1990). For example, in the absence of a ligature, relatively large volumes of blood collected from the femoral vein, from which no more than 5−10 ml can be collected if ligated (Jones, 2011), may be comingled with blood from the iliac vein, or blood collected from the subclavian vein may be comingled with blood from the vena cava, jugular vein, or perhaps even the right atrium. Peripheral vessels should not be "milked" in the collection procedure as this may cause analytes in muscle tissue to be transferred into the blood, potentially altering the blood concentration.[1,2]

The identity of a purported blood sample may be called into question if inappropriate collection methods are employed. An example of an unsatisfactory method of blood collection is the "scooping" of blood samples from body cavities, since the sample collected in this sample is likely to contain nonblood fluids in addition to blood. Another collection procedure that is problematic is the collection of blood from a cadaver in which the chest cavity is not opened, and samples are obtained by means of an external puncture or "blind stick." If not performed accurately, blood samples collected in such a manner may not be from a chamber of the heart, but rather from the chest cavity. The measured analyte concentrations in samples obtained by the "scooping" or "blind-stick" methods frequently will be artifactually increased or decreased as a consequence of contamination with nonblood fluids from the pericardial region or gastric contents, especially in cases of traumatic injuries (Jones, 2011; Logan and Lindholm, 1996). The problems generated by inappropriate or inaccurate methods of blood collection are compounded if no attempt is made to confirm, by a method such as the determination of hematocrit or hemoglobin concentrations of the samples, whether the red-colored fluid that has been collected is blood or a diluted or contaminated artifact thereof. Therefore, if used at all, these methods of collection are suitable only for qualitative analysis (Skoop, 2004), the results of which should not extend beyond concluding whether specific analytes are present.

Given that the distribution of analytes between the cellular and fluid components of blood often differs, concentrations determined from the analyses of these different fractions of blood can result in different interpretations. Alterations in the physical integrity of blood samples that can occur during storage periods may not result in a change in the total drug concentration, but rather may cause the redistribution of drugs within samples, possibly resulting in a change in the analyte concentration in the portion of sample used for analysis. For example, hemolysis of blood samples resulting from the use of improper collection methods, including the use of needles of extremely narrow diameter for collection (Lippi et al., 2006), the overly rapid filling and emptying of syringes, the excessive shaking of blood-containing tubes (Curry and Whelpton, 1981), elevated concentrations of EDTA, and prolonged centrifugation (Lippi et al., 2008), can alter the distribution of analytes within the sample if they are not homogeneously distributed between the RBC and the plasma. Also, the formation of a clot in a postmortem blood sample containing an analyte that is concentrated in erythrocytes will result in a decreased concentration of the drug in the plasma or serum fraction.

The administration of intravenous fluids to hospitalized patients can dilute the blood to the extent that there is a meaningful decrease in analyte concentrations following such administration, which can alter the interpretation of results. The determination of hemoglobin concentrations in samples that appear "watery" should be determined to ascertain whether analyte concentrations have been decreased due to sample dilution (Riley et al., 1996).

The use of intracranial, subdural, and epidural hematomas[2] as analytical samples often is valuable especially if the subject has survived for several hours after a traumatic injury. Drug concentrations determined in hematomas often are a more accurate representation of the blood concentration at the time of the trauma than blood collected from the general circulation because drug concentrations in hematomas often decrease at a slower rate; this is especially true for drugs that have relatively short half-life periods in blood (Hirsch and Adelson, 1973; McIntyre et al., 2000; Moriya and Hashimoto, 1998).

8.2 URINE

Because of the several advantages that urine affords as an analytical sample, it is used widely in both antemortem and postmortem cases for qualitative presumptive analyses ("screening tests"). Urine is perhaps the analytical sample most widely used by forensic toxicologists for the detection of drugs.

The widespread use of urine as an analytical sample, which was triggered initially as a method by which to monitor drug use by heroin addicts enrolled in methadone treatment programs (Dole and Nyswander, 1965), is now routinely used in several circumstances including preemployment evaluation, "for-cause" testing after an industrial or public transit incident, clinical evaluation of emergency cases, as a component of postmortem analytical protocols, for the supervision of persons on probation or parole and to facilitate testing of competitive athletes for the presumptive detection of prohibited substances. In these uses, the analysis of urine affords several benefits: it is readily available, numerous drugs and/or their metabolites are excreted and detectable in urine, the presence of drugs may be detected within hours after their use and continue to be detected for days after the last use, and the concentrations of drugs and their metabolites are frequently greater than in blood. Importantly, since urine is composed primarily of water, and only relatively small amounts of organic and inorganic substances, reasonably simple methods of analysis such as color tests and immunoassays may be used for the presumptive identification of drugs/metabolites, generally with little, if any, sample preparation.

The use of urine as an analytical sample in human-performance forensic toxicology and forensic urine drug testing presents problems of sample verification

---

[2]A hematoma is a pool of blood, often formed as a result of trauma that accumulates outside of the general circulation, forming a swelling or bump.

and adulteration. Persons submitting urine samples for drug analysis often attempt to mask their illegal use of drugs by preventing the detection of the drugs they are using (or their metabolites), since the consequences resulting from the detection of a controlled drug in their urine can be severe. Methods by which individuals may attempt to mask the presence of drugs and/or drug metabolites in their urine include the substitution of drug-free urine ("clean urine"), "synthetic" urine or other fluids in place of subject urine, the ingestion of large quantities of water ("water-loading"), and the adulteration of samples with substances intended to interfere with drug detection (Cook et al., 2000).

Urine donors who wish to avoid penalties associated with the detection of drugs in their urine may resort to the substitution of "clean," i.e., drug-free urine, obtained from nondrug using persons, which may be purchased from a number of online sites. Although the differentiation between urine from the test subject and another human is difficult, it may be achieved by means of DNA-short tandem repeat (DNA-STR) analysis (Thevis et al., 2007); however, this method is not widely employed. Certain animal urines and fruit juices that have creatinine[3] concentrations similar to those in human urine have been used as substitute urine samples. However, animal urines may be differentiated from human urine due to their distinctive odors (an unpleasant and unreliable method of detection), whereas the small number of fruit juices and energy drinks that have creatinine levels consistent with human urine is differentiable from human urine by the presence of colors and odors that are inconsistent with human urine (Villena, 2010).

Water loading is the process by which large amounts of water are ingested prior to the submission of urine samples in an attempt to dilute the urine, thereby decreasing the concentrations of analyte drugs and metabolites to levels below their detection limits. Although there is variance of acceptable ranges of normal creatinine concentrations and specific gravity values, these determinations are valuable for the identification of diluted urine samples. However, creatinine and specific gravity values must be considered in conjunction with the subject's history as several circumstances, other than water loading, may cause decreased creatinine concentrations and specific gravity values. Anemia, hyperthyroidism, muscular dystrophy, inflammatory diseases of the muscles, vegetarian diets, and advanced renal disease may cause decreased creatinine concentrations, whereas diabetes insipidus and various kidney diseases may decrease the specific gravity (Fischbach and Dunning, 2009; Tietz, 1992). The urine creatinine concentration also decreases with age, as a result of age-related decreased muscle mass. Since women generally have lower creatinine levels than men (Cook et al., 2000), it has been suggested that gender-specific creatinine cutoff limits should be established (Arndt, 2009). Increased creatinine concentrations may be produced by exercise and the ingestion of cooked meat (Cone et al., 2009).

---

[3]Creatinine is the breakdown product of creatine, which is involved in the production of energy in muscle tissue. It is found in normal urine at a relatively constant concentration.

The pH of urine samples is used as an additional check of their validity. Although the pH of freshly excreted urine normally is approximately 4.5, it is important to be aware that the pH of urine may not be within the normal range due to factors such as the time of day of collection, several diseases and drugs, and prolonged storage of samples at room temperature or greater (Cook et al., 2007).

A great many substances have been used in attempts to avoid drug detection. These substances usually are designed to cause drug degradation or to interfere with the methods employed in urine analysis, mainly immunoassays. Included among these substances are readily available commonplace materials such as bleach, ammonia, detergent, vinegar, alkali, and eye drops, as well as commercial substances such as "Klear" and "Whizzies" (potassium nitrite), "Urine Luck" (pyridinium chlorochromate), papain, "Clean X" (glutaraldehyde), and "Stealth" (peroxide and peroxidase) produced specifically for the purpose of minimizing or eliminating the detection of drugs in urine. There are numerous methods for the detection of many of these substances prior to analysis (Dasgupta, 2007). Analytical errors that may be caused by the undetected use of these adulterants are described in Chapter 13.

The criteria employed for the detection of substituted, diluted, and/or adulterated urine samples vary among various agencies and laboratories. However, because of widespread attempts to avoid detection, laboratories should follow standards of the *Mandatory Guidelines for Federal Workplace Drug Testing Programs*[4] *(Guidelines)* of the U.S. Department of Health and Human Services (DHHS) (Department of Health and Human Services, 2008), which contains procedures for the identification of samples that have been substituted, diluted, or adulterated. For example, specific methods and criteria are included to facilitate the identification of urine diluted by water-loaded (via the measurement of creatinine concentration and specific gravity and via the analysis of two characteristics consistent with water loading). Additionally, methods for the detection of several adulterants, including nitrites, chromium (VI), halogens, pyridine, aldehydes (for the detection of gluteraldehyde), and surfactants, may be found in the Guidelines.

In postmortem cases, all of the available urine should be collected, but urine can be obtained in only approximately 50% of postmortem cases (Jones, 2011). However, because the methods of detection that are used have low detection limits, even if the bladder is apparently empty, it should be rinsed with a small amount of water or saline to obtain any residual urine since the small amount of diluted urine collected may be sufficient for analysis (Isenschmid and Hepler, 2007).

---

[4]Although these guidelines are intended specifically to "establish the scientific and technical guidelines for Federal workplace drug testing programs and establish standards for certification of laboratories engaged in drug testing for Federal agencies," they are employed widely not only by laboratories conducting analyses for federal agencies, but also by laboratories conducting analyses for nonfederal clients, such as state and local governmental agencies and corporations.

8.3 BREATH

Traditionally, breath has been used as an analytical sample for the detection of ethanol in subjects suspected of driving while under the influence or driving while intoxicated. The manner of collection of breath samples for this purpose is dictated by state regulations. Included in many state regulations is an observation period of several minutes prior to the collection of a breath sample from a subject. This mandatory observation period is designed both to increase the likelihood that any residual ethanol remaining in the oral cavity will be cleared by normal salivation and to ensure that nothing is consumed by the subject during the immediate precollection period. These regulations are intended to decrease the possibility that any ethanol detected is from the oral cavity and not exhaled from the lungs.

In addition to the detection of ethanol in breath, several other drugs, including amphetamines, benzodiazepines, cocaine, opioids, and Δ9THC, may be detected in aerosol particles contained in exhaled breath for as long as 24 h after the last drug use Wang, et al., 2009; Beck, et al., 2010, 2011a, 2011b, 2013. The detection of these drugs in exhaled breath has the potential to become a valuable method for clinical and forensic screening and also for the possible identification of drug abusers.

8.4 VITREOUS HUMOR

Vitreous humor is the fluid-like gel, composed of approximately 98−99% water with trace amounts of hyaluronic acid, glucose, anions, cations, ions, and collagen, located in the posterior chambers of the eyes (Scott and Oliver, 2001). The relatively simple composition of vitreous humor allows it to be analyzed by methods that require little, if any, sample preparation.

Vitreous humor samples of approximately 2−3 mL can be collected from each eye (Forrest, 1993), and after collection, the samples collected from each eye should be stored separately (Flanagan et al., 2005). Samples should be collected using gentle aspiration in order to avoid contamination with nonvitreous substances (Isenschmid and Hepler, 2007). This is especially important because vitreous humor samples that are contaminated with blood as a result of existing pathology or improper collection may be unacceptable for analysis (Parsons et al., 2003).

Due to its location, which is relatively inaccessible and protected from trauma by the orbital bone and the eye, and its composition, vitreous humor is generally not susceptible to extensive postmortem microbial contamination. As a result, drugs distributed into the vitreous humor undergo little, if any, synthesis or degradation, and vitreous humor is therefore used commonly for the detection of drugs when other samples are unavailable due to trauma or putrefaction. In addition, vitreous humor, which is largely unaffected by embalming, is an excellent alternative to blood in bodies that have been embalmed (Forrest, 1993).

Although several drugs and metabolites such as cocaine and benzoylecgonine, morphine, codeine, 6-acetylmorphine, phencyclidine, and benzodiazepines are detectable in vitreous humor (Jenkins and Oblock, 2008; Peres et al., 2014; Rees et al., 2013; Scott and Oliver, 2001), other drugs and metabolites, such as Δ9THC and its metabolite, 9-carboxy tetrahydrocannabinol (THC COOH), are less likely to be detected in vitreous humor, even when present in urine or blood, presumably due to a high degree of protein binding in blood (Jenkins and Oblock, 2008; Peres et al., 2014). Esters such as 6-monoacetylmorphine (6MAM), a metabolite of heroin, have greater stability in vitreous humor, due to the lack of esterase activity in the fluid, than in many other samples (Dinis-Oliveira et al., 2010).

8.5 HAIR

The first demonstration that organic compounds could be detected in hair may have been the detection of barbiturates in guinea pig hair (Goldbaum et al., 1954). Notwithstanding this early experimental demonstration, the widespread use of hair as an analytical sample in forensic toxicology for the detection of therapeutic and abused drugs did not develop until the use of radioimmunoassay for the detection of opiates in hair was reported 25 years later (Baumgartner et al., 1979). Thereafter, the use of hair for the detection of drugs was advocated as an appropriate sample for drug screening (Baumgartner et al., 1989), and at present its use for this purpose is common.

Hair contains protein, water, lipids, pigments, and trace elements. The component present in the greatest quantity is protein, the quantity of which, approximately 65—95%, varies as a function of the amount of moisture in the hair (Gallardo and Queiroz, 2008; Robbins, 2002).

Hairs may exist in one of the following three different phases (Kintz, 2004):

1. The anagen phase: This is the period of active growth of the hair shaft.
2. The catagen phase: During this relatively short phase "the follicle begins to degenerate."
3. The telogen phase: Hair growth comes to a halt during this phase.

Drugs may be present both *in* and *on* hair shafts. The distribution of drugs and/or their metabolites *into* hair may be explained by a multicompartment model of diffusion that includes the diffusion of drugs and/or their metabolites from blood into the shaft during the growth phase (Henderson, 1993). The presence and concentration of specific drugs in hair are influenced largely by their degree of ionization at physiological pH, as determined by their acidic or basic nature, and the extent and type of pigmentation of the hair. A lesser extent of ionization and a greater concentration of melanin are consistent with increased drug concentrations in the hair shaft. Drugs may be detected *on* the hair shaft as a consequence of external contamination resulting from diffusion from sweat, sebum, and/or putrefactive fluids, or from passive exposure to volatile drugs in an environment in which the drug is being smoked; the drug in the vapor is adsorbed directly onto the shaft (Henderson, 1993).

The Society for Hair Testing has recommended that a "lock of hair or a pencil thickness of hair"[5] should be collected, preferably from the back of the head in the area known as the posterior vertex,[6] cut as close as possible to the skin, dried if wet, tied, and wrapped in an aluminum foil: if storage is necessary, hair samples should be stored in the dark, at room temperature, but they must not be refrigerated or frozen (Cooper et al., 2012).

Generally, hair collected from areas of the body other than the head, for example, axillary and pubic samples, is susceptible to greater contamination than is head hair due to its exposure to perspiration or urine, whereas samples from the chest, arms, and legs may be more reliable (Pianta et al., 2013; Pirro et al., 2011). Autopsy hair samples must be collected with care so that the samples are not contaminated with postmortem fluids.

Hair has several advantages as an analytical sample (Pragst and Balikova, 2006). It is suitable for the detection of both organic and inorganic analytes, it may be collected with ease and in a noninvasive manner, it may be stored at room temperature, it is resistant to adulteration either prior to or following its collection, and the distribution of analytes along the hair shaft may be used to approximate the long-term chronology of drug exposure. The storage and transmittal of hair samples present fewer problems than encountered with most other biological samples; drugs have been shown to have greater postmortem stability in hair than in most other samples (Chapter 7).

Although the advantages of hair as an analytical sample are substantial, there also are meaningful disadvantages associated with its use (Mussoff and Madea, 2007). A limiting disadvantage is that it is not a sample of choice for the determination of recent drug use because approximately 3 or more days are required for the distribution of drugs into hair in sufficient quantities to be detected (Wennig, 2000). Therefore, its use is limited to circumstances in which it is of importance to determine whether drug use occurred during a period exceeding the detection periods possible with the analysis of urine and blood.

Since the growth rate of head hair is somewhat predictable, the detection of a drug in sections of hair collected at various distances from the scalp may provide an indication of the chronology of drug use and an estimate of the time of use of detected drugs (Kintz, 2004). However, although an average growth rate of 1 cm/month has been suggested (Cooper et al., 2012), the rate at which head hair grows varies considerably and is dependent upon the location of the hair on the body, age, gender, and race (Harkey, 1993) and may range from 0.6−3.36 (Harkey, 1993) to 0.6−1.4 cm/month (Kintz, 2004).

---

[5]Several drugs of abuse have been detected in smaller samples collected from neonates (Kintz and Mangin, 1993; Koren et al., 1992).
[6]The density of hair in the anagen or growing phase in the posterior vertex is greater than in other areas of the head.

8.6 ORAL FLUID

Although the benefits of oral fluid as an analytical sample in forensic toxicology have been recognized for several years (Idowu and Caddy, 1981), only recently its use has become fairly widespread due to the several advantages it affords, among which are the ease of collection that can be accomplished without an invasion of privacy, the low potential for sample alteration, the opportunity for the collection of samples at the sites of incidents, and the detection of drugs within a short period after their use.

Oral fluid contains a number of secretions—saliva produced by the three major pairs of salivary glands (parotid, sublingual, and submandibular) and several minor salivary glands, crevicular fluid, and secretions from the pharynx and nasal cavity. The composition of oral fluid includes proteins such as enzymes and immunoglobulins, lymph, food debris, cells sloughed off from the gums, and mucosal lining of the mouth, bacteria, erythrocytes, and leukocytes (Aps and Martens, 2005; Lee and Huestis, 2014; Spiehler and Cooper, 2008).

Oral fluid may be collected with or without stimulation of the flow rate. Unstimulated oral fluid, collected by spitting, has the benefit of being undiluted, thus containing undiminished analyte concentrations. However, centrifugation may be required due to the presence of food debris and other substances, and frequently only relatively small samples of less than 1 mL are collectable and the high viscosity of the sample may present problems of analysis (Drummer, 2006). The collection of a suitable volume of an unstimulated sample may be difficult due to a decreased flow rate resulting from pathologic conditions, such as graft-versus-host disease, diabetes mellitus, alcoholic liver cirrhosis, and HIV, the effects of several anticholinergic or antiadrenergic drugs (Aps and Martens, 2005), and/or the development of "dry mouth" due to the anxiety of the situation (Kintz and Samyn, 2002).

The volume and flow of oral fluid may be stimulated by the movement of lips, tongue, or cheeks (Crouch, 2005) or by the use of several materials including Parafilm® wax (which is problematic since it may absorb lipophilic drugs) (Kintz and Samyn, 2002), Teflon, citric acid (which will alter the pH of the sample possibly altering the concentration of certain drugs, including codeine) (O'Neal et al., 2000), or chewing gum (Drummer, 2008; Idowu and Caddy, 1981; Kintz and Samyn, 2002). Analyte distribution into oral fluid is altered by the stimulation of the flow by nonacidic means, which increases the concentration of bicarbonate ions and the pH of oral fluid (Aps and Martens, 2005).

Subjects should be observed for several minutes prior to collection of an oral fluid sample to ensure that they do not introduce anything into their mouths and to minimize the likelihood that contaminants from foods may be present when the sample is collected (Spiehler, 2011).

The devices that are utilized for the collection of oral samples (Drummer, 2006; Spiehler and Cooper, 2008) contain materials that absorb oral fluid, after which the drug in the collected fluid can be extracted for analysis. However, since different collection devices demonstrate meaningful intra- and interdevice variations in sample volumes collected and recovery of specific drugs (Crouch, 2005; Langel et al., 2008), the choice of a collection device and its subsequent storage following sample collection can influence the measured concentration of specific drugs of abuse (Walsh et al., 2007). For example, depending upon the type of collection device utilized, large differences in the concentrations of codeine (O'Neal et al., 2000), nitrobenzodiazepines (Kempf et al., 2009), and Δ9THC (Dickson et al., 2007) may be measured. Therefore, because it cannot be assumed that the data obtained from different devices are comparable, the use of each collection device must be validated prior to its use.

Oral fluid may be analyzed rather easily by commonly used presumptive and confirmatory methods, such as immunoassays and GC/MS, respectively. The use of common beverages, foods, and mouth rinses,[7] including those purportedly capable of producing negative results, has no direct effect on specific immunoassays designed for the detection of drugs in oral fluid (Cooper et al., 2005; Wong et al., 2005). However, the presence of cellular debris, food particles, and residues of orally administered or inhaled drugs may influence drug concentrations.

The European Workplace Drug Testing Society has published guidelines for the use of oral fluid in workplace testing (Cooper et al., 2011) and the U.S. Department of Health and Human Services is evaluating the inclusion of oral fluid in the *Mandatory Guidelines for Federal Workplace Drug Testing Programs* (Department of Health and Human Services, 2008).

8.7 NAILS

Arsenic may have been the first analyte to have been detected in nails for forensic purposes. Several years later, methamphetamine and amphetamine were reported to be the first drugs of abuse detected in nails (Suzuki et al., 1984). Since then, several other common drugs of abuse including cannabinoids, opiates, cocaine, phencyclidine, benzodiazepines, and methadone have been detected in nails (Kim et al., 2010; Palmeri et al., 2000).

Generally, the advantages of fingernails and toenails as analytical samples are similar to those described above for hair. For example, because fingernails and toenails grow at somewhat predictable rates of approximately 3 mm/month and 1 mm/month, respectively, a chronology of drug use may be estimated from the longitudinal distribution of the drug in the nails. This determination is especially useful when hair is not available (Dinis-Oliveira et al., 2010). However, the rate of growth may be influenced by age, cold, and malnutrition (Palmeri et al., 2000). As is the case with hair, drug concentrations in nails remain relatively constant for prolonged periods, possibly longer than in hair (Dinis-Oliveira et al., 2010).

---

[7]Mouth rinses can decrease drug concentrations in oral fluids as a result of sample dilution.

Additionally, in both ante- and postmortem cases, an abnormality in the appearance of fingernails and toenails may be consistent with the exposure to certain substances. This is demonstrated by the presence in nails of transverse white lines, known as Mees lines, which are consistent with a number of pathological conditions, as well as exposure to several chemicals including arsenic, thallium, and carbon monoxide. The presence of Mees lines should prompt the analysis for these substances in the nails as well as in other samples such as blood and hair (Daniel et al., 2004; Fawcett et al., 2004; Saddique and Peterson, 1983).

Generally, 50−100 mg of a nail sample is an adequate analytical sample, which should be protected from light and stored in plastic bags at room temperature (Madej, 2010).

8.8 SWEAT

Sweat offers several advantages as an analytical sample. Its collection is simple and noninvasive, alterations of samples are difficult, drug use may be detected over an entire period of collection of hours to days (Huestis et al., 2000), and drugs in sweat will be retained and concentrated as the fluid evaporates from a collection device such as the PharmChek Sweat Patch™, which is placed on the skin for the collection of the sweat sample (Liberty et al., 2004). However, concerns have been raised concerning the meaning of analytical results detected in samples collected in these devices as it is possible that the sample collected may originate, not from sweat, but rather from skin, subcutaneous adipose tissues (Levisky et al., 2000), or drug vapors (especially in the case of cocaine and methamphetamine) (Kidwell and Smith, 2001). Also, the recommended use of 70% isopropanol to clean the skin prior to application of the PharmChek Sweat Patch™ may not be sufficient to remove drugs that have been on the skin prior to application of the patch (Kidwell and Smith, 2001). The location on the body where the collection patch is placed is also significant, as is has been shown that sweat samples collected from different areas of the body contain unequal concentrations of analytes and metabolites (Thieme et al., 2003).

In addition to the intentional collection of sweat samples, there may be occasions in which drugs may be detected in sweat collected coincidentally. For example, the methadone metabolite, ethylene-1,5-dimethyl-3,3-dimethyl-diphenylpyrrolidine, and continine, a nicotine metabolite, have been detected in incidental sweat from fingerprints (Hazarika, et al., 2009; Rowell et al., 2009; Leggett, et al., 2007), and morphine, codeine, and 6MAM have been detected in the incidental sweat on clothing (Tracqui et al., 1995).

8.9 GASTRIC CONTENTS

Gastric contents are useful samples for the detection of recently ingested drugs because these drugs may be present in milligram or even gram quantities rather than in the microgram or nanogram quantities found in blood and urine. This is notably the case with "body packers," who attempt to smuggle illicit drugs, such as cocaine, by ingesting packets containing the drugs, or "body stuffers," who ingest illicit drugs to evade arrest (Sporer and Firestone, 1997; Wetli and Mittlemann, 1981). The ingestion of drugs in an attempt to evade detection results in the release of large amounts of drugs into the gastric and intestinal contents.

The collection and analysis of gastric contents is appropriate even if there is evidence that the drug was administered by a route other than the oral route since basic drugs may be detected in gastric contents regardless of the route of administration as a result of ion trapping.[8] The total stomach contents should be collected and homogenized prior to analysis since the contents are not homogeneous (Jones, 2011).

8.10 LIVER

There are several reasons that liver frequently is selected for postmortem toxicological analysis. Liver is the first major organ to which drugs are distributed after they have been absorbed from the gastrointestinal tract following oral administration, and the liver is the major organ of drug metabolism in the body. As a result, many drugs and their metabolites are found in greater concentrations in the liver than in blood and other samples. In addition, often when other, more desired, samples are not available due to putrefaction and decomposition, ample liver tissue is available for collection.

In both experimental animals and humans, drugs are distributed heterogeneously in the liver. Often the greatest concentrations of drugs are found in the left lobe, likely due to the postmortem redistribution of drugs from gastric contents, which is more likely to occur into the left lobe because it is located closer to the stomach than the right lobe (Hilberg et al., 1992, 1993; Kugelberg and Jones, 2007; Pounder et al., 1996a, 1996b). Because of this, the protocols for liver sampling should be formalized so that liver samples are collected from deep within the right lobe of the liver (Pounder et al., 1996a). Forensic pathologists must be informed of the significance of the liver site from which samples are collected and of the necessity of following established collection guidelines (Morley and Bolton, 2012).

8.11 BILE

Prior to the advent of modern methods of analysis in the mid- to late-twentieth century, the use of bile in forensic toxicology was commonplace because drug concentrations often are greater in this sample than in blood and urine and, therefore,

---

[8]Ion trapping in gastric contents occurs when nonionized drugs enter the gastric contents, the pH of which is lower than that of blood and lower than the pK_a of many basic drugs. This causes a greater percentage of these basic drugs to be ionized, minimizing their ability to cross membranes, thus becoming "trapped" as ions in the gastric contents.

were detectable using the available analytical methods, which had relatively high detection limits.

Because bile is a surfactant containing aqueous matrix with both hydrophilic and hydrophobic characteristics (Fabritius et al., 2012), it may be a route for the excretion of both ionized and neutral drug species with molecular weight of approximately 500—600 Da (Fabritius et al., 2012). The glutathione and glucuronide conjugates (Rozman and Klaassen, 2001) of drugs that are extensively conjugated, for example, opioids, cannabinoids, and benzodiazepines (Fabritius et al., 2012; Kerrigan, 2011), are found in greater concentrations in bile than in blood (Agarwal and Lemos, 1996; Fabritius et al., 2012; Spiehler et al., 1978). As a result of the extensive distribution into bile, these drugs and metabolites may be detected in bile not only when they are detectable in blood and urine, but, importantly, also when they are not (Tassoni et al., 2007; Vanbinst et al., 2002). For this reason, bile can be an important screening sample for the identification of drug use when the desired samples, e.g., blood and urine, are not available due to embalming or the passage of prolonged periods of time between the last drug use and death (Alunni-Perret et al., 2003; Tassoni et al., 2007).

A disadvantage of bile as an analytical sample is that the extraction of drugs from bile is somewhat more complicated than from other samples because of the presence of fatty acids and bile salts (Kerrigan, 2011).

8.12 BRAIN

Although both abused and therapeutic drugs that exert effects on the brain are of interest to forensic toxicologists, the use of the brain as an analytical sample has not been a principal analytical focus. This is due to the high fat content in the brain that makes the analysis somewhat more difficult than for other samples; because of the composition of brain tissue, the interpretation of results obtained from the analysis of brain samples is dependent upon the section of the brain that is analyzed, and often the analytical results do not correlate with the physiological effects produced.

It is reasonable to assume that the distribution of drugs within the brain would be heterogeneous because of the anatomical dissimilarity of the structures comprising the brain and the heterogeneous distribution of drug receptors among these structures. However, the effect of sampling site on drug concentrations is inconsistent. Little difference has been reported in the concentrations of methamphetamine, cocaine, and their metabolites in 15 regions of brains obtained from users of these drugs (Kalasinsky et al., 2000, 2001). In contrast to this, the distributions of morphine (Spiehler et al., 1978; Pare et al., 1984; Stimpfl and Reichel, 2007) and antipsychotics (Rodda et al., 2006) in different regions of the brain vary with no obvious trends. Regardless of these inconsistencies, recording the specific areas of the brain from which analytical samples are collected is consistent with good laboratory practice, although it is not always done.

An advantage of the brain as an analytical sample is that certain drugs or their metabolites are detectable for a longer period than in other tissues such as the blood and liver (Stimpfl, 2008). For example, the half-life of 6MAM, the ester metabolite of heroin, is longer in the brains than in the blood of experimental animals, presumably due to lower esterase activity in the brain than in blood (Gottas et al., 2013). http://www.ncbi.nlm.nih.gov/pubmed/23245263—comments. As a result, 6MAM often may be detectable in the brain for longer periods of time than it is detectable in blood.

8.13 LUNG

The lungs are served by an extensive blood supply from which nonionized, lipophilic drugs can diffuse readily into the lungs; drugs without these characteristics may rely on specialized transport systems to enter the lungs (Bend et al., 1985). As a result, lungs are a repository for many drugs, including phenothiazines, opioids, antihistamines, and tricyclic antidepressants, which may be present in greater concentrations in lung than in blood and other tissues, independent of the route of administration (Brown, 1974; Pounder et al., 1996; Spiehler et al., 1978).

It has been suggested that lung samples should be collected from the apical lobes rather than from the basal lobes because postmortem diffusion from gastric contents into the basal lobes, particularly the basal lobe of the right lung, which is in close proximity to the stomach, may lead to elevated drug concentrations (Pounder et al., 1996).

8.14 ADIPOSE TISSUE

Although adipose tissue is not a sample of first choice for forensic analyses, in the absence of preferred samples, its use as an analytical sample may be valuable for the detection of highly lipid soluble drugs, such as thiopental, glutethimide, THC, propofol (Colucci et al., 2013; Hikiji et al., 2010), polychlorinated biphenyls, organochlorine, and organophosphate pesticides (Colucci et al., 2010). Due to their lipophilicity, these compounds are sequestered in relatively greater concentrations in adipose tissue than in blood and may be detectable in adipose tissue for prolonged periods of time following their intentional or unintentional exposure (Colucci et al., 2010).

The anatomical site from which adipose tissue is collected has an unpredictable effect on the qualitative or quantitative detection of drugs. The postmortem insulin concentrations detected in subcutaneous fat samples obtained from the area of injection sites on the arms and thighs from a subject whose death was attributed to insulin overdose showed meaningful variation (Dickson et al., 1977). However, only minor differences in the concentrations of cocaine and benzoylecgonine have been reported in adipose samples collected from either the thigh or abdomen (Levisky et al., 2001).

8.15 BONE AND BONE MARROW

Bone is heterogenous, consisting primarily of two different tissues types—cortical bone, which is dense and compact, and cancellous bone, which is spongy and more porous; this difference in the anatomy of bone may result in the differential distribution of a drug along a bone, such as the femur, that consists of both types of bone (Watterson, 2006). Therefore, both the intra- and interbone distribution of drugs may be variable.

Although bone is not commonly collected for analysis, it is a valuable sample because specific drugs may be detectable in bone for prolonged periods.

There are two types of bone marrow—red and yellow. Red marrow is capable of producing hematopoietic cells and is located in the bones of the lower skull, vertebrae, shoulder and pelvic girdles, ribs, and sternum, whereas yellow marrow consists largely of fat cells and is located in the bones of the hands, feet, legs, and arms (Koury and Lichtman, 2010). Differences in the distribution of drugs in marrow collected from different bone types, as well as concentration differences in marrow from the same bone type, may be expected due to several factors including differences in the composition of the types of marrow, age of the subject, postmortem redistribution, and postmortem degradation or synthesis (Cartiser et al., 2011a, 2011b).

8.16 SKELETAL MUSCLE

An important benefit of skeletal muscle is its availability in large amounts from several different sites—often when other samples are not available due to trauma, incineration, or putrefaction (Williams and Pounder, 1997). Although in most cases, drugs present in blood are also present in muscle, occasionally drugs detected in blood are not detected in muscle (Garriott, 1991; Hargrove and Molina, 2014). Because of this, it has been suggested that muscle should be included as a routine postmortem screening sample; however, the use of muscle samples for this purpose is not a standard procedure in forensic toxicology laboratories (Christensen et al., 1985). Whereas skeletal muscle generally is an anatomically homogeneous sample, the distribution of drugs in randomly collected portions of muscle tissue from the same leg muscle may be heterogeneously distributed as reflected by an extensive variance in the concentrations of the same drug detected in these samples (Williams and Pounder, 1997).

8.17 BREAST MILK (ANDERSON, 1979; FRIGULS ET AL., 2010; KERRIGAN AND GOLDBERGER, 2008)

Breast milk contains high concentrations of lipids and proteins and has a pH of 6.35—7.35, which is somewhat lower than that of plasma. Many drugs being used by the mother that are present in her plasma are likely to be present in her breast milk, often at concentrations greater than those in her plasma. Therefore, the presence of drugs in breast milk is a marker for the likely presence of these drugs in the breast-fed infant.

Drugs most likely to be distributed into breast milk are small molecules, characterized by low plasma protein binding and high lipophilicity. Drugs such as nicotine, Δ9THC, buprenorphine, and tramadol that distribute into breast milk may be concentrated there due to its high lipid content and/or in the case of basic drugs, as a result of ion trapping. Since the concentration of lipids in breast milk may vary during the day and within different fractions of the breast milk expressed, drug concentrations in breast milk may also vary depending on these variables.

8.18 NEONATAL SAMPLES

The results obtained from the analysis of neonatal samples are valuable for the determination of whether in utero drug exposure had occurred. Several drugs of abuse including cocaine, opiates, methadone, and amphetamines are detectable in meconium, umbilical cord, and placenta (Lozano et al., 2007).

A minimum of 0.5 g meconium can be collected from the diaper of a newborn during the first 5 days of birth and stored frozen for several months without any meaningful effect on matrix or drug stability (Madej, 2010). Since meconium is not a homogeneous sample, it must be mixed as thoroughly as possible before it is analyzed (Kintz and Samyn, 2000).

8.19 MISCELLANEOUS HUMAN SAMPLES

Although the samples of choice for a toxicological analysis generally are available in both antemortem and postmortem cases, in some postmortem cases, they may not be available for reasons described above, and therefore it would be necessary to rely on the use of the so-called unconventional or alternative samples, i.e., samples that are not used frequently. Examples of several drugs that have been detected in alternative samples are presented in Table 8.2.

8.20 NONHUMAN SAMPLES
8.20.1 INSECTS

When human postmortem samples are not available, insect samples, such as larvae, pupae, adults, puparial cases, and exuviae, collected from cadavers, have been used for the detection of drugs (Gagliano-Candela and Aventaggiato, 2001). The initial report of the use of insects in forensic toxicology may have been the detection of

Table 8.2 Selected Drugs Detected in Alternative Samples[a]

Samples	Drugs Detected	References
Amniotic fluid	Cocaine and metabolites	Ripple et al. (1992), Moore et al. (1992), De Giovanni and Marchetti (2012)
Antecubital fossae (injection sites)	Morphine and codeine	Druid and Holmgren (1999)
Bloodstains[b]	Morphine	Moller et al. (1977), Smith et al. (1980)
	Diphenylhydantoin	Shaler et al. (1978)
	Digoxin	Smith (1981)
	Phenobarbital	Smith and Pomposini (1981)
	Cocaine/ Benzoylecgonine	Smith and Liu (1986), Sosnoff et al. (1996)
	Amitriptyline	Noguchi et al. (1978)
Bone	Benzodiazepines	Gorczynski and Melbye (2001)
	Opioids	Guillot et al. (2007), Raikos et al. (2001)
Bone marrow	Ethanol	Winek and Jones (1980)
	Amitriptyline	Noguchi et al. (1978)
Cremation ashes	Arsenic	Brachet et al. (2006)
Nails	Arsenic	Pounds et al. (1979)
	Cocaine	Skopp and Potsch (1997), Ropero-Miller et al. (2000)
	Methamphetamine	Suzuki et al. (1984),
Placenta	Several drugs of abuse	Joya et al. (2010)
Pleural effusions[c]	Several drugs	Sims et al. (1999)
Putrefactive blisters	Ethanol	Grellner and Iffland (1997)
Umbilical cord	9-Carboxy tetrahydrocannabinol	Chittamma et al. (2013)
Synovial fluid	Ethanol Several drugs of abuse	Sutheimer et al. (1992), Winek et al. (1993), Buyuk et al. (2009) Felscher et al. (1998)
Tears	Amphetamine and acetaminophen	Madej (2010)

[a] Except as noted, results from experimental animal studies are not included.
[b] The data are from experimental studies using prepared stains.
[c] Blood containing fluids that accumulates in the pleural cavity.

Table 8.3 Drugs Detected in Larvae

Amitriptyline and nortriptyline (Sadler et al., 1997a)
Amphetamine (Sadler et al., 1997b)
Cocaine and benzoylecgonine (Goff et al., 1989; Nolte et al., 1992)
3,4-Methylenedioxymethamphetamine (Goff et al., 1997)
Malathion (Gunatilake and Goff., 1989)
Morphine and codeine (Kintz et al., 1994)
Phencyclidine (Goff et al., 1994)
Phenobarbital (Beyer et al., 1980)
Temazepam (Sadler et al., 1995)
Triazolam (Kintz et al., 1990)

phenobarbital in maggots that had fed on the decomposing body of a young female (Beyer et al., 1980). Subsequently, it has been shown that several drugs including barbiturates, tricyclic antidepressants, opioids, and cocaine can be absorbed by insects feeding on decomposing bodies (Introna et al., 2001). The most desirable insect stage for use as analytical samples are feeding larvae, since the rapid elimination of drugs in nonfeeding larvae and pupae results in lower drug concentrations; these larvae must be washed thoroughly to eliminate surface drug contamination (Sadler et al., 1995, 1997c).

Examples of drugs that have been detected in larvae are listed in Table 8.3.

8.20.2 SOIL

Barbiturates (Dunnett et al., 1979) and several other drugs (Wyman et al., 2011) have been detected in the soil beneath the decomposing bodies of humans and experimental animals, and several—amitriptyline, diazepam, and pentobarbital—were detected after 2 years. Precursors and by-products associated with the illegal production of methamphetamine also have been detected in soil (Pal et al., 2012).

8.20.3 HOUSEHOLD AND PERSONAL SAMPLES

Occasionally, forensic toxicologists will be asked to analyze samples such as household chemicals, the contents of aerosol containers, vials of prescription medication, syringes, cigarettes, and clothing obtained from the scenes of homicides, suicides, automobile accidents, or the scenes of other incidents of interest (Tracqui et al., 1995).

Because containers often do not contain the substance listed on the labels, the contents of containers, even prescription vials, must be identified by analysis. The analysis of these samples often provides insights into the type of drugs or chemicals that might have been involved in the incident.

REVIEW QUESTIONS

1. Describe the major advantages and disadvantages of the use of blood as an analytical sample.
2. Describe the major advantages and disadvantages of the use of urine as an analytical sample.
3. Describe the major advantages and disadvantages of the use of breath as an analytical sample.
4. Describe the major advantages and disadvantages of the use of hair as an analytical sample.
5. Describe the major advantages and disadvantages of the use of vitreous humor as an analytical sample.

APPLICATION QUESTIONS

1. Discuss the reasons why urine and blood are often considered to be the most desirable samples for analysis. Under what conditions would these samples not be appropriate for use as analytical samples?
2. Describe two scenarios in which nonhuman samples might be analyzed by a forensic toxicologist. Are there any special considerations that you, as a forensic toxicologist, must be aware of when analyzing nonhuman samples? How would your interpretations be affected if the analytical sample is of nonhuman origin?
3. Forensic toxicologists may be called upon to perform both antemortem and postmortem analyses. Discuss the challenges associated with each type of analysis, in terms of choice of analytical sample, sample collection, sample analysis, and interpretation.
4. Assume that you are a forensic toxicologist who has analyzed blood, urine, liver, and adipose tissue samples in a postmortem case. You have detected drug X in each sample, but the concentrations of drug X vary among the samples. Why? What characteristics of the samples and/or drug X might explain these findings? How would you explain these results in your report?

REFERENCES

Agarwal, A., Lemos, N., 1996. Significance of bile analysis in drug-induced deaths. J. Anal. Toxicol. 20 (1), 61–63.

Alunni-Perret, V., Kintz, P., Ludes, B., Ohayon, P., Quatrehomme, G., 2003. Determination of heroin after embalmment. Forensic Sci. Int. 134 (1), 36–39.

Anderson, P.O., 1979. Drugs and breast feeding. Semin. Perinatol. 3 (3), 271–278.

Aps, J.K.M., Martens, L.C., 2005. Review: the physiology of saliva and transfer of drugs into saliva. Forensic Sci. Int. 150, 119–131.

Arndt, T., 2009. Urine–creatinine concentration as a marker of urine dilution: reflections using a cohort of 45,000 samples. Forensic Sci. Int. 186, 48–51.

Baumgartner, A.M., Jones, P.F., Baumgartner, W.A., Black, C.T., 1979. Radioimmunoassay of hair for determining opiate abuse histories. J. Nucl. Med. 20, 748−752.

Baumgartner, W.A., Hill, V.A., Blahd, W.H., 1989. Hair analysis for drugs of abuse. J. Forensic Sci. 34, 1433−1453.

Beck, O., Leine, K., Palmskog, G., Franck, J., 2010. Amphetamines detected in exhaled breath from drug addicts: a new possible method for drugs-of-abuse testing. J. Anal. Toxicol. 34 (5), 233−237.

Beck, O., Sandqvist, S., Dubbelboer, I., Franck, J., 2011a. Detection of Delta9-tetrahydrocannabinol in exhaled breath collected from cannabis users. J. Anal. Toxicol. 35 (8), 541−544.

Beck, O., Sandqvist, S., Franck, J., 2011b. Demonstration that methadone is being present in the exhaled breath aerosol fraction. J. Pharm. Biomed. Anal. 56 (5), 1024−1028.

Beck, O., Stephanson, N., Sandqvist, S., Franck, J., 2013. Detection of drugs of abuse in exhaled breath using a device for rapid collection: comparison with plasma, urine and self-reporting in 47 drug users. J. Breath Res. 7 (2), 026006−7155/7/2/026006. Epub 2013 Apr 25.

Bend, J.R., Serabjit-Singh, C.J., Philpot, R.M., 1985. The pulmonary uptake, accumulation, and metabolism of xenobiotics. Ann. Rev. Pharmacol. Toxicol. 25, 97−125.

Beyer, J.C., Enos, W.F., Stajic, M., 1980. Drug identification through analysis of maggots. J. Forensic Sci. 25 (2), 411−412.

Brachet, R., Harzer, K., Helmers, E., Wippler, K., 2006. Arsenic content of cremation ash after lethal arsenic poisoning. In: Proceedings of the 1994 Joint TIAFT/SOFT International Meeting, Tampa, Florida, pp. 315−317.

Brown, E.A.B., 1974. The localization, metabolism and effects of drugs and toxicants in the lung. Drug Metab. Rev. 3, 33−87.

Buyuk, Y., Eke, M., Cagdir, A.S., Karaaslan, H.K., 2009. Post-mortem alcohol analysis in synovial fluid: an alternative method for estimation of blood alcohol level in medico-legal autopsies? Toxicol. Mech. Methods 19 (5), 375−378.

Cartiser, N., Bevalot, F., Chatenay, C., Le Meur, C., Gaillard, Y., Malicier, D., et al., 2011a. Postmortem measurement of caffeine in bone marrow: influence of sample location and correlation with blood concentration. Forensic Sci. Int. 210 (1−3), 149−153.

Cartiser, N., Bevalot, F., Fanton, L., Gaillard, Y., Guitton, J., 2011b. State-of-the-art of bone marrow analysis in forensic toxicology: a review. Int. J. Legal Med. 125 (2), 181−198.

Chittamma, A., Marin, S.J., Williams, J.A., Clark, C., McMillin, G.A., 2013. Detection of in utero marijuana exposure by GC-MS, ultra-sensitive ELISA and LC-TOF-MS using umbilical cord tissue. J. Anal. Toxicol. 37 (7), 391−394.

Christensen, H., Steentoft, A., Worm, K., 1985. Muscle as an autopsy material for evaluation of fatal cases of drug overdose. J. Forensic Sci. Soc. 25 (3), 191−206.

Colucci, A.P., Aventaggiato, L., Centrone, M., Gagliano-Candela, R., 2010. Validation of an extraction and gas chromatography-mass spectrometry quantitation method for cocaine, methadone and morphine in post-mortem adipose tissue. J. Anal. Toxicol. 34, 342−346.

Colucci, A.P., Gagliano-Candela, R., Aventaggiato, L., DeDonno, A., Leonardi, S., Strisciullo, G., et al., 2013. Suicide by self-administration of a drug mixture (propofol, midazolam, and zolpidem) in an anesthesiologist: the first case report in Italy. J. Forensic Sci. February 3.

Cone, E.J., Caplan, Y.H., Moser, F., Robert, T., Shelby, M.K., Black, D.L., 2009. Normalization of urinary drug concentrations with specific gravity and creatinine. J. Anal. Toxicol. 33, 1−7.

Cook, J.D., Caplan, Y.H., LoDico, C.P., Bush, D.M., 2000. The characterization of human urine for specimen validity determination in workplace drug testing: a review. J. Anal. Toxicol. 24, 579–588.

Cook, J.D., Strauss, K.A., Caplan, Y.H., Lodico, C.P., Bush, D.M., 2007. Urine pH: the effects of time and temperature after collection. J. Anal. Toxicol. 31 (8), 486–496.

Cooper, G., Wilson, L., Reid, C., Baldwin, D., Hand, C., Spiehler, V., 2005. Validation of the Cozart microplate EIA for analysis of opiates in oral fluid. Forensic Sci. Int. 154 (2–3), 240–246.

Cooper, G., Moore, C., George, C., Pichini, S., European Workplace Drug Testing Society, 2011. Guidelines for European workplace drug testing in oral fluid. Drug Test. Anal. 3 (5), 269–276.

Cooper, G.A., Kronstrand, R., Kintz, P., Society of Hair Testing, 2012. Society of hair testing guidelines for drug testing in hair. Forensic Sci. Int. 218 (1–3), 20–24.

Crouch, D.J., 2005. Oral fluid collection: the neglected variable in oral fluid testing. Forensic Sci. Int. 150, 165–173.

Curry, S.H., Whelpton, R., 1981. Critical factors in drug analysis. In: Reid, E. (Ed.), Trace-organic Sample Handling. John Wiley & Sons, New York.

Daniel III, C.R., Piraccini, B.M., Tosti, A., 2004. The nail and hair in forensic science. J. Am. Acad. Dermatol. 50 (2), 258–261.

Dasgupta, A., 2007. The effects of adulterants and selected ingested compounds on drugs-of-abuse testing in urine. Am. J. Clin. Path. 128, 491–503.

Department of Health and Human Services, November 25, 2008. Mandatory Guidelines for Federal Workplace Drug Testing Programs. Federal Register, Part V, 73, No. 228 71858.

Dickson, S.J., Cairns, E.R., Blazey, N.D., 1977. The isolation and quantitation of insulin in post-mortem specimens—a case report. Forensic Sci. 9 (1), 37–42.

Dickson, S., Park, A., Nolan, S., Kenworthy, S., Nicolspn, C., Midgley, J., et al., 2007. The recovery of illicit drugs from oral fluid sampling devices. Forensic Sci. Int. 165, 78–84.

Dinis-Oliveira, R.J., Carvalho, F., Duarte, J.A., Remiao, F., Marques, A., Santos, A., et al., 2010. Collection of biological samples in forensic toxicology. Toxicol. Mech. Methods 20 (7), 363–414.

Dole, V.P., Nyswander, M., 1965. A medical treatment for diacetylmorphine (heroin) addiction. JAMA 193, 646–650.

Drummer, O.H., 2001. The Forensic Pharmacology of Drugs of Abuse. Arnold, London.

Drummer, O.H., 2006. Drug testing in oral fluid. Clin. Biochem. Rev. 27, 147–159.

Drummer, O.H., 2008. Introduction and review of collection techniques and applications of drug testing of oral fluid. Ther. Drug Monit. 30, 203–206.

Druid, H., Holmgren, P., 1999. Fatal injections of heroin. Interpretation of toxicological findings in multiple specimens. Int. J. Legal Med. 112 (1), 62–66.

Dunnett, N., Ashton, P.G., Osselton, M.D., 1979. The use of enzymes as an aid to release drugs from soil following the exhumation of a skeleton. Vet. Hum. Toxicol. (Suppl. 21), 199–201.

Fabritius, M., Staub, C., Mangin, P., Giroud, C., 2012. Distribution of free and conjugated cannabinoids in human bile samples. Forensic Sci. Int. 223 (1–3), 114–118.

Fawcett, R.S., Linford, S., Stulberg, D.L., 2004. Nail abnormalities: clues to systemic disease. Am. Fam. Physician 69 (6), 1417–1424.

Felscher, D., Gastmeier, G., Dressler, J., 1998. Screening of pharmaceuticals and drugs in synovial fluid of the knee joint and in vitreous humor by fluorescence polarization immunoassay (FPIA). J. Forensic Sci. 43 (3), 619–621.

Fischbach, F.T., Dunning III, M.B., 2009. A Manual of Laboratory and Diagnostic Tests, eighth ed. Lippincott Williams and Wilkins, Philadelphia.

Flanagan, R.J., Connally, G., Evans, J.M., 2005. Analytical toxicology: guidelines for sample collection postmortem. Toxicol. Rev. 24, 63−71.

Forrest, A.R.W., 1993. Obtaining samples at post mortem examination for toxicological and biochemical analysis. J. Clin. Pathol. 46, 292−296.

Friguls, B., Joya, X., Garcia-Algar, O., Pallas, C.R., Vall, O., Pichini, S., 2010. A comprehensive review of assay methods to determine drugs in breast milk and the safety of breast feeding when taking drugs. Anal. Bioanal. Chem. 397, 1157−1179.

Gagliano-Candela, R., Aventaggiato, L., 2001. The detection of toxic substances in entomological specimens. Int. J. Legal Med. 114, 197−203.

Gallardo, E., Queiroz, J.A., 2008. The role of alternative samples in toxicological analysis. Biomed. Chromatogr. 98, 795−821.

Garriott, J.C., 1991. Skeletal muscle as an alternative specimen for alcohol and drug analysis. J. Forensic Sci. 36 (1), 60−69.

De Giovanni, N., Marchetti, D., 2012. Cocaine and its metabolites in the placenta: a systematic review of the literature. Reprod. Toxicol. (Elmsford, N.Y.) 33 (1), 1−14.

Goff, M.L., Omori, A.I., Goodbrod, J.R., 1989. Effect of cocaine in tissues on the development of *Boettcherisca peregrina* (Diptera, Sarcophagidae). J. Med. Entomol. 26 (2), 91−93.

Goff, M.L., Brown, W.A., Omori, A.I., LaPointe, D.A., 1994. Preliminary observations of the effects of phencyclidine in decomposing tissues on the development of *Parasarcophaga ruficornis* (Diptera, Sarcophagidae). J. Forensic Sci. 39 (1), 123−128.

Goff, M.L., Miller, M.L., Paulson, J.D., Lord, W.D., Richards, E., Omori, A.I., 1997. Effects of 3,4-methylenedioxymethamphetamine in decomposing tissues on the development of *Parasarcophaga ruficornis* (Diptera, Sarcophagidae) and detection of the drug in postmortem blood, liver tissue, larvae, and puparia. J. Forensic Sci. 42 (2), 276−280.

Goldbaum, R.W., Goldbaum, L.R., Piper, W.N., 1954. Barbiturate concentrations in the skin and hair of guinea pigs. J. Invest. Dermatol. 22, 121−128.

Gottas, A., Oiestad, E.L., Boix, F., Vindenes, V., Ripel, A., Thaulow, C.H., et al., 2013. Levels of heroin and its metabolites in blood and brain extracellular fluid after I.V. heroin administration to freely moving rats. Br. J. Pharmacol. 170 (3), 546−556.

Gorczynski, L.Y., Melbye, F.J., 2001. Detection of benzodiazepines in different tissues, including bone, using a quantitative ELISA assay. J. Forensic Sci. 46 (4), 916−918.

Grellner, W., Iffland, R., 1997. Assessment of postmortem blood alcohol concentrations by ethanol levels measured in fluids from putrefactive blisters. Forensic Sci. Int. 90 (1−2), 57−63.

Guillot, E., de Mazancourt, P., Durigon, M., Alvarez, J.C., 2007. Morphine and 6-acetylmorphine concentrations in blood, brain, spinal cord, bone marrow and bone after lethal acute or chronic diacetylmorphine administration to mice. Forensic Sci. Int. 166 (2−3), 139−144.

Gunatilake, K., Goff, M.L., 1989. Detection of organophosphate poisoning in a putrefying body by analyzing arthropod larvae. J. Forensic Sci. 34 (3), 714−716.

Hargrove, V.M., Molina, D.K., 2014. Morphine concentrations in skeletal muscle. Am. J. Forensic Med. Pathol. 35 (1), 73−75.

Harkey, M.R., 1993. Anatomy and physiology of hair. Forensic Sci. Int. 63, 9−18.

Hazarika, P., Jickells, S.M., Russell, D.A., 2009. Rapid detection of drug metabolites in latent finger marks. Analyst 134 (1), 93−96.

Henderson, G.L., 1993. Mechanisms of drug incorporation into hair. Forensic Sci. Int. 63, 19—29.

Hikiji, W., Kudo, K., Usumoto, Y., Tsuji, A., Ikeda, N., 2010. A simple and sensitive method for the determination of propofol in human solid tissues by gas chromatography-mass spectrometry. J. Anal. Toxicol. 34, 389—393.

Hilberg, T., Bugge, A., Beylich, K.M., Morland, J., Bjorneboe, A., 1992. Diffusion as a mechanism of postmortem drug redistribution: an experimental study in rats. Int. J. Legal Med. 105 (2), 87—91.

Hilberg, T., Bugge, A., Beylich, K.M., Ingum, J., Bjorneboe, A., Morland, J., 1993. An animal model of postmortem amitriptyline redistribution. J. Forensic Sci. 38 (1), 81—90.

Hirsch, C.S., Adelson, L., 1973. Ethanol in sequestered hematomas. Am. J. Clin Path. 59, 429—433.

Huestis, M.A., Cone, E.J., Wong, C.J., Umbricht, A., Preston, K.L., 2000. Monitoring opiate use in substance abuse treatment patients with sweat and urine drug testing. J. Anal. Toxicol. 24 (7), 509—521.

Idowu, O.R., Caddy, B., 1981. A review of the use of saliva in the forensic detection of drugs and other chemicals. J. Forensic Sci. Soc. 22, 123—135.

Introna, F., Campobasso, C.P., Goff, M.L., 2001. Entomotoxicology. Forensic Sci. Int. 120 (1—2), 42—47.

Isenschmid, D.S., Hepler, B.R., 2007. Specimen selection, collection, preservation and security. In: Karch, S.B. (Ed.), Postmortem Toxicology of Abused Drugs. CRC Press, Boca Raton, FL.

Kintz, P., 2004. The value of hair in postmortem toxicology. For. Sci. Int. 142, 127—134.

Jenkins, A.J., Oblock, J., 2008. Phencyclidine and cannabinoids in vitreous humor. Leg. Med. (Tokyo, Japan) 10 (4), 201—203.

Jones, G., 2011. Postmortem toxicology. In: Moffat, A.C., Asselton, M.D., Widdop, B. (Eds.), Clarke's Analysis of Drugs and Poisons, fourth ed. Pharmaceutical Press, Chicago.

Jones, G.R., Pounder, D.J., 1987. Site dependence of drug concentrations in postmortem blood—a case study. J. Anal. Toxicol. 11, 186—190.

Joya, X., Pujadas, M., Falcon, M., Civit, E., Garcia-Algar, O., Vall, O., et al., 2010. Gas chromatography-mass spectrometry assay for the simultaneous quantification of drugs of abuse in human placenta at 12th week of gestation. Forensic Sci. Int. 196 (1—3), 38—42.

Kalasinsky, K.S., Bosy, T.Z., Schmunk, G.A., Ang, L., Adams, V., Gore, S.B., et al., 2000. Regional distribution of cocaine in postmortem brain of chronic human cocaine users. J. Forensic Sci. 45 (5), 1041—1048.

Kalasinsky, K.S., Bosya, T.Z., Schmunkb, G.A., Reiberd, G., Anthony, R.M., Furukawae, Y., et al., 2001. Regional distribution of methamphetamine in autopsied brain of chronic human methamphetamine users. Forensic Sci. Int. 116, 163—169.

Kempf, J., Wuske, T., Schubert, R., Weinmann, W., 2009. Pre-analytical stability of selected benzodiazepines on a polymeric oral fluid sampling device. Forensic Sci. Int. 186, 81—85.

Kerrigan, S., 2011. Sampling, storage and stability. In: Moffat, A.C., Osselton, M.D., Widdop, B., Watts, J. (Eds.), Clarke's Analysis of Drugs and Poisons, fourth ed. Pharmaceutical Press, Chicago.

Kerrigan, S., Goldberger, B.A., 2008. Specimens of maternal origin: amniotic fluid and breast milk. In: Jenkins, A.J., Caplan, Y.H. (Eds.), Drug Testing in Alternate Biological Specimens. Humana Press, Totowa, NJ.

Kidwell, D.A., Smith, F.P., 2001. Susceptibility of PharmChek drugs of abuse patch to environmental contamination. Forensic Sci. Int. 116 (2—3), 89—106.

Kim, J.Y., Shin, S.H., In, M.K., 2010. Determination of amphetamine-type stimulants, ketamine and metabolites in fingernails by gas chromatography-mass spectrometry. Forensic Sci. Int. 194 (1−3), 108−114.

Kintz, P., Mangin, P., 1993. Determination of gestational opiate, nicotine, benzodiazepine, cocaine and amphetamine exposure by hair analysis. J. Forensic Sci. Soc. 33, 139−142.

Kintz, P., Samyn, N., 2000. Unconventional samples and alternative matrices. In: Bogusz, M.J. (Ed.), Forensic Science: Handbook of Analytical Separations. Elsevier.

Kintz, P., Samyn, N., 2002. Use of alternative specimens: drugs of abuse in saliva and doping agents in hair. Therap. Drug Monit. 24, 239−246.

Kintz, P., Tracqui, A., Mangin, P., 1994. Analysis of opiates in fly larvae sampled on a putrefied cadaver. J. Forensic Sci. Soc. 34 (2), 95−97.

Kintz, P., Godelar, B., Tracqui, A., Mangin, P., Lugnier, A.A., Chaumont, A.J., 1990. Fly larvae: a new toxicological method of investigation in forensic medicine. J. Forensic Sci. 35 (1), 204−207.

Koren, G., Klein, J., Forman, R., Graham, K., Phan, M., 1992. Biological markers of intrauterine exposure to cocaine and cigarette smoking. Dev. Pharmacol. Ther. 18, 228−236.

Koury, M.J., Lichtman, M.A., 2010. Structure of the marrow and the hematopoietic microenvironment. In: Lichtman, M.A., Kipps, T.J., Seligsohn, U., Kaushansky, K., Preston, K.L. (Eds.), Williams Hematology, eighth ed. McGraw-Hill, New York.

Kugelberg, F.C., Jones, A.W., 2007. Interpreting results of ethanol analysis in postmortem specimens. Forensic Sci. Int. 165, 10−29.

Langel, K., Engblom, C., Pehrsson, A., Gunnar, T., Ariniemi, K., Lillsunde, P., 2008. Drug testing in oral fluid-evaluation of sample collection devices. J. Anal. Toxicol. 32 (6), 393−401.

Lee, D., Huestis, M.A., 2014. Current knowledge on cannabinoids in oral fluid. Drug Test. Anal. 6 (1−2), 88−111.

Leggett, R., Lee-Smith, E.E., Jickells, S.M., Russell, D.A., 2007. Intelligent fingerprinting: simultaneous identification of drug metabolites and individuals by using antibody-functionalized nanoparticles. Angew. Chem. Int. Ed. Engl. 46 (22), 4100−4103.

Levisky, J.A., Bowerman, D.L., Jenkins, W.W., Karch, S.B., 2000. Drug deposition in adipose tissue and skin: evidence for an alternative source of positive sweat patch tests. Forensic Sci. Int. 110 (1), 35−46.

Levisky, J.A., Bowerman, D.L., Jenkins, W.W., Johnson, D.G., Karch, S.B., 2001. Drugs in postmortem adipose tissue: evidence of antemortem deposition. For. Sci. Int. 121, 157−160.

Liberty, H.J., Johnson, B.D., Fortner, N., 2004. Detecting cocaine use through sweat testing: multilevel modeling of sweat patch length-of-wear data. J. Anal. Toxicol. 28 (8), 667−673.

Lippi, G., Salvagno, G.L., Montagnana, M., Brocco, G., Guidi, G., 2006. Influence of the needle bore size used for collecting venous blood samples on routine clinical chemistry testing. Clin. Chem. Lab. Med. 44, 1009−1014.

Lippi, G., Blanckaert, N., Green, S., Kitchen, S., Paicla, V., Plebani, M., 2008. Haemolysis: an overview of the leading cause of unsuitable specimens in clinical laboratories. Clin. Chem. Lab. Med. 46, 764−772.

Logan, B.K., Lindholm, G.M., 1996. Gastric contamination of postmortem blood samples during blind-stick sample collection. Am. J. Forensic Med. Pathol. 17, 109−111.

Lozano, J., Garcia-Algar, O., Vall, O., de la Torre, R., Scaravelli, G., Pichini, S., 2007. Biological matrices for the evaluation of in utero exposure to drugs of abuse. Ther. Drug Monit. 29 (6), 711−734.

Madej, K.A., 2010. Analysis of meconium, nails and tears for determination of medicines and drugs of abuse. Trends Anal. Chem. 29, 246−259.

McIntyre, L.M., King, C.V., Boratto, M., Drummer, O.H., 2000. Post-mortem drug analyses in bone and bone marrow. Ther. Drug Monit. 22 (1), 79−83.

Moller, M.R., Tausch, D., Biro, G., 1977. Radiological detection of morphine in stains of blood and urine. Z. Rechtsmed 79 (2), 103−107.

Moore, C., Browne, S., Tebbett, I., Negrusz, A., Meyer, W., Jain, L., 1992. Determination of cocaine and benzoylecgonine in human amniotic fluid using high flow solid-phase exaction columns and HPLC. For. Sci. Int. 56, 177−181.

Moriya, F., Hashimoto, Y., 1998. Medicolegal implications of drugs and chemicals detected in intracranial hematomas. J. Forensic Sci. 43 (5), 980−984.

Morley, S.R., Bolton, J., 2012. Variation in postmortem liver sampling: implications for postmortem toxicology interpretation. J. Clin. Pathol. 65 (12), 1136−1137.

Musshoff, F., Madea, B., 2007. Analytical pitfalls in hair testing. Anal. Bioanal. Chem. 388, 1475−1494.

Noguchi, T.T., Nakamura, G.R., Griesemer, E.C., 1978. Drug analyses of skeletonizing remains. J. Forensic Sci. 23 (3), 490−492.

Nolte, K.B., Pinder, R.D., Lord, W.D., 1992. Insect larvae used to detect cocaine poisoning in a decomposed body. J. Forensic Sci. 37 (4), 1179−1185.

O'Neal, C., Crouch, D.J., Rollins, D.E., Fatah, A.A., 2000. The effects of collection methods on oral fluid codeine concentrations. J. Anal. Toxicol. 24, 536−542.

Pal, R., Megharaj, M., Naidu, R., Klass, G., Cox, M., Kirkbride, K.P., 2012. Degradation in soil of precursors and by-products associated with the illicit manufacture of methylamphetamine: implications for clandestine drug laboratory investigation. Forensic Sci. Int. 220 (1−3), 245−250.

Palmeri, A., Pichini, S., Pacifici, R., Zuccaro, P., Lopez, A., 2000. Drugs in nails: physiology, pharmacokinetics and forensic toxicology. Clin. Pharmacokinet. 38 (2), 95−110.

Pare, E.M., Monforte, J.R., Thibert, R.J., 1984. Morphine concentrations in brain tissue from heroin-associated deaths. J. Anal. Toxicol. 8 (5), 213−216.

Parsons, M.A., Start, R.D., Forrest, A.R.W., 2003. Concurrent vitreous disease may produce abnormal vitreous humor biochemistry and toxicology. J. Clin. Path. 56, 720.

Peres, M.D., Pelicao, F.S., Caleffi, B., De Martinis, B.S., 2014. Simultaneous quantification of cocaine, amphetamines, opiates and cannabinoids in vitreous humor. J. Anal. Toxicol. 38 (1), 39−45.

Pianta, A., Liniger, B., Baumgartner, M.R., 2013. Ethyl glucuronide in scalp and non-head hair: an intra-individual comparison. Alcohol Alcohol (Oxford, Oxfordshire) 48 (3), 295−302.

Pirro, V., Di Corcia, D., Pellegrino, S., Vincenti, M., Sciutteri, B., Salomone, A., 2011. A study of distribution of ethyl glucuronide in different keratin matrices. Forensic Sci. Int. 210 (1−3), 271−277.

Pounder, D.J., Adams, E., Fuke, C., Langford, A.M., 1996a. Site to site variability of postmortem drug concentrations in liver and lung. J. Forensic Sci. 41 (6), 927−932.

Pounder, D.J., Fuke, C., Cox, D.E., Smith, D., Kuroda, N., 1996b. Postmortem diffusion of drugs from gastric residue: an experimental study. Am. J. Forensic Med. Pathol.: Off. Publ. Natl. Assoc. of Med. Exam. 17 (1), 1−7.

Pounds, C.A., Pearson, E.F., Turner, T.D., 1979. Arsenic in fingernails. J. For. Sci. 19, 165−173.

Pragst, F., Balikova, M.A., 2006. State of the art in hair analysis for detection of drug and alcohol abuse. Clin. Chem. Acta 370, 17–49.

Prouty, R.W., Anderson, W.H., 1990. The forensic science implications of site and temporal influences on postmortem blood–drug concentrations. J. Forensic Sci. 35, 243–270.

Raikos, N., Tsoukali, H., Njau, S.N., 2001. Determination of opiates in postmortem bone and bone marrow. Forensic Sci. Int. 123 (2–3), 140–141.

Rees, K.A., Pounder, D.J., Osselton, M.D., 2013. Distribution of opiates in femoral blood and vitreous humour in heroin/morphine-related deaths. Forensic Sci. Int. 226 (1–3), 152–159.

Reese, J.J., 1874. Textbook of Medical Jurisprudence and Toxicology. P. Blakiston, Son & Co, Philadelphia, 22.

Riley, D., Wigmore, J.G., Yen, B., 1996. Dilution of blood collected for medicolegal alcohol analysis by intravenous fluids. J. Anal. Toxicol. 20 (5), 330–331.

Ripple, M.G., Goldberger, B.A., Caplan, Y.H., Blitzer, M.G., Schwartz, S., 1992. Detection of cocaine and its metabolite s in human amniotic fluid. J. Analyt. Tox. 16, 328–331.

Robbins, C.R., 2002. Chemical and Physical Behavior of Hair, fourth ed. Springer-Verlag, New York.

Rodda, K.E., Dean, B., McIntyre, I.M., Drummer, O.H., 2006. Brain distribution of selected antipsychotics in schizophrenia. Forensic Sci. Int. 157 (2–3), 121–130.

Ropero-Miller, J.D., Goldberger, B.A., Cone, E.J., Joseph Jr., J.E., 2000. The disposition of cocaine and opiate analytes in hair and fingernails of humans following cocaine and codeine administration. J. Analyt. Tox. 24, 496–508.

Rowell, F., Hudson, K., Seviour, J., 2009. Detection of drugs and their metabolites in dusted latent fingermarks by mass spectrometry. Analyst 134 (4), 701–707.

Rozman, K.K., Klaassen, C.D., 2001. Absorption, distribution and excretion of toxicants. In: Klaassen, C.D. (Ed.), Casarett and Doull's Toxicology, the Basic Science of Poisons, sixth ed. McGraw-Hill, New York. pp. 107.

Saddique, A., Peterson, C.D., 1983. Thallium poisoning: a review. Vet. Human Toxicol. 25 (1), 16–22.

Sadler, D.W., Fuke, C., Court, F., Pounder, D.J., 1995. Drug accumulation and elimination in *Calliphora vicina* larvae. Forensic Sci. Int. 71 (3), 191–197.

Sadler, D.W., Richardson, J., Haigh, S., Bruce, G., Pounder, D.J., 1997a. Amitriptyline accumulation and elimination in *Calliphora vicina* larvae. Am. J. Forensic Med. Pathol. 18, 397–403.

Sadler, D.W., Robertson, L., Brown, G., Fuke, C., Pounder, D.J., 1997b. Barbiturates and analgesics in *Calliphora vicina* larvae. J. Forensic Sci. 42 (3), 481–485.

Sadler, D.W., Chuter, G., Seneveratne, C., Pounder, D.J., 1997c. Barbiturates and analgesics in *Calliphora vicina* larvae. J. Forensic Sci. 42 (6), 1214–1215.

Scott, K.S., Oliver, J.S., 2001. The use of vitreous humor as an alternative to whole blood for the analysis of benzodiazepines. J. Forensic Sci. 46 (3), 694–697.

Sims, D.N., Lokan, R.J., James, R.A., Felgate, P.D., Felgate, H.E., Gardiner, J., et al., 1999. Putrefactive pleural effusions as an alternative sample for drug quantification. Am. J. Forensic Med. Pathol. 20 (4), 343–346.

Shaler, R.C., Smith, F.P., Mortimer, C.E., 1978. Detection of drugs in a bloodstain. I: diphenylhydantoin. J. For. Sci. 23 (4), 701–706.

Skoop, G., 2004. Preanalytic aspects in postmortem toxicology. Forensic Sci. Int. 142, 75–100.

Skopp, G., Potsch, L., 1997. A case report on drug screening of nail clippings to detect pre-natal drug exposure. Ther. Drug Monit. 19 (4), 386−389.

SOFT/AAFS, 2006. Forensic Toxicology Laboratory Guidelines. Retrieved November 3, 2012 from http://www.soft-tox.org/files/Guidelines_2006_Final.pdf.

Smith, F.P., Shaler, R.C., Mortimer, C.E., Errichetto, L.T., 1980. Detection of drugs in a blood-stain. II: morphine. J. For. Sci. 25 (2), 369−373.

Smith, F.P., 1981. Detection of digoxin in bloodstains. J. For. Sci. 26 (1), 193−197.

Smith, F.P., Pomposini, D.A., 1981. Detection of phenobarbital in bloodstains, semen, seminal stains, saliva, saliva stains, perspiration stains, and hair. J For. Sci. 26 (3), 582−586.

Smith, F.P., Liu, R.H., 1986. Detection of cocaine metabolite in perspiration stain, menstrual bloodstain and hair. J. For. Sci. 31 (4), 1269−1273.

Sossnoff, C.S., Ann, Q., Bernet Jr., J.T., Powell, M.K., Miller, B.B., Henderson, L.O., Hannon, W.H., Fernhoff, P., Sampson, E.J., 1996. Analysis of benzoylecgonine in dried blood spots by liquid chromatography-atmospheric pressure chemical ionization tandem mass spectrometry. J. Analyt. Tox. 20 (3), 179−184.

Spiehler, V., 2011. Drugs in saliva. In: Moffat, A.C., Osselton, M.D., Widdop, B. (Eds.), Clarke's Analysis of Drugs and Poisons, fourth ed. Pharmaceutical Press, Chicago.

Spiehler, V., Cooper, G., 2008. Drugs-of-abuse testing in saliva or oral fluid. In: Jenkins, A.J. (Ed.), Drug Testing in Alternate Biological Specimens. Humana Press, Totowa, NJ.

Spiehler, V.R., Cravey, R.H., Richards, R.G., Elliott, H.W., 1978. The distribution of morphine in the brain in fatal cases due to the intravenous administration of heroin. J. Anal. Toxicol. 2, 62−67.

Sporer, K.A., Firestone, J., 1997. Clinical course of crack cocaine body stuffers. Ann. Emerg. Med. 29 (5), 596−601.

Stimpfl, T., 2008. Drugs-of-abuse testing in brain. In: Jenkins, A.J., Caplan, Y.H. (Eds.), Drug Testing in Alternative Biological Specimens. Human Press, Totowa, NJ.

Stimpfl, T., Reichel, S., 2007. Distribution of drugs of abuse within specific regions of the human brain. Forensic Sci. Int. 170 (2−3), 179−182.

Sutheimer, C.A., Lavins, E., King, T., 1992. Evaluation of the Syva ETS-PLUS ethyl alcohol assay with application to the analysis of antemortem whole blood, routine postmortem specimens, and synovial fluid. J. Analyt. Tox. 16, 119−124.

Suzuki, O., Hattori, H., Asano, M., 1984. Nails as useful materials for detection of metham-phetamine or amphetamine abuse. Forensic Sci. Int. 24 (1), 9−16.

Tassoni, G., Cacaci, C., Zampi, M., Froldi, R., 2007. Bile analysis in heroin overdose. J. Forensic Sci. 52 (6), 1405−1407.

Thevis, M., Geter, H., Mareck, U., Sigmund, G., Henke, J., Henke, L., et al., 2007. Detection of manipulation in doping control urine sample collection: a multidisciplinary approach to determine identical urine samples. Anal. Bioanal. Chem. 388, 1539−1543.

Thieme, D., Anielski, P., Grosse, J., Sachs, H., Mueller, R.K., 2003. Identification of anabolic steroids in serum, urine, sweat and hair: comparison of metabolic patterns. Anal. Bioanal. Chem. 483, 299−306.

Tietz, N.W. (Ed.), 1992. Clinical Guide to Laboratory Tests, second ed. W. B. Saunders Company, Philadelphia.

Tracqui, A., Kintz, P., Ludes, B., Jamey, C., Mangin, P., 1995. The detection of opiate drugs in nontraditional specimens (clothing): a report of ten cases. J. Forensic Sci. 40 (2), 263−265.

Vanbinst, R., Koenig, J., Di Fazio, V., Hassoun, A., 2002. Bile analysis of drugs in postmortem cases. Forensic Sci. Int. 128 (1−2), 35−40.

Villena, V.P., 2010. Beating the system: a study of a creatinine assay and its efficacy in authenticating human urine specimens. J. Anal. Toxicol. 34, 39–44.

Walsh, J.M., Crouch, D.J., Danaceau, J.P., Cangianelli, L., Liddicoat, L.A.R., 2007. Evaluation of ten oral fluid point-of-collection drug-testing devices. J. Anal. Toxicol. 31, 44–54.

Wang, H., Li, E.Y., Xu, G.W., Wang, C.S., Gong, Y.L., Li, P., 2009. Intravenous fentanyl is exhaled and the concentration fluctuates with time. J. Int. Med. Res. 37 (4), 1158–1166.

Watterson, J., 2006. Challenges in forensic toxicology of skeletonized human remains. Analyst 131 (9), 961–965.

Wennig, R., 2000. Potential problems with the interpretation of hair analysis results. For. Sci. Int. 107, 5–12.

Wetli, C.V., Mittlemann, R.E., 1981. The "body packer syndrome"-toxicity following ingestion of illicit drugs packaged for transportation. J. Forensic Sci. 26 (3), 492–500.

Williams, K.R., Pounder, D.J., 1997. Site-to-site variability of drug concentrations in skeletal muscle. Am. J. Forensic Med. Pathol. 18 (3), 246–250.

Winek, C.L., Jones, T., 1980. Blodd versus bone marrow ethanol concentrations in rabbits and humans. For. Sci. Int. 16, 101–109.

Winek, C.L., Bauer, J., Wahba, W.W., Collom, W.D., 1993. Blood versus synovial fluid ethanol concentrations in humans. J. Analyt. Tox. 17, 233–235.

Wong, R.C., Tran, M., Tung, J.K., 2005. Oral fluid drug tests: effects of adulterants and foodstuffs. Forensic Sci. Int. 150 (2–3), 175–180.

Wyman, J.F., Dean, D.E., Yinger, R., Simmons, A., Brobst, D., Bissell, M., et al., 2011. The temporal fate of drugs in decomposing porcine tissue. J. Forensic Sci. 56 (3), 694–699.

Sample Preparation

Thus, in some recent French trials, the medical witnesses have not hesitated to boil up and evaporate the whole of the human body with many gallons of water and acids in large iron cauldrons …

Alfred Swaine Taylor, 1848

Taylor, who decried the boiling of an entire body in cauldrons as an "enthusiastic" analysis, relates one such example, the LaFarge affair, in which the body of the victim, Monsieur LaFarge, after having been disinterred was boiled in a cauldron in the courtyard outside of the court in which his wife Marie was on trial for his murder! Fortunately, such draconian measures of sample preparation are not necessary in the modern forensic toxicology laboratory. However, depending on the analyte, the sample type, and the analytical method, some sample preparations may be required before the methods of detection, identification, and quantitation are implemented.

These preparatory procedures include:

- *Decontamination*: The unintentional environmental exposure to analyte vapors of smoked drugs can result in the adsorption of these analytes onto the surface of hair. This eventuality requires the decontamination of the hair by washing it thoroughly with various solvents.
- *Physical alteration of samples*: These procedures are intended to alter sample structures so that the analytes are more accessible to extraction solvents.
- *Protein and lipid removal*: These "cleanup" procedures are intended to remove substances such as proteins and lipids that may either interfere with or complicate subsequent methods of analysis.
- *Hydrolysis*: Analytes may be released from protein–drug complexes or conjugated drug metabolites by hydrolysis when it is desired to increase the concentrations of detectable analytes or to determine the total (free and protein-bound) analyte concentrations.
- *Extraction*: Following any of the previous procedures, extraction of analytes from samples often is necessary for partially isolating and concentrating the analyte. The type of extraction employed depends upon the physical/chemical characteristics of the analytes and the methods of analysis to be employed.

Forensic Toxicology. http://dx.doi.org/10.1016/B978-0-12-799967-8.00009-8

Regardless of the sample preparation method(s) selected, there must be an evaluation to determine the extent of any analyte losses during preparation due to the analyte:

- being unstable in acids or bases,
- becoming "trapped" in and discarded with a protein precipitate,
- forming insoluble compounds,
- binding to ultrafiltration membranes (Kataoka and Lord, 2002b), or
- being removed by wash solutions.

9.1 DECONTAMINATION (SCHAFFER ET AL., 2005; PRAGST AND BALIKOVA, 2006; AGIUS AND KINTZ, 2010; MUSSHOFF AND MADEA, 2007)

The decontamination of hair samples is essential in order to remove contaminants including sweat, sebum, dust, and cosmetic products that may interfere with subsequent analyses. Decontamination procedures are also vital to the determination of whether analytes are *in* the hair shaft as a result of systematic absorption or are *on* the surface of the hair shaft after being adsorbed as a result of environmental exposure. The removal of analytes from the surface of hair shafts is essential so that their detection does not cause a misinterpretation of the analytical results, that is, positive results may be erroneously interpreted to be the result of active drug use rather than passive exposure.

A number of solvents have been used in various protocols for the decontamination of hair. The most common method for the removal of analytes from the surface of hair samples is by means of a series of washes, consisting of organic solvents and/ or aqueous buffers to remove analytes adsorbed to the surface of the hair without removing them from within the hair shaft (Drummer, 2001). A variety of solvents such as methanol, dichloromethane, or acetonitrile, or mixtures thereof, surfactants such as Tween 80 or sodium dodecyl sulfate, or buffers (Wada et al., 2010) have been employed in various combinations of volumes, washing periods, and number of washes (Kintz, 2012). The effectiveness of decontamination procedures depends upon the specific washing procedure employed, the type of external contaminants adsorbed onto the surface of the hair, and the source of the contamination, e.g., aqueous samples or smoke (Kintz, 2012). Nonprotic solvents[1] such as acetone and acetonitrile may be more suitable than protic solvents such as methanol since the former, unlike the latter, do not cause swelling of the hair resulting in extraction of analytes from the interior of the shaft (Pragst and Balikova, 2006).

---

[1]Protic solvents possess donatable hydrogen from functional groups such as —OH and —NH and can form hydrogen bonds, whereas nonprotic solvents do not possess —OH or —NH groups.

9.2 PHYSICAL ALTERATION

The structural alteration of samples, such as liver, muscle, brain, and kidney, facilitates the handling of these samples and also increases the efficiency of liquid—liquid extractions (LLE) or solid-phase extractions (SPE) by making the analytes more accessible to the solvents used in those extractions. A sufficient alteration of samples may be achieved by means of mincing or chopping, or more commonly, by homogenization or digestion.

Homogenization is commonly employed to disrupt the matrix of tissues to produce a fluid suspension of samples. The selection of a solution to be used for homogenization, which may include water, buffers, weak acids, and weak bases, depends upon the stability of the analytes in the various fluids. The volume ratio of the homogenizing fluid to the amount of sample usually is no greater than 5:1 or 10:1, ratios that improve the handling of samples without excessively decreasing analyte concentrations. The manner of homogenization will depend upon the character of the tissues, for example, brain is soft and relatively easy to homogenize, whereas skeletal muscle requires a more vigorous treatment (Maickel, 1973). Depending on the homogenizing fluid used and its pH, the hydrolysis of protein-bound analytes and conjugated drug metabolites may occur.

Instead of homogenization, samples may be treated with nonspecific proteolytic enzymes such as subtilisin Carlsberg (Osselton et al., 1977), neutrase, papain, trypsin (Shankar et al., 1987), or strong acids. The digestion by these enzymes produces a fluid sample that is easier to handle during analysis and may liberate drugs from their protein-binding sites. The choice of the appropriate method will depend on the stability of analytes at the pH values of the digestion and the efficiency of drug release. For example, although the optimum pH for subtilisin Carlsberg is greater than 10, a pH at which esters such as acetylsalicylic acid and cocaine are unstable, the recovery of these drugs is increased at a pH of 7.4; the recovery of other drugs, for example, amobarbital, diazepam, and dextromethorphan, is as efficient at a pH of 7.4 as it is at a pH of 10.3 (Hammond and Moffat, 1981), making them better candidates for recovery via subtilisin Carlsberg treatment.

The structure of keratinous samples, i.e., hair and nails, may be reduced by cutting samples into smaller segments or, perhaps more commonly, by either particle size reduction via milled pulverization at low temperatures (Monch et al., 2013) or by enzymatic or chemical digestion.

9.3 PROTEIN REMOVAL

It is often desirable to remove protein from samples or homogenates so that the resulting protein-free filtrates are more amenable to subsequent sample preparation methods. Although proteins may be removed from samples by heating or subjecting the samples to several freeze—thaw cycles, the efficiency of these methods is poor and, therefore, they are not used regularly. An alternative method of protein removal is by precipitation by means of the process of salting out, which is achieved by the addition of relatively large quantities of salts to samples (Scopes, 1994, p. 80). The added salt ions become hydrated, thus depriving the protein molecules of sufficient water of hydration to maintain them in solution, causing them to precipitate. Generally, salts best suited for this purpose are those with anions that carry charges greater than one, e.g., sulfates, and cations that are monovalent, e.g., ammonium.

Protein precipitation may also be achieved by the use of organic solvents such as acetone and alcohols; acids such as perchloric and trichloroacetic acid; or reagents such as sodium tungstate, zinc hydroxide, and aluminum chloride. The precipitated proteins can be removed by centrifugation or filtration.

Ultrafiltration, the process by which membranes restrict the passage of substances based on their molecular weights, can be used to separate proteins from lower molecular weight analytes. Ultracentrifugation enables the concentrations of analytes that are protein-bound and those that are free, i.e., not protein-bound, to be determined independently from each other and from the total analyte concentration, i.e., protein-bound plus free analytes. The separation may be achieved by use of membranes, often contained in a cone-shaped plastic housing that contains a space for the collection of the filtrate (Cheryan, 1998, p. 173). These membrane-containing units are fit into tubes and centrifuged, causing the analytes to pass through the membrane and be collected in the filtrate, whereas the proteins are retained within the membrane container to be discarded.

The method selected for protein removal must be evaluated to determine whether certain drugs may be lost due to their instability in acids or bases, e.g., cocaine may be lost in alkaline solutions, being "trapped" in the precipitate or forming insoluble compounds, e.g., tungstate salts (Stevens et al., 1977). In each case, the concentration of the drug will be decreased and subsequent quantitation errors will result, possibly leading to errors of interpretation.

9.4 FAT REMOVAL

Emulsions may form when samples containing a large amount of fat are extracted with organic solvents. Often these emulsions are extremely stable and difficult to break even with prolonged and vigorous centrifugation. To minimize or avoid the formation of emulsions, it is advisable to remove the fat from the sample prior to extraction of drugs. Fat removal may be achieved by an initial extraction of the sample, usually without pH adjustment, with a highly nonpolar solvent such as hexane. In such solvents, fats can be extracted and then discarded, but most drugs of interest are not soluble and will not be extracted. However, because hexane can cause peripheral neuropathy, a substitute such as "isohexane," a mixture of hexane isomers with a low *n*-hexane concentration, is advisable (Flanagan et al., 2007, p. 59). Fortunately, the fat-related problem of emulsion formation has been largely eliminated as smaller samples than previously necessary are now used for analyses (Jones, 2008).

9.5 HYDROLYSIS

The hydrolysis of conjugated drug metabolites is often a component of analytical methods utilized to increase the concentration of the free drug fraction in a sample. This is advantageous if only the free drug is detectable by the method of analysis. Also, analysis prior to and after hydrolysis allows the free, total (free plus conjugated metabolites), and conjugated metabolite concentrations of the drug to be determined. However, the release of drugs either from protein-binding sites or from inactive metabolic conjugates in blood or other tissues in which drug concentrations may be correlated with effects may lead to erroneous conclusions because the concentration of the free drug, the toxicologically active form of the drug, is greater than it was in the sample.

Often the hydrolysis of conjugated metabolites occurs as the result of the nonenzymatic and enzymatic procedures used in the homogenization and digestion of samples. However, specific enzymes such as esterases and glucuronidases are still used frequently for the hydrolysis of conjugated metabolites. For example, morphine glucuronides may be hydrolyzed either by HCl, with and without boiling or autoclaving, or enzymatically by β-glucuronidase.

9.6 EXTRACTION

Following sample preparation, most methods include an extraction component by which analytes are separated from the matrix and as many nonanalyte substances in the sample as possible. The three principal methods used for the extraction of analytes from analytical samples are volatilization, LLE, and SPE. By means of these methods, analytes are moderately isolated, partially purified, and concentrated.

9.7 VOLATILIZATION

Volatilization is achieved by relatively simple physical methods by which analytes are transferred from the aqueous–lipid environment of samples into a vapor phase. The analytes in the vapor phase may then be detected by colorimetric, chromatographic, or other appropriate methods. One of the major advantages of volatilization methods is that sample preparation procedures such as those described above generally are not required. The obvious disadvantage of the method is that it is applicable only to analytes that can be volatilized.

The use of steam distillation has been used in the past for the volatilization of several drugs including barbiturates, nicotine, amphetamines, and ethanol. In this method, steam is passed through liquid, minced, or homogenized samples, the pH values of which have been adjusted appropriately, that is, the pH of the samples is adjusted above the pK_a of basic drugs and below the pK_a of acid drugs, so that the majority of the drugs are in the unionized state. The resultant volatilized drug is passed through a condensation jacket, and the liquid condensate containing the analyte is collected for identification.

In the modern toxicology laboratory, the volatilization by means of steam distillation is no longer used. However, volatilization methods for the separation of volatile analytes from samples are commonly employed for the detection of volatile organic compounds such as ethanol. Volatilization separations coupled with methods of detection are described in Chapter 10.

9.8 LIQUID—LIQUID EXTRACTION

In the mid-nineteenth century, Jean Servais Stas developed a method for the extraction of nicotine in the Bocarme case (Chapter 1). The method developed by Stas may be summarized as follows (Witthaus and Becker, 1911, p. 130). Samples were mixed with alcohol acidified with either tartaric or oxalic acid and then warmed to 60—65 °C, following which the mixture was cooled, filtered, and the solvent evaporated. The residue, which contained the water-soluble salt of nicotine, was dissolved in a small amount of water. The aqueous solution was alkalinized with $NaHCO_3$ or $KHCO_3$ to convert the nicotine salt into its nonionized freebase form, which was then extracted with ether, in which the freebase nicotine dissolved. The ether was evaporated and the residue heated gently to detect whether the odor of the volatile nicotine could be detected. The method of Stas was subsequently modified by Frederick Julius Otto who added an initial extraction of the acidified material to remove fats (Otto, 1857). This modified procedure, which has since been known as the Stas—Otto method, serves as the foundation not only of the multitude of LLE protocols that have been developed subsequently and are employed today, but also of SPE methods.

The basis of LLE is that nonvolatile analytes can be transferred from the aqueous milieu of biological samples into organic solvents in which they have a high partition coefficient and thus a greater solubility than in water. Following this initial extraction of the analyte into an organic solvent, the analyte may be transferred or "back-extracted" into an aqueous solution (usually of smaller volume than the volume of the initial organic solvent extract) of appropriate pH in which they form water-soluble salts. Generally, the back-extraction is from a larger volume of organic solvent into a smaller volume of aqueous solution, e.g., a 25 mL organic extract may be back-extracted with 2 mL of aqueous solution. In addition to concentrating the analyte, back-extractions serve to eliminate additional potentially interfering compounds. If desired, an additional extraction of the analyte may be made from the aqueous solution into which it was back-extracted into a small volume of organic solvent.

Several factors that influence the efficiency of LLE are discussed below.

9.8.1 pH

The extraction of analytes into organic or aqueous solvents is achieved by altering the pH of samples, so that analytes are present predominantly in nonionized forms for extraction into an organic solvent and in the ionized form for extraction into an aqueous solution.

In order to optimize the extraction of drug analytes from their aqueous environment, the pH of the sample is adjusted so that analytes are present predominantly in the free nonionized forms that are soluble in organic solvents in which they have high partition coefficients. An acceptable first approximation of the relative concentrations of nonionized (free acids or freebases) and ionized forms of drug analytes **at equilibrium** may be determined by the Henderson—Hasselbach equations for weak acids and weak bases (Eqns (9.1) and (9.2)):

$$\text{For weak acids,} \quad \text{pH} = pK_a + \frac{\log [A^-]}{[HA]} \tag{9.1}$$

$$\text{For weak bases,} \quad \text{pH} = pK_a + \frac{\log [B]}{[BH^+]} \tag{9.2}$$

where

[A] = the concentration of the free acid form of a drug
$[A^-]$ = the concentration of the ionized form (conjugate base) of a drug
[B] = the concentration of the freebase form of a drug
[BH] = the concentration of the ionized form (conjugate acid) of a drug.

As is evident from the Henderson—Hasselbach equation, if the pH of the sample has been adjusted so that it is less than the pK_a of weak acids such as barbiturates, salicylic acid, and diphenylhydantoin, these drugs will be present largely in the nonionized, free acid form that is extractable into organic solvents. Weak bases such as opioids, amphetamines, benzodiazepines, phenothiazines, cocaine, and nicotine are extractable into organic solvents as freebases from aqueous samples, the pH of which has been adjusted so that it is greater than the pK_a of the drugs. The so-called neutral drugs, such as glutethimide, meprobamate, digitoxin, and dichlorodiphenyltrichloroethane (DDT), either do not possess ionizable acidic or basic functional groups or are weak acids or bases, with very large or very small pK_a values, respectively. Since these drugs are primarily nonionized at all pH values commonly used for extractions, they will be extracted from either acidic or alkaline aqueous solutions into organic solvents. Amphoteric drugs, e.g., morphine and phenylephrine, possess both acidic and basic functional groups and have an "effective" pK_a at which they are ionized to a minimum degree. These drugs are most efficiently extracted at a pH that is neither sufficiently low to cause significant protonation of the basic group nor sufficiently high to cause the acidic group to be significantly deprotonated. Examples of weak acid, weak base, neutral, and amphoteric drugs are presented in Table 9.1.

Table 9.1 Commonly Encountered Drugs and Their Approximate pK_a Values

Weak acids	pK_a
Diphenylhydantoin	8.3
Phenobarbital	7.3
Salicylic acid	3–4
Secobarbital	8.3
Theophylline	8.7
Weak bases	
Amitriptyline	9.4
Amphetamine	9.9
Chlorpheniramine	9.2
Chlorpromazine	9.3
Codeine	6.1
Cocaine	5.6
Imipramine	9.5
Neutrals	
Glutethimide	9.2
Meprobamate	9.2
Amphoterics	
Morphine	8.0, 9.6
Phenylephrine	8.9

Weak acids that have been extracted into organic solvents may be back-extracted into alkaline aqueous solutions, whereas weak bases and amphoterics can be extracted into acidic aqueous solutions. Since neutral drugs do not form salts readily, they are not extractable from organic solvents into either the acidic or alkaline solutions and therefore will remain in the organic solvent. For many of the drugs of interest, aqueous acid and base solutions with concentrations of 0.1–0.5 N are sufficient for the back-extraction. However, for very weak acids or bases, aqueous acidic or alkaline solution of greater concentration may be required, e.g., the back-extraction of the weak base diazepam requires an HCl concentration of 2–6 N.

Although the ionized salt forms of drugs generally have low solubility in organic solvents, the salts of several drugs are appreciably soluble in specific organic solvents. For example, the hydrochlorides of amitriptyline, dextropropoxyphene, meperidine, methadone, and several phenothiazines and the sulfates of diazepam and methaqualone have appreciable solubility in chloroform (Hackett et al., 1976) and as a result may not be back-extracted efficiently into the aqueous solution. Therefore, since these drugs may not be back-extracted effectively into aqueous hydrochloric or sulfuric acid solutions, acids or solvents other than chloroform should be used to achieve the desired back-extraction.

It must be kept in mind that the Henderson–Hasselbach equation describes the relative concentrations of ionized and nonionized weak acids and weak bases *at equilibrium*. In practice, when samples are extracted in separatory funnels or other containers, the equilibrium between the ionized and the nonionized will be altered. Because the organic and aqueous phases are mixed together, a virtually countless number of aqueous–organic interfaces are produced at which the nonionized analyte is transferred from the aqueous to the organic phase. As this transfer occurs, the equilibrium is stressed and shifts toward the nonionized form, thus causing more of the drug than predicted by the Henderson–Hasselbach equation to be extracted into the organic solvent. This equilibrium shift can result in a relatively efficient extraction of analyte from an aqueous sample in which the pH is not optimum. For example, phenobarbital, a weak acid with a pK_a of 7.4, may be effectively extracted into chloroform from an aqueous sample with a pH 9.

Care must be taken that extremes are avoided in the alteration of the sample pH in the initial or back-extractions since this may result in the physical alteration of the sample or the destruction of the drug. For example, the concentrations of esters such as cocaine will be decreased as a result of hydrolysis if the extraction is carried out at elevated pH values. Whole blood that is extracted at an excessively low pH may take on a coffee-ground consistency causing decreased extraction efficiency. A difference of 2–3 units between the pH of the samples and the pK_a values of the drugs generally is adequate.

9.8.2 SOLVENT CHARACTERISTICS

There are several criteria that influence the choice of solvents used in LLEs. These criteria include the polarity, density, safety, boiling point, and cost of the solvent. Commonly used solvents that meet most, if not all, of these criteria include chloroform, ether, dichloromethane, ethyl acetate, and various alcohols.

The efficiency with which a drug is extracted into the organic solvent is correlated with the partition coefficient of the drug in the organic solvent. The partition coefficient, which may be defined simply as the concentration of the analyte in the organic solvent divided by its concentration in the aqueous phase at equilibrium, is related to the polarity of the analyte and the polarity of the solvent (Nollet, 2004). As seen in Table 9.2, the polarity of an organic solvent is generally directly related to its dielectric constant and water solubility.

Since most organic analytes of interest to forensic toxicologists are somewhat polar, they are generally extracted more efficiently into solvents such as chloroform or ethyl acetate that possess moderate polarity than into nonpolar solvents such as hexane or heptane. When necessary, the polarity of solvents such as chloroform or ethyl acetate may be increased by preparing an admixture of these solvents with an alcohol to provide an extraction solvent of increased polarity that produces greater extraction efficiency. As a rule of thumb, the least polar solvent that is consistent with efficient

Table 9.2 Dielectric Constants and Polarity of Selected Organic Solvents

	Dielectric Constant	Solubility in Water (g/L)	Polarity
Heptane	1.92	0.5	0
Cyclohexane	2.03	0	0
Toluene	2.38	0.53	2.3
Dichloromethane	8.03	13	3.4
Ethyl acetate	6.02	83	4.3
Chloroform	4.81	8	4.4

extraction should be used as this will result in the least coextraction from the sample of polar endogenous substances, which may interfere with analyte detection.

Frequently, the organic solvents most appropriate for the extraction of analytes from aqueous samples may be those with which they are able to form hydrogen bonds (Siek, 1978). Therefore, proton-donating drugs are extracted more efficiently with proton-accepting solvents and vice versa. For example, the proton donor salicylic acid is extracted to a greater extent with proton acceptors such as ethyl acetate and 1-butanol than with the proton donor chloroform. This approach may have some utility as an initial identification of the solvents that would be most efficient, but its use should be tempered with the understanding that exceptions exist.

The density of the organic extraction solvent has certain practical consequences. Aqueous samples and solutions with densities less than that of organic solvents will form the lower layer when the immiscible aqueous and organic liquids separate and, therefore, will be conveniently removed from a separatory funnel. This enables a back-extraction of the organic extract remaining in the separatory funnel without a transfer.

Final organic extracts are often evaporated prior to detection in order to produce higher concentrations of analytes. Therefore, organic solvents with relatively low boiling points have the advantage of being more rapidly evaporated. In addition, lower boiling points minimize the loss of heat-labile or volatile analytes.

Emulsions are formed when the organic solvent and water have high mutual solubilities in each other and the interfacial tension is low. Generally, if emulsion formation is anticipated, solvents with densities that differ substantially from that of water should be used, or the ratio of organic solvent to aqueous sample should be greater than usual so that the likelihood of emulsion formation may be minimized. Although these emulsions once formed are extremely difficult to break, centrifugation with or without the addition of a salt may be successful.

Obviously, the use of exhaust hoods and explosion proof refrigerators, which can minimize the hazards associated with the use of organic solvents, is a laboratory necessity. However, the health hazards associated with organic solvents must be considered, because even when these appropriate precautions are taken, the potential exists for health hazards due to the chronic exposure to organic solvents experienced by many forensic toxicologists.

For purposes of economy, the least expensive solvent that produces the desired extraction efficiency will be used in laboratories that conduct a large number of LLEs yearly.

9.8.3 VOLUME OF SOLVENT

The effect of solvent volume on the fraction of analyte transferred into the organic phase may be estimated by the use of Eqn (9.3).

$$p = \frac{RU}{RU + 1} \tag{9.3}$$

where

p = fraction of analyte in organic phase
q = fraction of analyte in aqueous phase
R = partition coefficient
U = volume of organic phase/volume of aqueous phase.

The extraction efficiency of drugs from aqueous samples into organic solvents may be maximized by performing a single extraction using a large volume of organic solvent or by performing several extractions, each with a smaller volume. Using large volumes of organic solvents to increase efficiency leads to problems of cost, handling, and evaporation. Therefore, instead of using large volumes of solvent, increased extraction efficiency may be attained by making multiple extractions of the sample each with smaller volumes of solvent. If multiple extractions are performed using the same organic volume to aqueous volume in each, the total fraction extracted into the organic solvent may be determined by Eqn (9.4):

$$p_{total} = 1 - q^n \tag{9.4}$$

where

p_{total} = total fraction extracted into the organic phase
q = fraction remaining in the aqueous phase after the first extraction
n = number of extractions.

Examples of the effect of solvent volumes on extraction efficiency are presented in Of Interest 9.1.

9.8.4 IONIC STRENGTH

Increasing the ionic strength of an aqueous sample by addition of salts, such as NaCl or $NH_4(SO)_4$, commonly known as "salting-out," can be used to produce specific desired effects. Among these effects are:

- the increased transfer of a polar analyte such as benzoylecgonine into an organic solvent as a result of a deceased solubility in the aqueous phase (Sweeney et al., 1983);

OF INTEREST 9.1 EXTRACTION EFFICIENCY

If drug P has a chloroform: water partition coefficient of 4, and if a 5 mL blood sample is extracted with either 1 or 2, 20 mL volumes of chloroform or 1 to 3, 5 mL volumes of chloroform, the theoretical fraction of drug P extracted into the ether in each case, as calculated by the use of Eqns (9.3) and (9.4), is shown in the table below.

The data show that two extractions of 5 mL each would have a theoretical extraction efficiency greater than the extraction efficiency achieved by one extraction of 20 mL. Also, a theoretical extraction efficiency of approximately 99% requires two extractions of 20 mL each (a total of 40 mL), whereas the same extraction efficiency can be achieved with three extractions of 5 mL each (a total of 15 mL).

Therefore, in summary, multiple extractions with small volumes of solvent are more efficient, i.e., require less total solvent, than a smaller number of extractions with large solvent volumes.

Volume of Ether per Extraction (mL)	Number of Extractions	Total Volume of Ether Used (mL)	Amount of Drug P Extracted into Ether (%)
20	1	20	94.1
20	2	40	99+
5	1	5	80
5	2	10	96
5	3	15	99+

- the increased transfer of volatile analytes into the vapor phase; and
- the separation of azeotropes of water and relatively polar organic solvents such as acetonitrile, alcohols, and acetone into which drugs have been extracted.

9.8.5 A PROTOTYPICAL EXTRACTION PROTOCOL

An example of a prototypical extraction protocol is presented in Figure 9.1. In this protocol, the extraction of weak acid analytes (outlined in red) begins with the acidification of the sample (step 1) to convert the analyte predominantly into the nonionized form. This is followed by extraction with an organic solvent (step 2) by which the analyte is transferred into the organic solvent (fraction A). A back-extraction of fraction A with a solution such as 0.1 N NaOH (step 3) converts free acids to the sodium salts that are extracted into the aqueous alkaline solution (fraction C). However, neutral drugs in fraction A will not form salts and will remain in the organic phase (fraction B). Fraction C can be acidified and then extracted with an organic solvent (steps 4 and 5); the salts of the free acids will be converted into the free acid form and transferred to the organic solvent (fraction D). Organic fractions B and D can be reduced in volume and analyzed by appropriate methods. Weak bases are isolated and extracted by extractions and back-extractions as presented in the blue-outlined portions of Figure 9.1. Whereas weak acids are extracted into organic solvents from acidic aqueous solutions and back-extracted into alkaline aqueous solutions from organic solvents; weak bases are extracted into organic solvents from alkaline aqueous solutions and back-extracted into acidic aqueous solutions from

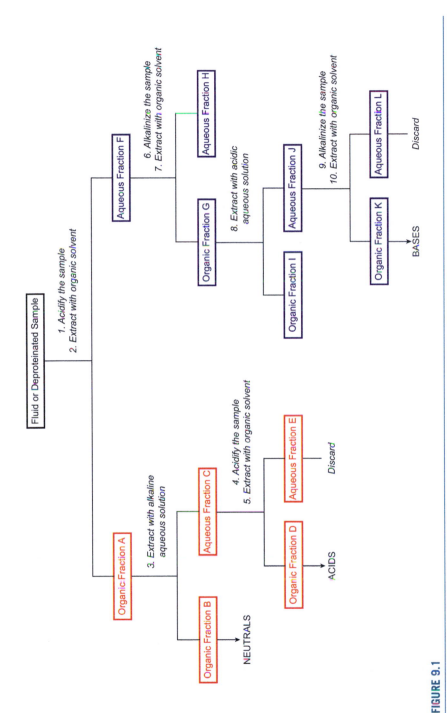

FIGURE 9.1

A prototypical extraction protocol.

organic solvents. In the case of either weak acids or weak bases, the adjustment of pH and the choice and volumes of organic solvents, and acids and bases should be consistent with the factors discussed above.

9.9 SOLID-PHASE EXTRACTION

Modern SPE, which was developed in the 1970s, is widely used by forensic toxicologists because of the several advantages it has compared to LLE (Supelco, 2004, accessed 04.12.11; Telepchak et al., 2004). These advantages include the following:

- separations are efficient, easy, and rapid
- phase separation and emulsions do not present problems
- small volumes of organic solvents are used
- expensive glassware is not necessary
- many columns may be used simultaneously for batch analysis
- several different drugs may be extracted with a single column.

A disadvantage of the use of SPE with postmortem samples, such as blood samples or homogenates, is that the frequent presence of clots and other solid matter in these samples may obstruct the flow of samples and solvents through the solid phase (Jones, 2008).

The basic principle of SPE is similar to that of LLE with the exception that the organic solvent used in LLE has been replaced by a solid phase to which the drug analytes will bond. The solid phase is usually contained in a disposable plastic tube that has a shape similar to that of a syringe barrel.

The solid phases consist of a silica (SiO_2) backbone to which are bonded sorbents of varying polarities—normal phase (hydrophilic), reverse phase (hydrophobic),[2] ionic (cationic or anionic), and copolymeric (having at least two types of sorbents).

The general procedure for SPE is as follows (Kataoka and Lord, 2002a):

1. *Conditioning*: The column is washed with alcohols and/or buffers to condition the column and to remove manufacturing residues.
2. *Loading*: The pH of the sample is adjusted appropriately so that, depending on the type of sorbent used, the drug analyte is either ionized (for ionic sorbents) or nonionized (for reverse phase sorbents). The sample is applied to the sorbent column and allowed to flow through.
3. *Rinsing*: The column is rinsed with solvent in order to remove unadsorbed materials and extraneous loading solvent.

---

[2]These phases may be uncapped, i.e., they contain unreacted exposed hydroxyl sites on the silanol groups that impart some degree of polarity to the phase or capped, i.e., the exposed hydroxyl sites have been reacted with a substituent that renders the phase less polar than the uncapped phase (Telepchak et al., 2004, pp. 14—15).

4. *Elution*: Eluting solvents are applied sequentially to elute the drugs from the sorbent. These solvents are selected so that the adsorbed drugs will transfer from the sorbent into the eluting solvent. For example, drugs that are bound to the solid phase by means of ionic bonds may be eluted by use of a solvent with a pH that converts the drugs into the nonionized nonpolar form, thus disrupting the bond between the drugs and the solid phase.
5. The eluting solvent is collected and subjected to the desired method of detection following additional preparatory steps, e.g., concentration of the drug analyte, evaporation of the solvent, and derivatization.

The flow rates of the sample, buffers, and solvents may be regulated by means of a vacuum system attached to the tube.

As an example, consider the extraction of a weak acid drug. The pH of the sample is adjusted to a value above the pK_a of the drug so that the drug is predominantly anionic. The sample is then applied to a column containing a cationic sorbent to which the anionic drug binds by means of electrostatic forces. The drug is eluted from the sorbent by means of an organic solvent containing a base that converts the anionic drug analyte into its nonionized form that is soluble in the organic eluting solvent.

9.10 SOLID-PHASE MICROEXTRACTION (LAFRENIERE AND WATTERSON, 2009; MULLETT, 2007; PEREIRA ET AL., 2014)

Solid-phase microextraction (SPME) is an adaptation of SPE in which the solid-phase column has been replaced by a microliter syringe-like device with a hollow needle and a plunger to which is attached a fused silica fiber coated with a suitable stationary phase polymer. As is the case with SPE, reverse, normal, and ionic phases are available.

Analytes may be extracted by two methods: headspace (HS) and direct immersion (DI) (Kataoka and Lord, 2002b). In the former method, the coated fiber is exposed to the HS in which volatile analytes may be present, whereas in the latter, the fiber is placed directly into a liquid sample. With the fiber drawn up into the needle, the needle can pierce the septum of a vial containing the sample (either liquid or vapor) and the fiber can be introduced into the sample where it will remain for several minutes until equilibrium has been established between the concentration of drug in the sample and on the solid phase (Supelco, 1998). Drugs adsorbed onto the fiber can be desorbed in the injection port of a gas chromatograph or in an SPME/HPLC interface. SPME is an equilibrium method and, therefore, analytes may not be exhaustively extracted from the sample. However, by standardizing the conditions of the extraction, e.g., pH, temperature, time of equilibration, etc., the results are reliably quantitative.

Among the advantages offered by SPME are ease of performance, applicability to small sample sizes, requirement of smaller solvent volumes than other extraction methods, and lowered cost. Several of the problems encountered with SPME in the extraction of drugs from postmortem samples, e.g., clots that clog the fibers, have been addressed with newer techniques and equipment.

9.11 MISCELLANEOUS EXTRACTION TECHNIQUES

The extraction of analytes from keratinous samples (hair and nails) and bone often requires modifications of the basic extraction protocols.

The extraction of drugs from bone may range from a relatively simple method of soaking bone tissue in water or methanol for 24 h (Horak and Jenkins, 2005) to a more involved procedure such as washing with sonication, pulverization, and prolonged extraction requiring more than 3 days (Lafreniere and Watterson, 2010).

Drugs can be extracted from dry blood spots with a number of solvents including methanol, methanol/acetone, ethyl acetate, phosphate, and borate buffers (Chace and Lappas, 2014).

REVIEW QUESTIONS

1. For what sample type(s) is decontamination most commonly necessary?
2. Why is sample pH sometimes altered during liquid-liquid extractions?
3. List and describe two methods by which protein can be removed from a sample.
4. The fat-related problem of emulsion formation has largely been eliminated by the use of small analytical samples. Why does the use of smaller samples reduce the likelihood of emulsion formation?
5. Describe what volatilization is.

APPLICATION QUESTIONS

1. Discuss the reasons why the physical alteration of a sample might be necessary. What are the advantages and disadvantages of utilizing homogenization as opposed to the enzymatic digestion to alter the structure of a sample? How would you make the determination as to whether a sample must be physically altered and if so, which method to use?
2. Describe the process of "salting out." When and why is this procedure utilized and how does it work?
3. Under what conditions would sample hydrolysis be performed? Are there specific sample types or analytes that most frequently require hydrolysis? Why or why not?
4. The three principle methods by which analytes are extracted from samples are volatilization, liquid-liquid extraction, and solid-phase extraction. Under what conditions (i.e., analyte, sample type, etc.) might each of these methods be utilized? What are the major advantages and disadvantages of each method of extraction?

REFERENCES

Agius, R., Kintz, P., 2010. Guidelines for European workplace drug and alcohol testing in hair. Drug Test. Anal. 2, 367−376.

Chace, D., Lappas, N.T., 2014. The use of dried blood spots and stains in forensic science. In: Li, W., Lee, M. (Eds.), Dried Blood Spots: Applications and Techniques. John Wiley & Sons, Hoboken, NJ.

Cheryan, M., 1998. Ultrafiltration and Microfiltration Handbook, second ed. CRC Press, Boca Raton, FL.

Drummer, O.H., 2001. The Forensic Pharmacology of Drugs of Abuse. Arnold, London.

Flanagan, R.J., Taylor, A., Watson, I.D., Whelton, R., 2007. Fundamentals of Analytical Toxiolcogy. John Wiley & Sons, Hoboken, NJ.

Hackett, L.P., Dusci, L.J., McDonald, I.A., 1976. Extraction procedures for some common drugs in clinical and forensic toxicology. J. For. Sci. 21, 263−274.

Hammond, M.D., Moffat, A.G., 1981. The stability of drugs to the conditions used in the enzymic hydrolysis of tissues using subtilisin carlsberg. J. For. Sci. Soc. 22, 293−295.

Horak, E.L., Jenkins, A.J., 2005. Postmortem tissue distribution of olanzapine and citalopram in a drug intoxication [Electronic version] J. For. Sci. 50 (3), 679−681.

Jones, G.R., 2008. Postmortem toxicology. In: Jickells, S., Negrusz, A. (Eds.), Clarke's Analyical Forensic Toxioclogy. Pharmaceutical Press, Chicago.

Kataoka, H., Lord, H.L., 2002a. Sampling and sample preparation for clinical and pharmaceutical analysis. In: Pawliszyn, J. (Ed.), Sampling and Sample Preparation for Field and Laboratory. Elsevier, New York.

Kataoka, H., Lord, H.L., 2002b. Sampling and sample preparation for clinical and pharmaceutical analysis. In: Pawliszyn, J. (Ed.), Wilson and Wilson's Comprehensive Analytical Chemistry: vol. XXXVII, Sampling and Sample Preparation for Field and Laboratory. New York.

Kintz, P., 2012. Segmental hair analysis can demonstrate external contamination in postmortem cases [Electronic version] For. Sci. Int. 215 (1−3), 73−76.

Lafreniere, N.M., Watterson, J.H., 2009. Detection of acute fentanyl exposure in fresh and decomposed skeletal tissues [Electronic version]. For. Sci. Int. 185 (1−3), 100−106.

Lafreniere, N.M., Watterson, J.H., 2010. Detection of acute fentanyl exposure in fresh and decomposed skeletal tissues, part II: the effect of dose-death interval [Electronic version]. For. Sci. Int. 194 (1−3), 60−66.

Maickel, R.P., 1973. Techniques for the microassay of drugs in biological materials. Crit. Rev. Clin. Lab. 4, 383−420.

Monch, B., Becker, R., Nehls, I., 2013. Quantification of ethyl glucuronide in hair: effect of milling on extraction efficiency [Electronic version]. Alcohol Alcohol. (Oxford, Oxfordshire) 48 (5), 558−563.

Mullett, W.M., 2007. Determination of drugs in biological fluids by direct injection of samples for liquid-chromatographic analysis. J. Biochem. Biophys. Methods 70 (2), 263−273.

Musshoff, F., Madea, B., 2007. Analytical pitfalls in hair testing. Anal. Bioanal. Chem. 388, 1475−1494.

Nollet, L.M.L., 2004. Handbook of Food Analysis: Residues and Other Food Component Analysis. Marcel Dekker, New York.

Osselton, M.D., Hammond, M.D., Twitchett, P.J., 1977. The extraction and analysis of benzodiazepines in tissues by enzymic digestion and high-performance liquid chromatography. J. Pharm. Pharmacol. 29, 460−462.

Otto, F.J., 1857. A Manual of the Detection of Poisons, by Medico-Chemical Analysis. H. Baillier, New York. http://books.google.com/books?id=Ho5n8eT3hPYC&printsec=frontcover&dq=%22friedrich+julius+otto%22&source=bl&ots=vt4Z4UkZuA&sig=7KttvOL6KiSVniiiMAVjw5V5CTQ&hl=en&ei=9u5zTL7aNoL-8Aav7PmFCQ&sa=X&oi=book_result&ct=result&resnum=6&ved=0CCUQ6AEwBQ#v=onepage&q=Stas&f=false.

Pereira, J., Camara, J.S., Colmsjo, A., Abdel-Rehim, M., 2014. Microextraction by packed sorbent: an emerging, selective and high-throughput extraction technique in bioanalysis [Electronic version]. Biomed. Chromatogr. BMC 28 (6), 839−847.

Pragst, F., Balikova, M.A., 2006. State of the art in hair analysis for detection of drug and alcohol abuse. Clin. Chem. Acta 370, 17−49.

Schaffer, M., Hill, V., Cairns, T., 2005. Hair analysis for cocaine: the requirement for effective wash procedures and effects of drug concentration and hair porosity in contamination and decontamination. J. Anal. Toxicol. 29 (5), 319−326.

Scopes, R.K., 1994. Protein Purification: Principles and Practice, third ed. Springer-Verlag, New York.

Shankar, V., Damodaran, C., Sekharan, P.C., 1987. Comparative evaluation of some enzymic digestion procedures in the release of basic drugs from tissue. J. Anal. Toxicol. 11, 164−167.

Siek, T.J., 1978. Effective use of organic solvents to remove drugs from biologic specimens. Clin.Toxicol. 13, 205−230.

Stevens, H.M., Owen, P., Bunker, V.W., 1977. The release of alkaloids from body tissues by protein precipitating reagents. J. For. Sci. Soc. 17, 169−176.

Supelco, 1998. Solid Phase Microextraction: Theory and Optimization of Conditions. Message posted to http://www.sigmaaldrich.com/catalog/Lookup.do?N5=All&N3=mode+matchpartialmax&N4=bulletin+923&D7=0&D10=bulletin+923&N1=S_ID&ST=RS&N25=0&F=PR (accessed 05.12.11).

Supelco, 2004. Guide to Solid Phase Extraction (Bulletin 910). Message posted to http://www.sigmaaldrich.com/etc/medialib/docs/Supelco/Bulletin/4538.Par.0001.File.tmp/4538.pdf (accessed 04.12.11).

Sweeney, W., Goldbaum, L.R., Lappas, N.T., 1983. Detection of benzoylecgonine in urine by means of UV spectrophotometry [Electronic version]. J. Anal. Toxicol. 7 (5), 235−236.

Telepchak, M.J., August, T.F., Chaney, G., 2004. Forensic and Clinical Applications of Solid Phase Extraction. Humana Press, Totowa, NJ.

Wada, M., Ikeda, R., Kuroda, N., Nakashima, K., 2010. Analytical methods for abused drugs in hair and their applications [Electronic version]. Anal. Bioanal. Chem. 397 (3), 1039−1067.

Witthaus, R.A., Becker, T.C., 1911. Jurisprudence, Forensic Medicine and Toxicology, vol. 4. William Wood and Company, New York.

Methods of Detection, Identification, and Quantitation

10

The three major tasks in analytical toxicology are to detect, identify and quantitate potentially harmful substances in biological or other relevant specimens.
Rokus A. De Zeeuw

10.1 CRITERIA FOR THE SELECTION OF METHODS

The literature of forensic and analytical toxicology is replete with methods for the detection and quantitation of drugs in virtually all tissues and fluids, thereby affording forensic toxicologists a wide variety and large number of analytical methods from which to choose. During the recent past, the sophistication of the methods of analysis has increased as has the ability to detect ever diminishing quantities of drugs. As a result of the advances in instrumental and immunological methods and their application to analytical toxicology, it is a fair assessment of the state of the art that virtually any analyte of interest may be detected at meaningful concentrations. This surfeit of available methods brings with it a problem—that of method selection. Regardless of the manner by which forensic toxicologists make their decision as to which method of analysis to use, as is the case with other decisions that they make, they must have a foundation for their choice and they must be able to explain and defend their selection. This requires that following the selection of a method that appears to meet their requirements, the method must meet stringent validation criteria to ensure that it performs in the manner described and expected.

The selection and use of methods of analysis by forensic toxicologists are determined in various ways. Most commonly employed methods are selected from those published in the refereed literature. The expansion of literature in forensic and analytical toxicology over the last several decades has resulted in an extensive literature of methods for the detection and quantitation of drugs and chemicals in antemortem and postmortem samples. The methods presented in the literature exemplify the advances in analytical instrumentation and methodology

Forensic Toxicology. http://dx.doi.org/10.1016/B978-0-12-799967-8.00010-4

that have enabled forensic toxicologists to detect relevant analytes in very low quantities in virtually all human tissues and fluids. In addition to methods selected from the literature, forensic toxicologist may use methods that have been recommended by colleagues, or methods that they themselves have developed or modified.

The many properties of analytical methods that should be evaluated may be distilled down to a handy few including safety, cost, ease of performance, sensitivity, and specificity. Of these, safety, cost, and ease of performance are of practical concern and, although important, do not bear as directly on the accuracy of the results obtained as do the sensitivity and specificity of the method.

10.1.1 PURPOSE OF THE ANALYSIS

The first step in the selection of a method is a clear understanding and statement of the purpose of the analysis. Without this knowledge, it is not possible to select the method that will provide the greatest likelihood of achieving analytical goals. Analytical goals within the framework of the standard analytical strategy in forensic toxicology, i.e., presumptive testing followed by confirmatory testing, require decisions as to the types of drugs to be detected and the limits of detection (LOD) and limits of quantitation (LOQ).

10.1.2 LIMITS OF DETECTION AND QUANTITATION

Generally, the methods employed by forensic toxicologists should be capable of the detection and quantitation of relevant concentrations in small samples, e.g., subtherapeutic concentrations in 1 mL or less. Fortunately, the detection of low analyte concentrations of virtually all analytes of interest in small samples is achieved by numerous available methods. That the LOD have decreased by orders of magnitude over the past several decades is borne out by displacement of the gram and milligram detection limits of the 1930s by the nanogram and picogram detection limits of today—as the earlier methods of distillation and precipitation have been replaced by immunoassay and mass spectroscopy.

As detection limits have decreased steadily over the last several decades, so too has the size of samples used for toxicological analysis. Methods of the past which required 50—100 mL or more, or several grams, of material have been replaced by newer methods requiring only a very small percentage of these quantities. It seems that future methods of analysis will allow for the use of even smaller samples. As these developments portend, the analytical and forensic toxicologists of the future will be able to obtain more information from smaller samples and, therefore, the sensitivity of methods should not be an obstacle to reliable drug detection in the future. An optimistic view of future sensitivity has envisioned in which the detection of 100 molecules of an analyte in a biological material will be a "routine procedure rather than an impossible dream" (Maikel, 1984).

The LOD is a measure of the lowest analyte concentration that can be detected reliably. The following are some of the many criteria that have been proposed for the determination of the LOD:

- A signal-to-noise ratio that is as low as 3:1 or 5:1 (Bramley et al., 2008), or at least as great as 10:1 (Finkle, 1983).
- The LOD "… is the lowest value for an analyte (usually expressed as concentration) that can be statistically distinguished from a blank" (Anderson, 1989).
- The LOD is "… the lowest concentration of an analyte that the analytical process can reliably differentiate from background levels," whereas the LOQ is "… the lowest concentration of an analyte that can be measured with a stated level of confidence" (Shah et al., 1992).

Several definitions of the LOD, which are dependent upon the method of analysis, are presented in the SOFT/AAFS Forensic Laboratory Guidelines (2006). For immunoassays, the mean value of a blank plus two or three standard deviations is acceptable, whereas for chromatographic methods it "… should not be less than the blank plus three standard deviations."

The LOQ is the lowest concentration that can be quantitated reliably; it is greater than the LOD. A number of definitions of the LOQ have been proposed:

- The concentration which has been determined from the analysis of samples fortified with known concentrations of the analyte drug ("spiked" samples) with a coefficient of variation of 20% or less (Chamberlain, 1978).
- The LOQ should be consistent with a signal-to-noise ratio from 5:1 to 10:1 (Bramley et al., 2008).
- "… the lowest concentration of an analyte that can be measured with a stated level of confidence" (Shah et al., 1992).
- "The LOQ is the minimum concentration of an analyte that can be distinguished from the assay background (i.e., the 'response' given by a blank sample known to be free of the analyte) at a specified level of confidence" (Lawson, 1994).
- Although it can be the concentration equal to the blank plus 10 standard deviations, the preferred method is an experimental determination of the lowest concentration that can be determined with an acceptable coefficient of variation (SOFT, 2006).

It is important to realize that although there are no consensus definitions for either the LOD or LOQ, any of these methods are preferable over the use of arbitrary methods, such as identifying a positive signal as any of which is twice as large as the blank signal. Therefore, forensic toxicologists must be able to demonstrate that the definition they use is not arbitrary, but rather one that has met validation criteria. It is also important to remember that the LOD and LOQ values of analytes are specific for the methods by which they have been determined.

In the case of certain analyses, instead of either the LOD or LOQ, a "cutoff" value is employed. This concentration, above which the sample is said to be positive for the analytes, frequently is equal to or greater than the LOD and less than the LOQ. Cutoff values may be established to meet a specific goal of interpretation, such as differentiating unintentional exposure from intentional use. For example, a cutoff concentration is established that is greater than the concentration expected to be detected in the urine of a passive inhaler of a drug—such as marihuana or cocaine—and below the concentration of an intentional user. To achieve this, the cutoff values established by the Department of Heart and Human Services for the detection of drugs and/or their metabolites in urine range from 10 ng/mL for 6-acetylmorphine to 2000 ng/mL for opioid metabolites (Department of Health and Human Services, 2008).

The LOD and LOQ of a method should be determined by the analysis either of analyte-fortified samples used as controls or calibrator samples that are made via the dilution of standard solutions that have been prepared by dissolving a weighed primary standard of the drug (one with stated concentrations of impurities) (Hadju and Chamberlin, 1984) in a small volume of solvent; drug-free sample standards of the same sample type that are anticipated in case work must also be analyzed. For cases in which it is difficult to replicate the sample, e.g., maggots and putrefied tissues, the use of the method of least additions is appropriate (Chapter 11).

Even the most careful and accurate preparation of controls and calibrators does not ensure that these in vivo samples are characterized by the same distribution and protein-binding patterns present in in vitro samples. Any such differences may cause a dissimilarity of analytical "behavior" between the in vivo and in vitro samples, such as disparate extraction efficiencies, and lead to analytical errors. In addition, errors in determining the LOD and LOQ of the method may arise from the use of unreliable standard solutions resulting from the evaporation of solvent, chemical instability of the drug, adsorption of the drug onto the surface of the container, impurities in the solvent or drug standard, or degradation by microorganisms (Uges, 1984).

The method selected should have LOD and LOQ values that are appropriate for the detection of drug analytes at "meaningful" concentrations in relatively small samples, e.g., 1 mL or less. A "meaningful" concentration of an analyte may range from the low concentrations that are produced following the therapeutic use of a drug or the casual environmental exposure to an industrial or commercial product, to the high concentrations that result from an intentional ingestion of a large quantity of a drug or the accidental exposure to an industrial compound following an accident.

10.1.3 SPECIFICITY

Biological samples contain a multitude of endogenous substances, many of which are present at concentrations that are orders of magnitude greater than the concentrations of analytes. In addition, numerous exogenous substances such as other drugs, chemicals, and their metabolites may also be present. This chemical complexity makes the identification of drug analytes in the presence of so many varied substances a daunting analytical task.

The specificity of the method is a measure of the degree to which the analyte is differentiated from the numerous other compounds that are present in the sample. A method must be sufficiently specific to account for the following considerations:

- *Substances from storage containers*: Compounds such as plasticizers from containers and from test tube stoppers may leech into the samples prior to analysis.
- *Analytical artifacts*: In the course of the analysis, the biological samples are often treated with acids or bases, extracted with one or more organic solvents, and possibly reacted with derivatizing agents. This may lead to the synthesis of compounds not present in the sample when it was collected.
- *Endogenous substances found in both healthy and diseased persons*: Since many drugs mimic the action and effects of endogenous substances, similarities between the drug analytes and these endogenous substances may be the cause of false-positive results.
- *Postmortem products*: The postmortem process of decomposition that includes autolysis (the digestion of cells by their own enzymes) and putrefaction (decomposition of biological material by microorganism) may result in the formation of substances not present in antemortem samples. For this reason, forensic toxicologists must be careful if they select methods of analysis that were not developed and validated for use with postmortem samples.
- *Drugs of different pharmacological classes and their metabolites*: The method must be able to differentiate classes of drugs, e.g., opioids from nonopioids. This level of specificity is generally attained in screening tests such as immunoassays.
- *Other drugs of the same pharmacological class and their metabolites*: The method should be able to differentiate between the drug analyte and other members of its pharmacological class, e.g., morphine must be distinguishable from other opioids such as oxycodone.
- *The analyte drug and its metabolites*: The differentiation between the drug analyte and its active and inactive metabolites, e.g., the differentiation of morphine from its metabolites morphine-3-glucuronide (inactive) and morphine-6-glucuronide (active), may be important for interpretation.

The use of an ideally specific method, one which would detect the drug analyte and **only** the drug analyte with absolute certainty, is not possible, but the method chosen should provide the lowest degree of interference from other substances—either endogenous or exogenous. Regardless of the degree of specificity afforded by the method employed, forensic toxicologists must be aware of the limits of the specificity so that they may take appropriate action, such as performing additional analyses, in order that these limits do not cause an error of interpretation.

10.1.4 COMPETENCE OF THE ANALYST

In addition to the identification of an acceptable analytical method, an additional and important factor which merits attention is the competence of the analyst. No method can be performed reliably unless the analyst possesses the requisite knowledge, skills, and/or experience to do so. Since it is the accuracy of a *specific* analytical result that is of interest, it is the competence of the *specific* forensic toxicologist who performed the *specific* analysis that must be evaluated. Therefore, evaluation programs that assess the overall performance of the laboratory, as evidenced, for example, by appropriate licenses and certifications as well as by a record of excellence in proficiency testing programs, are not sufficient to form an opinion as to the competence of the forensic toxicologist who performed the analysis that produced a specific result of interest. There are many ways by which a forensic toxicologist may attain the necessary competence to perform analyses and, therefore, the formal and practical experiences of forensic toxicologists will vary. However, all forensic toxicologists must possess both the knowledge of the theoretical aspects of analytical toxicology as well as the ability to perform analyses at the bench competently.

Short of either working closely with forensic toxicologists on a regular basis or administering proficiency tests to them, it is difficult to evaluate their competence reliably. It may be that identifying incompetent analysts is far easier than identifying those who are competent. However, by obtaining certain information, it is possible to gain some insights as to the competence of forensic toxicologists. Certain information relevant to the competency of an analyst can best be obtained through questioning, of the type that occurs in court on *voir dire*. For example: What is the individual's highest earned degree? What courses of study has the individual completed? What type of laboratory training has the individual received beyond his or her formal education? How much "hands-on" laboratory experiences does the individual have? Does the individual possess any special analytical skills or knowledge? How often has the individual performed this specific analysis? How has he or she performed on proficiency tests? Obviously the thrust of these questions is to identify the extent of theoretical knowledge and practical experience of the analyst. However, for any given case, it is virtually impossible to determine whether a valid method was employed in an appropriate manner in the analysis of a specific sample at a specific time of interest.

It may be that the competence of a forensic toxicologist is best evaluated by those who have developed competence themselves and are, therefore, presumably better able to identify it in others. However, in the final analysis, competence, as beauty, is in the eye of the beholder and each of us will establish our own criteria for judging competence. In so doing, we evaluate others in the light, however bright or dim, of our own abilities and if not careful we ultimately determine the professional competence of others by looking for ourselves in them.

10.1.5 RELIABILITY

The reliability of the method refers to the combination of the sensitivity, specificity, reproducibility, etc. that can be achieved by the use of a specific method. In other words, how well does the method achieve what it is expected to achieve? No method is perfect, and it is therefore important to know the limitations of the method. The most common problems of methodologies are associated with specificity, not sensitivity. The reliability of a method is determined by a validation process as discussed in Chapter 11.

10.2 METHODS OF DETECTION, IDENTIFICATION, AND QUANTITATION

A discussion of the theory of the various methods of detection and quantitation employed in forensic toxicology, and/or of the methods of analysis employed by forensic toxicologists for specific analytes, is beyond the scope and intent of this book. There are several excellent sources that provide the theoretical background for these methods that may be consulted for this information. What follows is a discussion of the criteria for choosing a method, the benefits and disadvantages, and the sources of error of several of the methods that are widely employed in forensic toxicology laboratories.

The "classic" wet-chemical analytical toxicology methods such as those developed and employed in Gettler's laboratory have given way in subsequent decades to a wide array of immunological and instrumental methods that are able to detect low concentrations of analytes with a high degree of specificity in human samples (Langman and Kapur, 2006). The development of modern methods has ranged from the early use of colorimetry and ultraviolet spectrophotometry to the presently employed methods such as gas chromatography (GC) and liquid chromatography (LC) coupled to single or tandem mass spectrometry (MS). Additionally, immunoassays such as radioimmunoassay (RIA), enzyme-multiplied immunoassay technique (EMIT), fluorescence polarization immunoassay (FPIA), and enzyme-linked immunoassay (ELISA) are used widely as screening tests for the detection of many drugs and metabolites in a variety of biological samples.

10.3 COLOR TESTS (SPOT TESTS)

Many of the earliest methods of identification were based upon the production of a product of specific color when the analyte, e.g., arsenic, reacted with specific reagents. Subsequently, these reagents, developed for the presumptive identification of organic compounds, have been used to detect drugs in urine, protein filtrates of blood and tissue, and on thin-layer chromatography (TLC) plates. The benefits of color tests are that they are simple to perform, are rapid, can be applied to certain samples without any sample preparation, require no instrumentation, and have LOD as low as 1 µg for certain drugs in dosage forms and standard solutions (O'Neal et al., 2000). Even in this age of sophisticated instrumentation, color reagents are effective for the presumptive identification of a number of drugs and have a place in the modern forensic toxicology laboratory (Siek, 2011). The reactions of several drugs with commonly used reagents have been described in the literature (O'Neal et al., 2000; Jeffery and Poole, 2008).

10.4 VOLATILIZATION

Compounds that can be volatilized can be extracted from the sample matrix by means of a simple method. A sample such as blood or urine, to which an internal standard (IS) has been added, is placed in a tube that is sealed tightly. The tube is warmed, during which a proportion of the analyte and the IS will be volatilized and transferred from the liquid phase of the sample into the vapor phase or "headspace" above the liquid sample. After a specific period of time, a sample of the headspace above the liquid sample is collected and analyzed, e.g., by GC. The degree to which volatile compounds partition between the aqueous and vapor phases is dependent upon the air–water partition value of the compound being partitioned, but it can be increased by increasing the temperature at which partitioning occurs and by the addition of salt to the liquid sample (Flanagan et al., 2007, p. 56). Under the specific conditions of the analysis, a proportionality will be established between the analyte concentration in the aqueous and vapor phases, which can be used to quantitate the concentration of the analyte when compared to the response of standard samples. A method such as this is widely used in forensic toxicology laboratories for the detection and quantitation of ethanol and other volatile organic compounds in samples such as blood and urine (Figure 10.1).

An alternative volatilization method may be performed with the use of a Conway diffusion chamber, a simple glass or porcelain device divided into two compartments by an interior ring that is lower than the exterior ring (Figure 10.2). An advantage of this procedure is that the analyte may be extracted from the sample and detected concurrently. The sample and a releasing reagent, which increases the volatility of the analyte, are placed together, without mixing, in the outer chamber, and a trapping agent is added to the center well. After the chamber has been made airtight by affixing a glass plate onto the outer wall of the chamber with stopcock grease or similar material, the sample and the releasing agent are mixed together. Upon reaction with the releasing agent, the analyte will be volatilized and react with the trapping agent to produce a colored product that may be detected visually or colorimetrically to obtain qualitative or quantitative results, respectively. The releasing agents and trapping agents used for the detection of cyanide, carbon monoxide, and ethanol are shown in Table 10.1.

10.5 IMMUNOASSAYS (HEARN AND WALLS, 2007; HAND AND BALDWIN, 2008)

The first immunoassay, RIA, was described by Yalow and Berson (1959) for the detection of the protein hormone insulin, using radioactively labeled insulin and antibodies produced against the insulin. The method was adapted subsequently for the detection of morphine, a nonprotein drug (Spector and Parker, 1970).

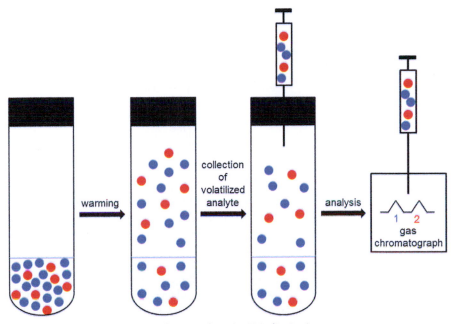

FIGURE 10.1 Gas Chromatographic Detection of a Volatile Analyte

A fluid sample such as blood or urine is placed along with an added internal standard in a vial. The vial is sealed and warmed. The volatile unknown analyte (●) and the internal standard (IS) (●) volatilize and transfer into the headspace from which an aliquot is collected and injected onto a gas chromatography column. In this example, the unknown volatile analyte (1) is identified by means of a comparison of its retention time relative to the IS (2) with that of a known analyte.

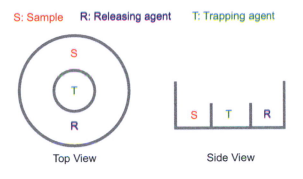

FIGURE 10.2

The Conway diffusion chamber.

Table 10.1 Examples of Analytes Detected by Volatilization in a Conway Diffusion Chamber

Analyte	Outer Chamber	Inner Chamber	End Point
Carbon monoxide	10% H_2SO_4	$PdCl_2$	Silver Pd film
		$PdCl_2 + CO + H_2O \rightarrow 2HCl + Pd$	
Cyanide	10% H_2SO_4	Pyridine-barbituric acid chloramines T in NaOH	Pink color
		$CN^- + NaOH \rightarrow NaCN$	
	$NaCN +$ pyridine-barbituric acid + chloramine T $\rightarrow$ pink product		
Ethanol	Saturated K_2CO_3	$K_2Cr_2O_7$	Green color of $Cr_2(SO_4)_3$
	$3C_2H_5OH + 2K_2Cr_2O_7 + 8H_2SO_4 \rightarrow 2Cr_2(SO_4)_3 + 2K_2SO_4 + 3CH_3COOH + 11H_2O$		

The foundation of RIA is the competitive binding of the radioactively labeled reagent drug and the analyte drug to antibodies produced against an epitope[1] on the drug molecule. The competition between the labeled reagent drug and the analyte drug can be determined and used to obtain qualitative and semiquantitative results. However, quantitative results rely on the method of curve fitting used (Hand and Baldwin, 2008) and generally are considered to be semiquantitative.

Due to problems such as monitoring and disposal of radioactive waste, several modifications of the basic RIA procedure have been developed in which the radioactive label has been replaced with nonradioactive labels, e.g., enzymes or fluorescence, that enable the unbound reagent drug to be detected. These immunoassays, which are available as kits, include EMIT, cloned enzyme donor immunoassay (CEDIA), FPIA, and ELISA (Appendix C).

Immunoassays are widely used in both forensic and clinical toxicology as presumptive (screening) methods for the detection of a wide variety of drugs because they are sensitive, possess detection limits at the ng/mL level, are easy to perform, lend themselves to automated batch analysis of large numbers of samples, are relatively inexpensive, and may be performed rapidly.

Depending on the method of antibody production, immunoassays may exhibit meaningful cross-reactivity with drugs with similar epitope structures, generally including those within the same pharmacological group as the reagent drug, e.g., morphine and codeine, but excluding those from different pharmacological groups. The extent of the cross-reactivity depends upon the specific method employed, the

---

[1]Epitopes, also known as antigenic determinants, are specific portions of a molecule recognized by a component of the immune system. Since the entire molecule is not recognized and since several drug molecules may have the same or very similar epitopes, antibodies used in the assay may recognize several different, but structurally related drugs.

manner in which the antibodies were prepared, and the manufacturer. However, unexpected cross-reactivity has been observed between the antibodies produced against the epitope of the analyte drug and drugs of a different pharmacological group that do not appear to have a similar epitope, e.g., ibuprofen has been shown to cause false-positive results for the detection of with cannabinoids by EMIT (Colbert et al., 1987).

The general lack of specificity observed with the use of immunoassays provides both an advantage and disadvantage. An advantage is that the lack of specificity may provide a broader spectrum of detectable analytes, e.g., several opioids and/or their metabolites may be detected instead of only morphine, allowing for the presumptive identification of a large number of drugs. This lack of specificity is a disadvantage because a positive result does not allow for the determination of the identity of the drug detected; this must be established by means of a confirmatory method using a more specific method, e.g., GC/MS or LC/MS/MS. The specificity of immunoassays is known to vary depending upon the analyte, for example, immunoassays exhibit greater specificity for phencyclidine than for amphetamines. Because of the potential for cross-reactivity and ambiguous results, forensic toxicologists should not report positive results unless both the immunoassay and the confirmatory test are positive. In the clinical use of immunoassays, the results often are used without further testing since the immunoassay results provide the information required, e.g., Is there evidence that drugs were used? Furthermore, often, time does not permit confirmation except for completion of the clinical record.

Although urine is the most frequently used sample for immunoassay analysis, immunoassays have been used as screening methods with blood and other fluids and tissues. However, if the method has been designed for use with urine, its use in other sample types may require precipitation of proteins or extraction of the drugs from these samples and requires the validation of the method for those samples (Drummer and Gerastamoulos, 2002).

10.6 CHROMATOGRAPHY (HEARN AND WALLS, 2007)

The birth of chromatography[2] is dated to 1903 with the presentation of a paper, "About a New Category of Adsorption Phenomena and Their Application for Biochemical Analysis" by Mikhail Semenovich Tswett who is credited with the development of the separatory method of chromatography (Berezkin, 1989), although other earlier workers had reported on similar methodologies. Modern chromatography used by forensic toxicologists has evolved from the column methods of Tswett and the paper chromatography used in early forensic toxicology laboratories, TLC, GC, and high-performance liquid chromatography (HPLC, or more commonly LC).

---

[2]The word chromatography, "color writing" in Greek, assigned by Tswett to his method was not novel as it had been used earlier in the nineteenth century by artists (Abraham, 2004).

All of the currently used methods of chromatography involve the separation of drugs and metabolites by introducing them into a mobile phase that passes over and/or through a stationary phase designed to affect their movement based on their partitioning between the two phases. Once separated, these compounds may be detected by various means depending upon the type of chromatography employed, e.g., color reagents with TLC and retention times and mass spectra with GC. Benefits of chromatographic methods include the ability to separate and differentiate drugs, including those with similar structures that belong to the same pharmacological class of drugs, and the ease and rapidity of their use. The vast number of permutations of stationary and mobile phases allows for the separation and presumptive identification of multiple drugs, i.e., drugs in the same drug class, other drug classes as well as their metabolites, often providing more information than immunoassays. The major disadvantage of chromatographic methods is that they are comparison methods, meaning that identifications are made by comparing the retention of drug standards on the stationary phase with that of the unknown analytes. Greater specificity may be achieved by coupling the chromatographic method with an appropriate detector, such as a mass spectrometer.

10.7 THIN-LAYER CHROMATOGRAPHY (JEFFERY AND POOLE, 2008)

TLC has been widely used in forensic toxicology laboratories for more than 50 years and although its use has diminished, it remains a valuable screening method as it provides toxicologists with a simple, rapid, easy method for the presumptive identification of several drugs simultaneously. Detection is based upon the mobility or retention factor of the analyte drug and its reaction with reagents that produce colored or fluorescent products, compared to drug standards analyzed simultaneously. Identification of an analyte drug by use of two or more different mobile phases may increase the reliability of the result.

10.8 GAS CHROMATOGRAPHY (DAWLING ET AL., 2008)

GC has been perhaps the most common form of chromatography used in forensic toxicology laboratories for several decades; it is faster than TLC and is amenable for the detection and quantitation of a large number of drugs and their metabolites. GC stationary phases are generally maintained in packed columns, or more popularly, in wall-coated open tubular columns, which due to a larger number of theoretical plates afford greater resolutions.

Stationary phases of varying polarity are available and may be characterized by the use of McReynolds constants that describe the relative retention of standard compounds including benzene, butanol-1,2-pentanone, 1-nitropropane, and pyridine that exemplify the retention characteristics of aromatics/olefins, alcohols, ketones/ethers/ esters/aldehydes, nitro and nitriles, and *N*-heterocyclics, respectively (Loconto, 2005, p. 374; Rotzsche, 1991, pp. 92—93). McReynolds constants may be used to select appropriate stationary phases for the separation of compounds similar to the elution sequence of these standard compounds.

One of the imitations of GC is that the mobile phase in GC is gaseous and, therefore, the drug analyte must be volatile. This eliminates the detection of compounds that either cannot be volatilized readily or are not stable at the temperatures needed for volatilization.

Several different types of detectors are available for GC and the selection of an appropriate detector depends on the characteristics of the analyte as summarized in the following list of detectors and the general type of compounds for which they are suitable (Stafford, 2003):

- flame ionization detectors (FID), for ethanol and other volatiles;
- electron capture detectors (EC), for electrophilic compounds such as halogens or compounds containing cyano or nitro groups;
- nitrogen—phosphorus detectors (NPD), for drugs containing nitrogen or phosphorus;
- mass spectrometry (MS), for numerous drugs and metabolites.

Of these detectors, MS is the most versatile as the use of the others is restricted to specific types of compounds with specific characteristics. Identification by means of FID, EC, and NPD is made on the basis of the GC retention time of the unknown analyte relative to that of an IS. Identification by means of MS is usually based on both the GC retention time of the unknown analyte relative to that of an IS and the presence of selected mass ions in appropriate ratios compared to those of a known analyte standard.

Identification by GC/MS methods generally includes a consideration of the following:

1. The GC retention time and shape of an analyte peak should be within acceptable tolerances.
2. The ions selected for monitoring should include the molecular ion as well as other ions that are characteristic of the structure of the compound and originate from different portions of the molecule.
3. The relevant abundance of monitored ions should be within acceptable tolerances.
4. Criteria 1 through 3 should be compared to simultaneously analyzed standards.

These criteria appear to be based largely on early work in which these criteria were found to be satisfactory for the identification of only one compound— diethylstilbestrol (de Zeeuw, 2004). In spite of this limited study, the use of similar criteria was reported in an early report for the confirmation of several drugs by GC/MS using a GC retention time within 1% and ion ratios within 20% of the drug standards (Mulé and Casella, 1988). Presently, the accepted tolerances for GC retention times, the minimum number of monitored ions, and the relative ion abundance vary among governmental agencies and professional organizations. For example, the confirmation criteria relative to appropriate standards suggested or required in the SOFT/AAFS Forensic Toxicology Laboratories Guidelines are GC retention times within 1−2% of the standard and a ratio of the relative abundance of at least 2 selected ions that is within ±20% of the standard for GC/MS and within ±25−30% of the standard for LC/MS (SOFT, 2006), whereas the World Anti-Doping Agency (WADA) requires a GC retention time within 1% and a ratio of 3 diagnostic ions within 20% of the standard (Cowan et al., 2008).[3] Unfortunately, the foundation for these criteria has not been provided by any of these organizations. It is not clear whether this lack of validation has ever been the basis of a Daubert challenge (Chapter 12). Clearly, additional work is required to validate identification criteria for each of the drugs for which they are employed.

Although GC/MS, which has long been considered the "gold standard" of identification in forensic toxicology laboratories, is being replaced by LC/MS, it remains an important method of confirmation.

10.9 LIQUID CHROMATOGRAPHY (AGILENT TECHNOLOGIES, 2001; GALLARDO ET AL., 2009; MAURER, 2010; PETERS, 2011)

LC affords several advantages over GC, including the analysis of a much greater number of compounds including thermolabile and nonvolatile drugs, detection of relatively polar drugs and metabolites without the need for derivatization, increased sensitivity, and shorter analysis time (Fritch et al., 2009). In addition, a variety of stationary phases such as ion exchange, and normal and reverse phases are available and are widely employed in forensic toxicology laboratories.

Although GC/MS has been the gold standard for analyte identification in the forensic toxicology laboratories for more than two decades, as a result of technical advances, LC/MS (MS) is becoming, or has become, the instrumental method of choice for identification in many laboratories. The traditional LC reliance on fluorescence, UV, and electrochemical detectors has been replaced to a large extent by MS. The use of LC/MS and LC/MS/MS in the forensic toxicology laboratory for the multianalyte analysis of drugs is being used to an ever-increasing extent (Peters et al., 2011).

Perhaps the most important limitation of LC/MS (MS) is the phenomenon commonly known as the matrix effect (Cote et al., 2009; Marchi et al., 2010; Matuszewski et al., 2003; Peters and Remane, 2012; Remane et al., 2010; Trufelli et al.,

---

[3]The Mandatory Guidelines for Federal Workplace Drug Testing programs of DHHS do not specify the criteria required for identification (Department of Health and Human Services, 2008).

2011). The matrix effect has been defined as "the direct or indirect alteration or interference in response due to the presence of unintended analytes (for analysis) or other interfering substances in the sample" (Shah, 2000). This phenomenon is caused by an interference with the ionization process of analytes resulting in either a decrease or increase in the ionization intensity of analytes, ion suppression, or ion enhancement, respectively.

Based on this definition cited above, the term "matrix effect" is misleading as it implies that the problem is due solely to the sample matrix, when in fact it may be caused by any substance that coelutes with the analyte (Peters and Remane, 2012). Substances that may cause a matrix effect may include those in the sample matrix, e.g., salts, amines, lipids, carbohydrates, peptides, and metabolic products, as well as those produced as a result of the analysis, e.g., organic acids, buffers, phthalates, and residues for solid-phase extractions (Trufelli et al., 2011).

The degree of the matrix effect may be influenced by:

- the type of ionization procedure employed—atmospheric pressure chemical ionization (APCI) or electrospray ionization (ESI);
- interspecies differences;
- intraspecies differences;
- the specific sample type in which the analyte is found;
- the method of sample preparation, especially the type of extraction.

Obviously, the significance of the matrix effect is that it may result in analyte concentrations determined by LC/MS (MS) being erroneously greater or lesser than the true concentrations in the sample, causing possible errors of interpretation. There is no single method for correcting the matrix effect, but the use of an extraction method that produces a "cleaner" extract and/or using the ionization method that produces the least effect are two of the most important steps to be taken. The matrix effect is of such importance that its magnitude in a specific method must be evaluated as a component of the validation of that method.

Several recently developed STA and multianalyte methods demonstrate the increasing utility and popularity of LC/MS and LC/MS/MS for the detection of a large number of drugs and their metabolites, not only in blood and urine, but also in other sample types, including placenta (de Castro et al., 2009), oral fluid (Fritch et al., 2009), hair, and meconium (Peters, 2011).

10.10 MASS SPECTROMETRY (DASS, 2007, PP. 17–28; GREAVES AND ROBOZ, 2014; WATSON ET AL., 2008, PP. 45–64)

The development and application of MS, a landmark in analytical and forensic toxicology, has allowed forensic toxicologists to obtain highly reliable identifications of a vast number of analytes at ever decreasing concentrations.

The basic components of a mass spectrometer are an inlet, ionization chamber, and a mass analyzer (MA). Samples are conveyed into an ion source of the mass spectrometer by means of the inlet. Generally, components of biological samples enter the mass spectrometer following a separatory method, for example, GC, LC, or capillary electrophoresis (CE), although solid samples may be introduced. An ionization chamber or ion source is the component of the MS in which the analytes are ionized. In the case of LC/MS (MS), both vaporization and ionization occur at the same time. Analytes can be ionized by one of several different mechanisms, as a result of which molecular ions and fragment ions are produced. The mechanisms widely employed in forensic toxicology include electron impact ionization, chemical ionization, APCI, and ESI. Each of these ionization mechanisms possesses advantages and disadvantages, a summary of which is presented in Table 10.2.

An MA separates analyte ions on the basis of their mass to charge (m/z) ratios. The types of MAs commonly employed in forensic toxicology laboratories include quadrupole, ion trap, and time-of-flight (TOF) instruments. MAs can be coupled to produce tandem instruments containing the same type of analyzers, e.g., TOF/TOF, or hybrid instruments containing different types of MAs, e.g., quadrupole TOF. Tandem and hybrid instruments are frequently used with soft ionization techniques to produce greater fragmentation that will generate spectra more consistent with specific molecules. Additionally, these MS/MS methods are able to produce an LOD as low as 1 ng/mL (0.1 ppb).

The data derived from MA analysis are displayed as a mass spectrum, a bar graph in which the m/z ratios of the analyte fragments (including the molecular ion) are plotted versus the peak height for each of the fragments, the height of the bar being proportional to the number of ions detected. The data in the mass spectrum are analyzed by computer systems that contain a library of mass spectra of thousands of compounds. A comparison of the spectrum of the unknown and the compounds in the computer library allows an identification to be made.

10.11 ADDITIONAL METHODS

Additional instrumental methods employed in forensic toxicology laboratories for specific classes of analytes include:

- Inductively coupled plasma—mass spectrometry for the detection of elements (Flanagan et al., 2007), which is replacing atomic absorption in clinical toxicology and forensic toxicology laboratories (Goulle et al., 2014) because it enables rapid and reliable multielement determinations with low detection limits.
- CE/MS methods for use in forensic toxicology laboratories have been developed including for the detection of drugs of toxicological interest in urine (Kohler et al., 2013) and hair (Gottardo et al., 2012).

Table 10.2 Ionization Mechanisms (Dass, 2007, pp. 17–28; Greaves and Roboz, 2014; Watson et al., 2008, pp. 45–64)

	Advantages	**Disadvantages**
Electron ionization (EI)	• Spectra are characteristic for specific molecules • Spectra may be compared to library spectra of known compounds for identification • Consistent predictable spectra that are generally reproducible from different instruments	• Analyte size of less than ~600–1000 Da • Absence of a molecular ion is common • Not used for nonvolatile or thermally unstable analytes
Chemical ionization (CI)	• Molecular ions produced with a limited number of ion fragments • Generally greater sensitivity than EI	• Analyte size of less than ~1000 Da • Analyte must be volatile • Lack of structural information • Identification by search of a library of spectra is not as suitable as EI
Atmospheric pressure chemical ionization	• Used with LC • Data similar to that of CI • Greater sensitivity that CI • Effective for the detection of analytes encountered in forensic toxicology laboratories	• Analyte size of less than ~1000 Da • Ion suppression may decrease detection limit • Not effective for analytes with poor thermal stability
Electrospray chemical ionization	• Used with LC • Does not require high-temperature volatilization of analytes • Can be used for the detection of polar compounds • Analyte size as large as 10^6 Da • Produces spectra similar to CI • May produce only molecular ions • Low detection limits	• Not effective with nonpolar analytes

REVIEW QUESTIONS

1. Why is it important to have a clear understanding of the purpose of an analysis before selecting a method of analysis?

2. Define limit of detection (LOD). How is an LOD different from a limit of quantitation (LOQ)? Why is knowledge of the LOD and LOQ of a method important?

3. Describe the ways in which the competence of a forensic toxicologist may be evaluated.
4. What are color tests? What are some of the benefits of utilizing color tests?
5. List the major components of a mass spectrometer and explain the purpose of each component.

APPLICATION QUESTIONS

1. When selecting a method of analysis, forensic toxicologists must consider both the specificity and the sensitivity of the method. Define sensitivity and specificity, in the context of an analytical method, and discuss the ways in which less than adequate specificity and sensitivity may cause errors in interpretation.
2. Describe the two major methods of analyte volatilization.
3. Immunoassays are commonly utilized as presumptive, or screening, tests. Discuss the characteristics of these tests that make them well suited for this purpose. Why are immunoassays not used as confirmatory tests? What are some shortcomings, or disadvantages of using immunoassays as presumptive tests?
4. LC/MS (MS) is becoming the instrumental method of choice in many forensic toxicologist laboratories. Describe how LC/MS (MS) works. What are some advantages of using LC/MS instead of GC/MS? Are there any disadvantages associated with using this method?

REFERENCES

Abraham, M.H., 2004. 100 years of chromatography-or is it 171? J. Chromatogr. A 1061, 113–114.

Agilent Technologies, 2001. Basics of LC/MS. From: http://ccc.chem.pitt.edu/wipf/Agilent%20LC-MS%20primer.pdf (retrieved 24.07.11).

Anderson, D.J., 1989. Determination of the lower limit of detection. Clin. Chem. 35 (10), 2152–2153.

Berezkin, V.G., 1989. Biography of Mikhail Semenovich Tswett and translation of Tswett's preliminary communication on a new category of adsorption phenomena. Chem. Rev. 89, 279–285.

Bramley, R.K., Bullock, D.G., Garcia, J.R., 2008. Quality control and assessment. In: Jickells, S., Negrusz, A. (Eds.), Clarke's Analytical Forensic Toxicology. Pharmaceutical Press, Chicago.

de Castro, A., Concheiro, M., Shkaleya, D.M., Huestis, M.A., 2009. Simultaneous quantification of methadone, cocaine, opiates, and metabolites in human placenta by liquid chromatography-mass spectrometry. J. Anal. Toxicol. 33, 243–252.

Chamberlain, J., 1978. Approaches to the evaluation of analytical methods. In: Reid, E. (Ed.), Blood, Drugs and Other Analytical Challenges. John Wiley & Sons, New York.

Colbert, D.L., Sidki, A.M., Gallacher, G., Landon, J., 1987. Fluoroimmunoassays for cannabinoids in urine. Analyst 112 (11), 1483–1486.

Cote, C., Bergeron, A., Mess, J.N., Furtado, M., Garofolo, F., 2009. Matrix effect elimination during LC-MS/MS bioanalytical method development [Electronic version]. Bioanalysis 1 (7), 1243–1257.

Cowan, D.A., Houghton, E., Jickells, S., 2008. Drugs abuse in sports. In: Jickells, S., Negrusz, A. (Eds.), Clarke's Analytical Forensic Toxicology. Pharmaceutical Press, Chicago.

Dass, C., 2007. Fundamentals of Contemporary Mass Spectrometry. John Wiley & Sons, Hoboken, NJ.

Dawling, S., Jickells, S., Negrusz, A., 2008. Gas chromatography. In: Jickells, S., Negrusz, A. (Eds.), Clarke's Analytical Forensic Toxicology. Pharmaceutical Press, Chicago.

Department of Health and Human Services, 2008. Mandatory guidelines for federal workplace drug testing programs. Fed. Regist. 73 (No. 228).

Drummer, O.H., Gerastamoulos, J., 2002. Postmortem drug analysis: analytical and toxicological aspects. Ther. Drug Monit. 24 (1), 199–209.

Finkle, B.S., 1983. Quality assurance in analytical toxicology. J. Anal. Toxicol. 7, 158–160.

Flanagan, R.J., Taylor, A., Watson, I.D., Whelton, R., 2007. Fundamentals of Analytical Toxicology. John Wiley & Sons, Hoboken, NJ.

Fritch, D., Blum, K., Nonnemacher, S., Haggerty, B.J., Sullivan, M.P., Cone, E.J., 2009. Identification and quantitation of amphetamines, cocaine, opiates and phencyclidine in oral fluid by liquid chromatography–tandem mass spectrometry. J. Anal. Toxicol. 33, 569–577.

Gallardo, E., Barroso, M., Queiroz, J.A., 2009. LC-MS: a powerful tool in workplace drug testing. Drug Test. Anal. 1, 109–115.

Gottardo, R., Miksik, I., Aturki, Z., Sorio, D., Seri, C., Fanali, S., et al., 2012. Analysis of drugs of forensic interest with capillary zone electrophoresis/time-of-flight mass spectrometry based on the use of non-volatile buffers. Electrophoresis 33 (4), 599–606.

Goulle, J.P., Saussereau, E., Mahieu, L., Guerbet, M., 2014. Current role of ICP-MS in clinical toxicology and forensic toxicology: a metallic profile. Bioanalysis 6 (17), 2245–2259.

Greaves, J., Roboz, J., 2014. Mass Spectrometry for the Novice. CRC Press, Boca Rato, FL.

Hadju, P., Chamberlin, J., 1984. Quality control systems for routine drug analyses. In: Reid, E., Wilson, I. (Eds.), Drug Determination in Therapeutic and Forensic Contexts. Plenum Press, New York.

Hand, C., Baldwin, D., 2008. Immunoassays. In: Jickells, S., Negrusz, A. (Eds.), Clarke's Analytical Forensic Toxicology. Pharmaceutical Press, Chicago.

Hearn, W.L., Walls, H.C., 2007. Common methods in post-mortem toxicology. In: Karch, S.B. (Ed.), Drug Abuse Handbook, second ed. CRC Press, New York.

Jeffery, W., Poole, C.F., 2008. Colour tests and thin-layer chromatography. In: Jickells, S., Negrusz, A. (Eds.), Clarke's Analytical Forensic Toxicology. Pharmaceutical Press, Chicago.

Kohler, I., Schappler, J., Rudaz, S., 2013. Highly sensitive capillary electrophoresis-mass spectrometry for rapid screening and accurate quantitation of drugs of abuse in urine. Anal. Chim. Acta 780, 101–109.

Langman, L.J., Kapur, B.M., 2006. Toxicology: then and now. Clin. Biochem. 39, 498–510.

Lawson, G.M., 1994. Defining limit of detection and limit of quantitation as applied to drug of abuse testing: striving for a consensus. Clin. Chem. 40 (7 Pt 1), 1218–1219.

Loconto, P.R., 2005. Trace Quantitative Environmental Analysis. CRC Press, Boca Raton, FL.

Maikel, R.P., 1984. Separation science applied to analyses on biological samples. In: Reid, E., Wilson, I.A. (Eds.), Drug Determination in Therapeutic and Forensic Contexts. Plenum Press, New York.

Marchi, I., Viette, V., Badoud, F., Fathi, M., Saugy, M., Rudaz, S., et al., 2010. Characterization and classification of matrix effects in biological samples analyses. J. Chromatogr. A 1217 (25), 4071−4078.

Matuszewski, B.K., Constanzer, M.L., Chavez-Eng, C.M., 2003. Strategies for the assessment of matrix effect in quantitative bioanalytical methods based on HPLC-MS/MS. Anal. Chem. 75 (13), 3019−3030.

Maurer, H.H., 2010. Perspectives of liquid chromatography coupled to low- and high-resolution mass spectrometry for screening, identification, and quantification of drugs in clinical and forensic toxicology. Ther. Drug Monit. 32, 324−327.

Mulé, S.J., Casella, G.A., 1988. Confirmation of marihuana, cocaine, morphine, codeine, amphetamine, methamphetamine, phencyclidine by GC/MS in urine following immunoassay screening. J. Anal. Toxicol. 12, 102−107.

O'Neal, C., Crouch, D.J., Fatah, A.A., 2000. Validation of twelve chemical spot tests for the detection of drugs of abuse. For. Sci. Int. 109, 189−201.

Peters, F.T., 2011. Recent advances of liquid chromatography-(tandem) mass spectrometry in clinical and forensic toxicology. Clin. Biochem. 44, 54−65.

Peters, F.T., Remane, D., 2012. Aspects of matrix effects in applications of liquid chromatography-mass spectrometry to forensic and clinical toxicology—a review. Anal. Bioanal. Chem. 403 (8), 2155−2172.

Peters, F.T., Maurer, H.H., Musshoff, F., 2011. Forensic toxicology. Anal. Bioanal. Chem. 400, 7−8.

Remane, D., Meyer, M.R., Wissenbach, D.K., Maurer, H.H., 2010. Ion suppression and enhancement effects of co-eluting analytes in multi-analyte approaches: systematic investigation using ultra-high-performance liquid chromatography/mass spectrometry with atmospheric-pressure chemical ionization or electrospray ionization. Rapid Commun. Mass Spectrom 24 (21), 3103−3108.

Rotzsche, H., 1991. Stationary Phases in Gas Chromatography. Elsevier, New York.

Shah, V.P., 2000. Bioanalytical method validation—a revisit with a decade of progress. J. Pharm. Res. 17, 1551−1557.

Shah, V.P., et al., 1992. Analytical methods validation: bioavailability, bioequivalence, and pharmacokinetic studies. J. Pharm. Res. 81, 309−312.

Siek, T.J., 2011. Classical Color Test for Today's Toxicology Lab. From: http://www.soft-tox. org/index.php?option=com_jdownloads&Itemid=109&view=finish&cid=19&catid=3 (retrieved 26.06.11).

SOFT/AAFS, 2006. Forensic toxicology laboratory guidelines. From: http://www.soft-tox. org/files/Guidelines_2006_Final.pdf (retrieved 03.11.12).

Spector, S., Parker, C.W., 1970. Morphine: radioimmunoassay. Science (New York, N.Y.) 168 (3937), 1347−1348.

Stafford, D.T., 2003. Chromatography. In: Levine, B. (Ed.), Principles of Forensic Toxicology, second ed. American Association for Clinical Chemistry, Washington, DC.

Trufelli, H., Palma, P., Famiglini, G., Cappiello, A., 2011. An overview of matrix effects in liquid chromatography-mass spectrometry. Mass Spectrom. Rev. 30 (3), 491−509.

Uges, D.R.A., 1984. The utility of lyophilized spiked serum as a standard in forensic and clinical toxicological analysis. In: Maes, R.A.A. (Ed.), Topics in Forensic and Analytical Toxicology. Elsevier, New York.

Watson, D., Jickells, S., Negrusz, A., 2008. Mass spectrometry. In: Jickells, S., Negrusz, A. (Eds.), Clarke's Analytical Forensic Toxicology. Pharmaceutical Press, Chicago.

Yalow, R., Berson, A., 1959. Assay of plasma insulin in human subjects by immunological methods. Nature 184, 1648−1649.

de Zeeuw, R.A., 2004. Substance identification: the weak link in analytical toxicology. J. Chromatogr. B 811, 3−12.

Quality Assurance and Quality Control

11

We are what we repeatedly do. Excellence, then, is not act but a habit.
Aristotle

It is quality rather than quantity that matters.
Marcus Annaeus Seneca

Quality means doing it right when no one is looking.
Henry Ford

11.1 INTRODUCTION

The functions of the forensic toxicology laboratory are unique for a number of reasons:

- The samples that are analyzed may be unusual, for example, liver, hair, maggots, and/or putrefied organs may be samples of interest.
- The results obtained from the analysis of samples often become the subject of a legal issue.
- The interpretation of results may lead to the deprivation of life or liberty of the subjects.

Because of the unique functions and responsibilities of forensic toxicology laboratories, the establishment, implementation, and documentation of procedures for the purpose of minimizing, or eliminating, errors is essential. The use of stringent quality assurance (QA) and quality control (QC) procedures facilitates the identification and correction of any defects in the operation and/or procedures of the laboratory, thus allowing both for the production of the most accurate results possible and the defense of the accuracy and reliability of the results in a courtroom under vigorous challenge.

The procedures employed to achieve the goals of accuracy and reliability within the forensic toxicology laboratory are contained within management plans known as QA and QC programs. The definitions of the terms QA and QC vary and are sometime used interchangeably. In this book, the following definitions will be used.

Forensic Toxicology. http://dx.doi.org/10.1016/B978-0-12-799967-8.00011-6

183

- QA refers to the procedures and policies that have been established by the laboratory management to ensure, to the greatest degree possible, that the analytical results are accurate and reliable.
- QC refers to the policies and procedures employed by the laboratory to ensure that the QA procedures are being implemented appropriately and effectively.

The National Research Council (2009) has made the following recommendation concerning quality control:

"Forensic laboratories should establish routine quality assurance and quality control procedures to ensure the accuracy of forensic analyses and the work of forensic practitioners. Quality control procedures should be designed to identify mistakes, fraud, and bias; confirm the continued validity and reliability of standard operating procedures and protocols; ensure that best practices are being followed; and correct procedures and protocols that are found to need improvement."

Although well-conceived and efficiently administered QA/QC programs are essential in a modern toxicology laboratory, they "… alone are not a means to achieving high quality laboratory analyses, but are important in maintaining the level of quality that can be achieved by a given laboratory" (Blanke, 1978). Without such a program, the accuracy and reliability of a laboratory's analyses may be suspect and potentially unpredictable.

The chief toxicologist, who is responsible for the development and implementation of a QA/QC program in a forensic toxicology laboratory, generally delegates the day-to-day responsibility of ensuring the proper functioning of the program to a member of the laboratory staff. Ideally, this laboratory staff member should not have any analytical functions in the laboratory and should report directly to the chief toxicologist. However, the assignment of a staff member solely to these nonanalytical, QA/QC duties may be feasible in laboratories with small staffs. Indeed, the implementation of such programs can be challenging as the oversight of a QA/QC program requires a significant commitment of time, effort, and resources, which may include as much as 5—15% of the laboratory's total personnel hours (Mason, 1981). Two of the conditions of Rule 702 of the Federal Rules of Evidence pertaining to the testimony of expert witnesses require that "… the testimony is the product of reliable principles and methods; and the expert has reliably applied the principles and methods to the facts of the case." A well-designed and implemented QA/QC program is of immense value in demonstrating that these requirements have been met.

It must be noted that QA/QC programs, even when well designed and well implemented, do not guard against or prevent the intentional tampering with or alteration of samples or the falsification of laboratory records by a person(s) authorized to handle and/or analyze samples who is determined to circumvent the established procedures. Unfortunately, such intentional and illegal activities do occur. Recently, the catastrophic effects of such activities were made evident when it was reported in 2012 that a forensic chemist employed in Massachusetts allegedly mishandled samples in thousands of cases. As a result, it is anticipated that several thousand persons who had been convicted (and protected against subsequent trial due to the protection of double jeopardy) or awaiting trial might be released or have the charges against them dropped. This apparent malfeasance led to the termination or resignation of several laboratory and agency administrators and the closing (at least temporarily) of the laboratory (Smith and Wedge, 2012). Ironically, the chemist allegedly involved in the mishandling of samples was in charge of the QC and QA programs of the laboratory (Associated Press, 2012)!

Although a comprehensive presentation of a QA/QC program is beyond the scope of this text, several salient components of such a program are presented below. More comprehensive resources describing the establishment and implementation of QA/QC programs are identified at the end of this chapter.

11.2 RECORDS

The hallmark of a QA/QC program is record keeping—the most relevant adage pertaining to QA/QC is "If it hasn't been recorded, it hasn't been done." This foundational principle of QA/QC requires that activities occurring within the laboratory, including staff training and evaluation, instrument calibration, certification and maintenance, method validation, control methods, and proficiency testing, fall under the purview of the QA/QC program and data pertaining to laboratory performance in each of these areas must be recorded. These records enable the performance of the staff members to be standardized and evaluated and can be used to establish the accuracy of the analytical results that are reported. In addition, these records provide a means for identifying potential sources of error. An important aspect of the records of a QA/QC program is the maintenance of a standard operating procedure (SOP) manual, which is an up-to-date record of the validated analytical methods employed for the detection, identification, and quantitation of analytes. The SOP manual is one of the most important components of a QA program and it is essential that all forensic toxicology laboratories maintain a document of this type. Specific information that should be contained in the SOP manual should include, but not be limited to, the following (Andollo, 2007; SOFT/AAFS, 2006):

- a detailed step-by-step description of each of the current methods employed by the laboratory, which includes the principles of the methods and appropriate literature references
- detailed descriptions of the instrumental components of the methods
- criteria for qualitative and quantitative detection utilizing each laboratory method, e.g., critical retention times and ion ratios
- descriptions of the limits of the methods, e.g., limits of detection (LOD), limits of quantitation (LOQ), limits of linearity and the standard curves with confidence intervals, and the statistical methods by which they were derived

- purity specifications of reagents and drug standards[1]
- methods for the preparation and labeling of all reagents utilized in each method, including standard solutions, blanks, and controls
- identification of the conditions and limits of storage of all reagents and samples
- descriptions of the types of samples for which each method is appropriate, as well as the preferred site and method of sample collection
- information pertaining to the date on which the use of each method was implemented or discontinued by the laboratory
- validation data for each method
- substances that may cause false-positive and false-negative results in each method
- descriptions of the methods by which results are reviewed prior to acceptance or rejection, including the identity of the specific persons authorized to conduct such a review
- descriptions of the methods for the storage, archiving, and accessing of data

Any other information that is deemed to be important should also be included in the SOP.

The SOP manual should be updated as frequently as required to remain up-to-date with current laboratory practice. All changes in the SOP must be archived in a manner that allows for the preservation of a record of the method employed for the analysis of a specific sample, even if that method is no longer used in the laboratory.

In addition to the SOP manual, all other activities related to the analysis of analytes must be recorded and retained for an extended period of time, for example, an up-to-date log book of instrument use, and maintenance and repair records should be retained for the life of the instrument, and then archived after the use of the instrument has been discontinued.

Although the maintenance of an SOP manual and records such as instrument log books, methods manuals, drug inventory records, proficiency test results, control charts, and personnel evaluations requires a major commitment of time and personnel, it may be the only method by which to demonstrate the validity of the laboratory product—the analytical result.

In addition to any other record-keeping measures of the laboratory, forensic toxicologists may maintain their own laboratory notebooks in which they preserve a chronological record of their daily activities, both analytical and administrative. The format of the notebook may take many forms, but the purpose is to create a permanent record of what was done, how it was done, and what was determined. A bound notebook with pages numbered by the manufacturer is the most appropriate

---

[1]Analytes used to prepare calibration curves should be certified drug standards or certified reference materials obtained from sources that meet stringent standards established by regulatory organizations, such as ISO. The Standard Reference Materials available from the National Institute of Standards and Technology (NIST) are examples of such materials.

type for this purpose. The description of analytical protocols should be described enough to be replicated by those who read the notebook. The identity of the analytical procedure used may be identified in the toxicologist's notebook by either the name of the method or the ID number identifier of the method as recorded in the SOP. If the method used is a modification of an SOP method, the modification must be described in detail. In order to protect the documentary nature of the data in the laboratory notebook, each entry should be handwritten using "permanent" paper and inks, described in the active voice in a clear and readable manner and read, signed, and dated by a witness (Kanare, 1985).

11.3 METHODS VALIDATION

Validation, the process by which an analytical method is determined to be reliable for its intended purposes, is a standard component of a laboratory's QA/QC program. Validation methods must be designed to assess the following general criteria of each analytical method utilized in the laboratory (Karnes et al., 1991):

- specificity: the detection of only one analyte;[2]
- selectivity: the ability to distinguish multiple analytes from one another;
- calibration: the determination between the analyte concentration and the analytical response;
- accuracy: the closeness of match between the analytically determined analyte concentration and the "true" analyte concentration;
- precision: the variation in the analytical analyte concentration determinations in several samples that are known to contain the same "true" analyte concentration;
- ruggedness: the agreement of analytical results produced by the same method on identical samples under varying conditions of time, environment, and analyst.

The Scientific Working Group for Forensic Toxicology (2013) (SWGTOX) has formulated specific standards for the validation of methods used in forensic toxicology laboratories. The following is a summary of several of the more significant of these standards. The reader is urged to consult the complete SWGTOX report for detailed explanations of all of the validation practices. Definitions are quoted from the SWGTOX standards (Scientific Working Group for Forensic Toxicology, 2013).

- Precision and bias must be determined. The acceptable values for each of these are between 10% and 20% and depend on the specific method being evaluated.
- Bias (also known as accuracy or trueness) is defined as "the closeness of agreement between the mean of the results of the measurements of a measurand

---

[2]Several of the components of validation such as sensitivity and specificity are discussed in Chapter 10.

and the true (or accepted true) value of a measurand. It is reported as a percent difference." Bias is defined mathematically as:

$$B = (GM - NC/NC) (100) \qquad (11.1)$$

where

      B = bias, expressed as a percentage at a specific concentration x
      GM = the grand mean of three separate samples at concentration x over five different runs
      NC = the nominal (expected) concentration of the samples used to determine GM

- Precision is defined as "the measure of the closeness of agreement between a series of measurements obtained from multiple samplings of the same homogeneous sample: it is expressed numerically as imprecision." Precision is defined mathematically as the coefficient of variation (CV), where CV = (standard deviation/mean) (100). It is recommended in the SWGTOX standard that CV determinations should be determined within and between analytical runs using the same data used for the determination of bias.
- A calibration model (standard curve or standard graph) must be established for quantitative methods. Calibration samples (control samples) should be prepared (see below) encompassing the range of values expected to be detected in case samples. The calibration model is prepared using the results of five or more replicate analyses conducted on separate occasions of six or more calibration samples and a blank sample. The calibration model shall be evaluated by means of a standardized residual analysis or another suitable method.
- The limit of detection (LOD), "an estimate of the lowest concentration of an analyte in a sample that can be reliably differentiated from blank matrix and identified by the analytical method," should be determined for all methods. The LOD may be determined by various methods. Commonly, the LOD is defined as the lowest analyte concentration that produces a signal exceeding the mean +3 standard deviations of blank samples.
- The limit of quantitation (LOQ), "an estimate of the lowest concentration of an analyte in a sample that can be reliably measured with acceptable bias and precision," should be determined for all methods. It may be determined by several methods, each of which requires that the LOQ meets acceptable criteria of detection, identification, bias, and precision criteria.
- Determination of the stability of analytes prior to and during analysis, following freeze—thaw cycles, and as a result of sample dilution.
- Evaluation of sources of interference including matrix effects, stale-isotope internal standards, and other analytes.

The SWGTOX recommendations are that validation methods should be applied to newly developed analytical methods, modified methods, existing methods that do not meet the criteria of these validation methods, and to determine the equivalence between new and existing methods.

11.4 CONTROL METHODS

Control methods are designed to determine whether the methods of analysis used in the laboratory are "in control." That is, whether they are producing the results that they are designed to produce.

Commonly, the ability of a laboratory to detect, identify, and quantitate a specific analyte in a specific matrix is achieved by the use of control samples that are prepared to contain a known analyte concentration. Control samples are prepared in a matrix that is as similar as possible to that of the unknown samples.[3] The preparation of control samples requires the use of standard solutions prepared by dissolving a weighed primary standard of the drug, one with analytically determined concentrations of analyte and impurities, into a suitable solvent such as water or methanol (Hadju and Chamberlin, 1984). Small volumes of this standard are diluted with the appropriate matrix, which has been analyzed to ensure the absence of analytes and to produce fortified ("spiked") samples with known analyte concentrations.

Control samples are stored frozen and then thawed to be analyzed together with a group of unknown samples as described below. In addition to fortified control samples, blank samples (negative controls) should also be prepared in a manner identical to that used for the preparation of the control samples with the exception that the analyte is not included. For samples in which it is difficult to prepare control samples and blanks because the sample matrix cannot be replicated, or a substitute matrix is not reliable, the method of standard additions is an acceptable method (Of Interest 11.1).

Even the most careful and accurate preparation of controls and calibrators does not ensure that these in vitro control samples are characterized by the same distribution and protein-binding patterns as seen in in vivo case samples. Any such differences may cause a dissimilarity of analytical "behavior," such as disparate extraction efficiencies and lead to analytical errors.

The Society of Forensic Toxicologists/American Academy of Forensic Sciences (SOFT/AAFS) Laboratory Guidelines (SOFT/AAFS, 2006) do not specify the number of controls and calibrators that should be used for each batch of case samples, but rather make the following vague statement: "Each batch should contain a sufficient number of calibrators and controls, the total number of which will depend on the size of the batch and the nature of the tests." However, the Guidelines of the Department of Health and Human Services (2008) have specific requirements for the number of controls that should be included in batch analyses or urine: a minimum of 10% of the urine samples in a batch of samples must be calibrators or controls, including negative controls (blanks) and controls with analyte concentrations at the cutoff concentration and 25% above and at least 40% below the cutoff value.

---

[3]The matrices of test and control samples do not have to be the same, but it must be demonstrated that the bias and precision are the same in all matrices to be analyzed by the method.

OF INTEREST 11.1 METHOD OF STANDARD ADDITION

The methods of standard addition are designed for use in forensic toxicology when it is not possible to prepare blank and control samples with a matrix identical or similar to that of the test sample. The basis of this method is that the test sample will serve as the matrix for the preparation of control and blank samples in the preparation of a standard curve.

The method consists of processing the test sample, e.g., homogenizing a putrefied liver, and then spiking aliquots of the homogenate with a known quantity of the analyte standard to produce a range of final test sample concentrations that are expected to bracket the anticipated concentration of the test sample. No standard drug is added to one aliquot of the test sample that acts as a blank.

The table below is an example of a standard addition in which five aliquots of the test sample were spiked with a standard analyte solution to produce four spiked samples with known analyte concentrations and one blank.

Unknown Sample Aliquot	Sample Volume (mL)		Volume of Analyte Standard Solution Added[a] (µL)	Final Added Analyte Concentration of the Spiked Standards (µg/L)	Instrument Response
	Initial	Final			
1	1	1	0	0	0.75
2	0.98	1	20	3	1.2
3	0.96	1	40	6	1.65
4	0.94	1	60	9	2.10
5	0.92	1	80	12	2.55

[a] The concentration of analyte standard solution is 150 µg/L.

When the instrument response is plotted against the blank and the final concentrations of the spiked standards, as shown below, the analyte concentration in the test sample is equal to the absolute value of the x-intercept, i.e., |−4.43 µg/L| or 4.43 µg/L.

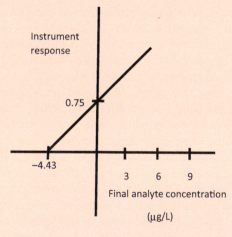

One of the several methods employed to determine whether a method is in control is the use of a Levey–Jennings chart, a graphical representation of the control data that can be used in conjunction with the so-called Westgard rules (Westgard, 2003, 2009) which provide criteria for the identification of out-of-control methods. This approach, widely used in clinical laboratories, also is appropriate for use in forensic toxicology laboratories. The initial analytical results of control samples, which are analyzed as soon as possible after their preparation, are plotted in chronological order; these results are meant to represent the optimal performance of the method. Subsequently, the results of the stored control samples analyzed along with unknown samples are also plotted on the same graph. After a sufficient number of control samples, e.g., 20, have been analyzed, the mean and standard deviation of the results are determined and plotted graphically in the form of a Levey–Jennings chart. This chart is constructed by placing control limit lines at the mean value and at ± 1, ± 2, and ± 3 standard deviations (s.d.) from the mean, and the Westgard rules are employed to determine whether the method is in control. A summary of several of the common Westgard rules is presented in Table 11.1 and an example of their use is illustrated in Figure 11.1.

11.5 PROFICIENCY TESTING

A proficiency testing program is essential to assess the performance of the laboratory. The proficiency program, which is a valuable component of the QA/QC program, is an effective means by which the performance of laboratory personnel and instrument function can be evaluated. Frequently, participation in a proficiency test program may be required by laboratory accrediting organizations. Any deficiencies in personnel performance or instrument function that are detected as a result of proficiency test results should be immediately subjected to appropriate remedial action.

The proficiency program should include the analysis of samples prepared by both the laboratory (internal proficiency tests) and nonlaboratory organizations (external proficiency tests). Both internal and external proficiency tests should include

Table 11.1 Selected Westgard Rules Indicating that the Method Is Out of Control[a]

Rule#	Rule
1_{3s}	The value of a single control analysis exceeds the mean ± 3 s.d.
2_{2s}	The values of two consecutive control analyses are greater than the mean ± 2 s.d.
10_x	The values of 10 consecutive control analyses are greater or smaller than the mean.
R_{4s}	The difference between two control analyses is greater than the difference between the mean $+2$ s.d and the mean -2 s.d.

[a] Adapted from Westgard (2009).

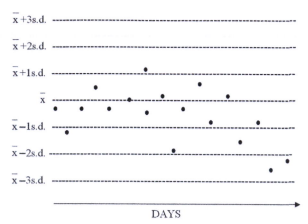

FIGURE 11.1 Results of Chronologically Analyzed Control Samples

This plot represents a method that is considered to be out of control according to the Westgard rules. The results from the last two chronologically analyzed control samples are a violation of Westgard rule 2_{2s}, which states that the values of the two consecutive control analyses must not be greater than the mean plus or minus 2 standard deviations ($\bar{x} \pm 2$ s.d). The last two results exceed the mean -2 s.d. The source of the error must be identified and corrective measures instituted.

samples that are identified as proficiency test samples (open samples) and unidentified as proficiency test samples (blind samples). These samples should be prepared, stored, and transported in such a manner that drug concentrations are not altered before the samples arrive at the testing laboratory as a result of transport conditions such as excessive temperatures (Kelly and Sunshine, 1976; McCloskey and Finkle, 1977). Since external proficiency samples are received infrequently during the course of a year, e.g., quarterly, both blind and open internal proficiency samples should be used on a more frequent basis. Although the use of lyophilized (freeze-dried) blood (Osselton et al., 1990) and urine (Jimenez et al., 2004) samples has been recommended for proficiency testing, the concentration of volatile analytes may be decreased as a result of the lyophilization process, and the pH of reconstituted lyophilized samples may increase by as much as 1 pH unit, which may cause stability problems for certain analytes.

An apparently outstanding performance in proficiency testing may be misleading since often there is no general accord as to what constitutes acceptable results in a proficiency study. External proficiency test results may be considered to be acceptable if they compare favorably with the results of other laboratories, that is, within a specific statistical or percentile deviation from the mean of all reported results. For example, a quantitative result that is within ± 2 standard deviations of the mean result of all responding laboratories often is considered to be an acceptable performance, since it is thought to represent the general reliability of laboratory results. However, this may not be a sufficiently rigorous standard because standard deviations as great as or greater than 25% of the mean reported value have been reported by a meaningful number of laboratories participating in proficiency tests (Chaturvedi et al., 2009; Wallace, 2010). Similarly, quantitative results that are within an arbitrary range, for example, 5% or 20%, of the mean may be considered to represent an acceptable performance. However, although quantitative errors of as great as 20% may not influence interpretations, acceptance of such errors may engender shoddy laboratory performance, which can jeopardize the overall reliability of the laboratory. More rigorous standards may require that acceptable results must be within 2 standard deviations or a stated percentage of either the weighed-in concentration of the drug analyte or the results reported by selected laboratories of demonstrated high proficiency.

An additional potential problem with proficiency testing is that the drug concentrations in the test samples often are greater than the laboratory's stated detection limits. This may result in a decreased rate of false-positive results and lower quantitative errors than would incur at concentrations near or at the detection limit reported by the laboratory. In addition, the proficiency samples often are prepared in a matrix more pristine than those encountered in postmortem case samples, thus circumventing several of the analytical problems that are often encountered in forensic toxicology laboratories. Many laboratories expend an extraordinary amount of time and effort on the analysis of proficiency open test samples, often analyzing the sample multiple times and using more sophisticated and reliable methods than those routinely employed for case samples. As a result, proficiency test results may often closely resemble the very best of what the laboratory is capable but not its routine day-to-day performance. Thus, under these circumstances, proficiency testing may not be an accurate representation of the laboratory's proficiency. Nonetheless, proficiency testing must be considered to be a vital component of any QA/QC program.

11.6 ANALYST COMPETENCE

In addition to the development of a validated analytical method, an additional and important factor which merits attention is the competence of the analyst. No method can be performed reliably unless the analyst possesses the requisite knowledge, skills, and experience to do so. As described in Chapter 10, it is often difficult to reliably assess the competence of a specific analyst. However, the American Board of Forensic Toxicology (ABFT) offers four different categories of certification in forensic toxicity: fellow of forensic toxicology and three diplomate level certifications (ABFT; ABFT 1; ABFT 2). The qualifications that a forensic toxicologist must possess to sit for the required examinations differ for the two levels of certification. For the fellow of forensic toxicology certification, the PhD degree and formal courses and/or documented training in pharmacology and toxicology are required, whereas for the three diplomate certifications a bachelor's degree and optional training in pharmacology and toxicology are required.

All levels require 3 years of professional experience, acceptable performance on a written examination,[4] and evidence of continuing education in forensic toxicology following certification.

11.7 SECURITY

Because of the confidential nature of the analyses being conducted and due to the professional and legal requirements to protect samples against the possibility of tampering, procedures must be in place to ensure the security of the forensic toxicology laboratory. At a minimum, access to laboratories should be restricted to authorized personnel, and all refrigerators and freezers should be locked with access limited to specifically designated persons. An alarm system capable of detecting unauthorized entry to the laboratory should be in place.

All drug standards must be stored in a locked safe together with a log in which the following must be recorded for each drug: the amount of drug received, the name and address of the supplier, the date the drug was received, the names of persons using the standard, the purpose(s) for which the standard was used, the dates on which the standard was used, the quantities of standard used on each date, the date and method of disposal of outdated standard and standard container, and the signatures of the persons who witnessed the disposal. Controlled substances should be ordered by one person who has the only authorized signature and stored in a safe to which another person has the combination; this procedure ensures that a single person cannot both order and access to the controlled substances.

11.8 ACCREDITATION

In the twenty-first century, one of the most important administrative activities in a forensic toxicology laboratory is obtaining and maintaining accreditation and/or certification. Accreditation requires that the laboratory must meet requirements encompassing the full scope of laboratory activities, including management, analytical proficiency, QC, etc., and certification usually refers to the process by which a laboratory has demonstrated that it possesses the ability to perform specific analyses in forensic toxicology, for example, drug detection in urine, or blood ethanol analysis. There are several organizations, including those in Table 11.2, by which forensic toxicology laboratories may be accredited or certified as having met specific standards. In addition to the organizations that offer formal accreditation, there are organizations such as the SWGTOX, SOFT, and AAFS (SOFT/AAFS, 2006) that identify standards necessary for the operation of forensic toxicology laboratories,

---

[4]A study guide for examination preparation is available at http://abft.org/index.php?option=com_content&view=article&id=50&Itemid=59.

Table 11.2 Accrediting Organizations

The American Board of Forensic Toxicology (ABFT)
(ABFT 5)
Eligible laboratories must be performing postmortem forensic toxicology and/or human performance toxicology.
Accreditation requires demonstrated proficiency in the following three programs of the College of American Pathologists (CAP, 2012): CAP Whole Blood Alcohol, CAP Whole Blood Forensic Toxicology (FTC), and the CAP T-series.
As of September 18, 2012, 30 laboratories were accredited.
The program is outlined and a detailed manual is available.

College of American Pathologists (CAP)
CAP provides a wide range of extensive proficiency programs for both clinical and forensic toxicology laboratories.
Proficiency samples prepared in both urine and blood are available.

The International Standardization for Organizations (ISO, 2012)
Provides standards of performance for a number of laboratory types and functions.
ISO standards employed by forensic toxicology laboratories include ISO17025.

Mandatory Guidelines for Federal Workplace Drug Testing Programs
(Department of Health and Human Services, 2008)
These guidelines apply to selected US federal agencies
The guidelines may also apply to those who supply services to these agencies including collectors of samples, medical review officers, and laboratories.

---

including accreditation. A 2010 survey of forensic toxicology laboratories by the Forensic Toxicology Council (FTC) determined that forensic toxicology laboratories had been accredited by several accreditation agencies including the ABFT, The International Organization for Standardization (ISO), the College of American Pathologist (CAP), and the National Laboratory Certification Program (NLCP). Some laboratories were accredited by more than one agency, whereas 12% of the laboratories were not accredited by any organization. In 2013, the Department of Justice and the National Institute of Standards and Technology announced plans to establish a commission to establish guidelines in order "… to strengthen and enhance the practice of forensic science" and "… to standardize national guidance for forensic science practitioners" (Department of Justice, 2012).

11.9 ADDITIONAL RESOURCES

There are a number of excellent sources that should be referred to for more detailed information on the establishment and implementation of QA/QC programs: Andollo (2007), Dux (1986), CFR (2012), Thoma (1977), Blanke (1978), Field (1981), Finkle (1983), Hadju and Chamberlain (1984), Ferrara et al. (1998), Flanagan et al. (2007), Aderjan (2008), GTGCH (2009).

REVIEW QUESTIONS

1. Define quality assurance and quality control.
2. Who is generally responsible for the development and implementation of a QA/QC program in a forensic toxicology laboratory? Who is often responsible for the day-to-day functioning of the program?
3. What are the Westgard rules and to what specific purpose are they applied in a QA/QC program?
4. What is the difference between an internal proficiency test and an external proficiency test?
5. Why is it important that a forensic toxicology laboratory be accredited?

APPLICATION QUESTIONS

1. Accurate record keeping is a vital component of an effective QA/QC program. Describe two types of records that must be mainlined within a forensic toxicology laboratory. Who (i.e., what laboratory personal) is responsible for maintaining these records? What information must be included in the records? What are some potential ramifications of improper and/or inaccurate record keeping in a forensic toxicology laboratory?
2. Methods validation is of the utmost importance in forensic toxicology laboratories. Discuss two standards that have been established for the validation of methods.
3. Describe the major similarities and differences in purpose and procedure between the use of fortified (spiked) samples and the use of the method of standard additions as a control method. Under what conditions would you use each of the control methods? Is one method more accurate and/or more reliable than the other, why or why not?
4. You are in charge of the proficiency testing of a forensic toxicology laboratory. Describe the actions that you would take if your data suggest that the function of an instrument has been compromised. What action would you take if your proficiency data suggest that a specific analyst is not competent to perform his/her job?

REFERENCES

ABFT. Certification Categories. Retrieved May 23, 2015 from http://abft.org/index.php?option=com_content&view=article&id=46&Itemid=55.

ABFT 1. Certification As a Diplomate of the Board. Retrieved October 5, 2012 from http://abft.org/index.php?option=com_content&view=article&id=46&Itemid=2.

ABFT 2. Certification As a Forensic Toxicology Specialist. Retrieved October 5, 2012 from http://abft.org/index.php?option=com_content&view=article&id=47&Itemid=2.

ABFT 5, November 4, 2012. ABFT Accredited Forensic Toxicology Laboratories. Retrieved December 4, 2012, 2012 from http://abft.org/index.php?option=com_content&view=article&id=55&Itemid=64.

Aderjan, R.E., 2008. Aspects of quality assurance in forensic toxicology. In: Bogusz, M.J. (Ed.), Forensic Science Handbook of Analytical Separations, vol. 6. Elsevier B.V., New York.

Andollo, W., 2007. Quality Assurance in Post-mortem Toxicology. In: Karch, S.B. (Ed.), Drug Abuse Handbook. CRC Press, New York.

Associated Press, 2012. Chemist Claimed Lab Oversight. Boston Herald.Com.

Blanke, R.V., 1978. Quality control in the toxicology laboratory. Clin. Toxicol. 13, 141−151.

CAP. Toxicology. Retrieved November 3, 2012 from http://www.cap.org/apps/cap.portal?_nfpb=true&cntvwrPtlt_actionOverride=%2Fportlets%2FcontentViewer%2Fshow&_windowLabel=cntvwrPtlt&cntvwrPtlt%7BactionForm.contentReference%7D=committees%2Ftoxicology%2Ftoxicology_index.html&_state=maximized&_pageLabel=cntvwr.

CFR- Code of Federal Regulations−Title 21-Part 58, 2012.

Chaturvedi, A.K., Craft, K.J., Cardona, P.S., Rogers, P.B., Canfield, D.V., 2009. The FAA's postmortem forensic toxicology self-evaluated proficiency test program: the second seven years. J. Anal. Toxicol. 33, 229−236.

Department of Health and Human Services, November 25, 2008. Mandatory guidelines for federal workplace drug testing programs. Fed. Regist. Part V 73 (No. 228), 71858.

Department of Justice, 2012. Department of Justice and National Institute of Standards and Technology Announce Launch of National Commission on Forensic Science. Retrieved Februray 15, 2013 from http://www.justice.gov/opa/pr/2013/February/13-dag-203.html.

Dux, J.P., 1986. Handbook of Quality Assurance for the Analytical Chemistry Laboratory. Van Nostrand Reinhold Company, New York.

Ferrara, D.S., Tedeschi, L., Frison, G., Brusisni, G., 1998. Quality control in toxicological analysis. J. Chromatogr. B 713, 227−243.

Field, P.H., 1981. Quality assurance and proficiency testing. In: Cravey, R.H., Baselt, R.C. (Eds.), Introduction to Forensic Toxicology. Biomedical Publications, Davis, California.

Finkle, B.S., 1983. Quality assurance in analytical toxicology. J. Anal. Toxicol. 7, 158−160.

Flanagan, R.J., Taylor, A., Watson, I.D., Whelton, R., 2007. Fundamentals of Analytical Toxiolcogy. John Wiley & Sons, Hoboken, NJ.

FTC. What Is Forensic Toxicology? Retrieved November 3, 2012 from http://www.abft.org/files/WHAT%20IS%20FORENSIC%20TOXICOLOGY.pdf.

GTGCH, 2009. Guideline for Quality Control in Forensic-toxicological Analyses. Retrieved November 12, 2012 from http://www.gtfch.org/cms/images/stories/files/Guidelines%20for%20quality%20control%20in%20forensic-toxicological%20analyses%20(GTFCh%2020090601).pdf.

Hadju, P., Chamberlain, J., 1984. Quality control systems for routine drug analyses. In: Reid, E., Wilson, I. (Eds.), Drug Determination in Therapeutic and Forensic Contexts. Plenum Press, New York.

ISO. International Organization for Standardization. Retrieved November, 2012 from www.iso.org.

Jimenez, C., Ventura, R., Segura, J., de la Torre, R., 2004. Reference materials for analytical toxicology including doping control: freeze-dried urine samples. Analyst 129, 449−455.

Kanare, H.M., 1985. Writing the Laboratory Notebook. American Chemical Socity, Washington, DC.

Karnes, H.T., Shiu, G., Shah, V.P., 1991. Validation of bioanalytical methods. Pharmaceut. Res. 8, 421–426.

Kelly, R.C., Sunshine, I., 1976. Proficiency testing in forensic toxicology: criteria for experimental design (letter). Clin. Chem. 22, 1413–1414.

Mason, M.F., 1981. Some realities and results of proficiency testing of laboratories performing toxicological analyses. J. Anal. Toxicol. 5, 201–208.

McCloskey, K.L., Finkle, B.S., 1977. Proficiency testing in forensic toxicology. J. Forensic Sci. 22, 675–678.

National Research Council, 2009. Strengthening Forensic Science in the United States: A Path Forward. National Academies Press, Washington, DC.

NIST. Definitions. Retrieved November 10, 2012 from http://www.nist.gov/srm/definitions. cfm.

Osselton, M.D., et al., 1990. Whole blood quality assurance control samples for forensic toxicology. J. Anal. Toxicol. 14, 318–319.

Scientific Working Group for Forensic Toxicology, 2013. Scientific working group for forensic toxicology (SWGTOX) standard practices for method validation in forensic toxicology. (Electronic version). J. Anal. Toxicol. 37 (7), 452–474.

Smith, E., Wedge, D., 2012. Bosses Who Lost Jobs at Drug Lab Missed "red Flags". Boston Herald.Com.

SOFT/AAFS, 2006. Forensic Toxicology Laboratory Guidelines. Retrieved November 3, 2012 from http://www.soft-tox.org/files/Guidelines_2006_Final.pdf.

Thoma, J.J., 1977. Quality assurance in toxicology. In: Thoma, J.J., Bondo, P.B., Sunshine, I. (Eds.), Guidelines for Analytical Toxicology Programs, vol. 1. CRC Press, Cleveland.

Wallace, J., 2010. Proficiency testing as a measure for estimating uncertainty of measurement: application to forensic alcohol and toxicology quantitations. J. Forensic Sci. 55, 767–773.

Westgard, J.O., 2003. Internal quality control: planning and implementation strategies. Ann. Clin. Biochem. 40, 593–611.

Westgard, J.O., 2009. Westgard Rules and Multirules. Retrieved November 19, 2012 from http://www.westgard.com/mltirule.htm#westgard.

Types of Interpretations

Life would be much simpler for the toxicologist if his task ended when he was able to report that in the material submitted to him he had found such-and-such a poison and that the concentration was so-and-so

C. Stewart and A. Stolman

12.1 INTRODUCTION

The statement of Stewart and Stolman (1960) is one with which forensic toxicologists generally agree, that is, of the three major functions of forensic toxicologists—analysis, interpretation, and reporting—the interpretation of analyte concentrations in either antemortem or postmortem samples is the most challenging.

Although ultimate issues, such as the cause of death of an individuals or the state of sobriety of a driver, are determined by others such as forensic pathologists or juries, forensic toxicologists have the important role of providing an interpretation of analytical drug results in cases in which a wide variety of questions may be asked. Examples of these questions include:

- Is the blood concentration of oxycodone in a 22-year-old unconscious male who was brought to the hospital Emergency Department by his friends consistent with his condition?
- Was the driver of a car drunk at the time that the car he was driving crossed the highway center line and caused an accident?
- Is the concentration of anesthetic in the blood of a patient who died during surgery consistent with an overdose of the drug?
- Is the presence of the detected drug consistent with naïve or chronic use of that drug?

When possible, answers to these questions should be based upon several factors, including:

- data obtained from investigative and medical reports
- a knowledge of the pharmacokinetics, pharmacodynamics, and pharmacogenomics of the detected analyte
- results obtained from the analysis of samples collected from subjects.

Forensic Toxicology. http://dx.doi.org/10.1016/B978-0-12-799967-8.00012-8

12.2 **REASONING IN FORENSIC TOXICOLOGY INTERPRETATION**

The variables and uncertainties in many forensic toxicology cases are numerous and because information essential to the formulation of an accurate interpretation may be uncertain, unknown, or unknowable, differing opinions often are offered by competent forensic toxicologists. In these cases of "conflicting systems" (Paul and Elder, 2008), which involve competing perspectives and opinions, a clear-cut interpretation may not be possible due to incomplete evidence or opposing interpretations of the evidence. However, an interpretation meeting the standard of a reasonable scientific probability or certainty often is possible. The development of well-reasoned interpretations and, ultimately, expert opinions must be based upon the application of the *relevant principles and concepts* of forensic toxicology to the totality of the *available evidence*, both toxicological and nontoxicological, and *only this evidence*. This requires that there can be no "cherry-picking" of selected evidence and no exclusion of probative evidence and/or reliable literature that either is not consistent with, or conflicts with, predetermined conclusions. Additionally, and of absolute importance, the interpretations of a forensic toxicologist must be impartial and devoid of contextual or confirmation bias.

As is the case with all scientific reasoning, theories and concepts relied upon by forensic toxicologists have been developed by means of inductive reasoning—the use of data from specific instances to formulate general principles or theories. Deductive reasoning, or the application of these theories to specific instances, is valid only if the theory thus formulated is valid. Unfortunately, the principles and theories of interpretation formulated by inductive reasoning in forensic toxicology generally are the result of studies of small groups of subjects whose physical and biological characteristics are highly diverse, often not thoroughly described and frequently not representative of the population as a whole. Databases containing information such as the correlation of blood levels with effects, the rate of metabolism of drugs, and/or the effect of gender on interpretation have often been developed from such limited studies or even from a compilation of several such studies. Such databases are therefore often not applicable in specific cases in which subjects do not have the same biological traits and/or characteristics as the population upon which the databases are grounded, or in cases in which there are conditions not encompassed by the foundational studies. In other words, the populations studied in the foundational studies may not be sufficiently large or varied to represent either the population at large or the specific circumstances that may be encountered in a given case. Because of this, the range of blood concentrations of a drug in a database considered to be consistent with a specific effect such as lethality serves only as a guide—it may not apply to a subject who has developed tolerance to the drug, is a geriatric subject, and has kidney and liver pathologies, all of which may contribute to a difference between the blood concentration consistent with death in this subject and the concentrations consistent with death presented in a database.

12.3 NONANALYTICAL CASE-RELATED EVIDENCE

In addition to the analytical results, evidence such as the medical history of the subject and investigative reports of the case must be reviewed and considered by forensic toxicologists in order to make informed interpretations.

12.3.1 MEDICAL HISTORY

The medical history of the subject, including pharmacy records, notes of treating physicians, and records of hospitalizations, should be reviewed to obtain a history of prior conditions requiring medical attention, treatment received, drugs and doses of drugs prescribed, frequency of drug use, duration of drug use, and any adverse reactions caused by drugs. Relevant additional medical information including blood pressure, heart rate, respiratory status, the Glasgow coma score,[1] and the initial diagnoses are available in the reports of emergency medical personnel and emergency room physicians and nurses, who treated the subject following an incident.

In fatal cases, forensic toxicologists must review the autopsy reports as they may include findings that are consistent with the use of specific drugs or drug classes, e.g., pulmonary edema, and nasal and oral foaming, that are consistent with CNS depression.

12.3.2 INVESTIGATIVE REPORTS

Investigations by police and medicolegal investigators often provide important information as to the date, time, location, and circumstances of the incident, as well as witness statements describing the actions and/or behavior of the subject. For example, investigative reports may answer pertinent questions such as the following:

- Did the subject faint, convulse, act groggy, have slurred speech, or complain of any abnormal symptoms?
- Was the subject driving erratically? Did the subject act aggressively toward another person?
- Was the subject a known drug abuser?

Pictures and sketches of the scene generally are available, as are the results of the analyses of drugs, syringes, and/or other drug-related paraphernalia obtained from the subject, the victims, or the scene; all such information should be reviewed.

Well-trained medicolegal investigators often are able to identify drug-related fatalities, and the types of drugs involved in the fatality, with a high degree of accuracy prior to an autopsy having been performed (Ernst et al., 1982). The availability of this information to forensic pathologists and toxicologists is valuable in directing the analytical strategy for the case.

---

[1]The Glasgow coma score is a numerical rating, from a low of 3 to a high of 15, of the neurological status of a patient determined by the evaluation of visual, verbal, and motor responses.

12.4 INTERPRETATIONS

Although the ultimate opinion as to whether a specific drug was the cause of death is the responsibility of the medical examiner, the judgment of the forensic toxicologist, which develops as a result of experience, is an important opinion. This judgment is brought to bear in the evaluation of the evidence in the case and the evaluation of the reliability of the databases—both of which are crucial in determining whether blood concentrations are consistent with specific effects. Such scientific judgment (Paul and Elder, 2008) is often the ultimate action of forensic toxicologists in situations of a complex nature.

Often, analytical results alone are sufficient to conclude with "a reasonable scientific probability" whether a drug caused, or contributed to, the signs and symptoms of a subject. However, in specific instances, the analytical results may not be sufficient, due to several factors summarized below:

- *Accuracy of the results*: All interpretations are based on the analytical results, the accuracy of which is often difficult or impossible to determine after the fact except by reanalysis, which may not be possible due to the improper storage or disposal of samples.
- *Lack of appropriate and reliable evidence*: Evidence, including the size and frequency of drug doses, the time of the last dose, as well as evidence of the presence and extent of tolerance of the detected drugs often is not available.
- *Biological factors*: Specific personal characteristics of the subject including gender, age, ethnicity, genome, and physical condition may have bearing on the effect(s) caused by the concentration of the detected drug.

Forensic toxicologists may be asked a variety of questions by interested parties such as the police, attorneys, and family members. These frequently asked toxicology questions (FATQs) are related to the presence of drugs or chemicals in the body of specific persons. Several FATQs typical of the types of interpretations requested of forensic toxicologists are considered below.

12.5 WAS A PERSON EXPOSED TO A SPECIFIC DRUG?

It is generally true that the accurate detection of either exogenous substances or their unique metabolites is a proof of exposure to these substances. Although there are notable exceptions to this principle, the identification of such substances by a qualitative analysis designed to determine whether a specific drug and/or one or more of its unique metabolites is present in one or more samples obtained from the body of a subject may be the simplest type of analysis performed by forensic toxicologists, and often serves to establish exposure. Positive results obtained from this type of analysis frequently are sufficient evidence to establish the use of a drug in an inappropriate, unauthorized, or illegal manner and may have meaningful repercussions. For example:

- The presence of a prohibited drug in athletes following a competition may be grounds for their disqualification.
- The presence of an illegal or unprescribed drug in a minor may lead to a charge of reckless endangerment and/or child abuse being leveled against the parent or other caregiver.
- The detection of banned drugs in pilots may lead to suspension or revocation of their licenses.

In addition, the detection of drugs and chemicals in clinical cases is significant as it may influence or alter the treatment of a patient.

Under conditions in which the quantitation of analytes is not required to establish exposure, but rather a qualitative analysis will suffice, the samples selected for analysis should be those in which there is a great likelihood that the drug or its metabolite(s) will be found if the drug has been used, those that can be analyzed in as simple a manner as is consistent with reliable results and those that are readily available and easily collected. As described in Chapter 8, the samples that meet these criteria, and are therefore most commonly used, are urine, saliva, and hair.

It is important to note that caution must be exercised in interpreting the presence of a drug as an indication that a specific detected drug was used by the subject because certain drugs are not only used and abused, but also are metabolites of other drugs. For example, the detection of morphine, amphetamine, and/or methamphetamine may not be only due solely to the use of these drugs, but also to metabolism since they are metabolites of heroin and selegiline, respectively. Also, the unintended presence of drugs produced in the manufacturing process of other drugs may be detected in samples obtained from subjects who used these medications, e.g., hydrocodone and codeine in oxycodone (West et al., 2011) and morphine (West et al., 2009) medications, respectively.

The detection of metabolites in the absence of parent compounds is often used as a means by which to establish the use of the parent compounds. An important example of this is the detection of ethanol metabolites. In the absence of ethanol in samples, the detection of the minor metabolites of ethanol, (EtG), or ethyl sulfate (EtS), which together constitute less than 1% of the total amount of ethanol consumed (Albermann et al., 2012), may be used as biomarkers verifying prior ethanol use. These metabolites may be detected in blood for hours after ethanol use, in urine for hours to days after ethanol use (Walsham and Sherwood, 2012), and in hair for months to centuries after ethanol use (Musshoff et al., 2013). However, there are potential problems with the reliance upon the detection of these metabolites as an indicator of ethanol use. EtG concentrations in urine greater than the cutoff values deemed to be consistent with ethanol use also may be detected following the use of mouthwash (Costantino et al., 2006) and hand sanitizers (Reisfield et al., 2011), albeit excessive use of these agents would be required (Rohrig et al., 2006). It is possible that with the repeated use of mouthwash over a short period of time EtS, but not EtG may be detected in urine, but unlikely that either would be detected in blood or oral fluid (Hoiseth et al., 2010). In urine samples contaminated with *Escherichia coli*, low concentrations of EtG may be hydrolyzed to ethanol (at concentrations that are undetectable by commonly employed methods of detection) by β-glucuronidase, which is present in a majority of *E. coli* strains and to a lesser extent in other bacteria (Helander et al., 2007). Although a false-negative result for EtG and ethanol would be obtained in this circumstance, since neither EtG nor ethanol would be detected, the determination of prior ethanol use may be made by the detection of EtS, which is not converted into ethanol by β-glucuronidase (Helander and Dahl, 2005; Baranowski et al., 2008).

In postmortem toxicology, determining whether the detection of ethanol in a sample is due to antemortem ingestion or postmortem synthesis due to microbial synthesis (Chapter 7) can be problematic. Several considerations may aid in the analysis of this problem:

- The presence of ethanol in the blood but not other fluids and/or tissues of the body would be suggestive of postmortem synthesis.
- The presence of other alcohols may be used as markers of decomposition. Several volatile compounds, including alcohols, are synthesized during postmortem putrefaction. Among these, several of which are present in low concentrations in alcoholic beverages, elevated concentrations of *n*-propanol have been detected most consistently in cases in which the postmortem synthesis of ethanol is thought to be likely (Ziavrou et al., 2005; Boumba et al., 2008).
- The effect of ethanol consumption on the metabolism of serotonin has been proposed as a means of differentiating between antemortem consumption and postmortem production of ethanol (Helander et al., 1995; Beck and Helander, 2003). In the absence of ethanol, serotonin is metabolized to 5-hydroxy indole acetaldehyde and then to either 5HTOL (pathway #1) by aldehyde dehydrogenase (ADH) or to the major end metabolite, 5HIAA (pathway #3), by aldehyde dehydrogenase (AlDH) (Figure 12.1). When ethanol has been ingested, it competes with aldehyde dehydrogenase for the utilization of NAD, a necessary cofactor for the enzymatic activity of AlDH, thereby decreasing the metabolism of serotonin to 5HIAA via pathway #3. Via its competition for NAD, ethanol also effectively increases the levels of available NADH, a necessary cofactor for the enzymatic activity of ADH, thereby enhancing the metabolism of serotonin to 5HTOL via pathway #1. As a result, the conversion of 5-hydroxy indole acetaldehyde to 5HIAA is decreased and its conversion into 5HTOL is increased, i.e., the ratio of the concentrations of 5HTOL to 5HIAA increases compared to normal values. Because the metabolism of serotonin in urine is not altered, even in the presence of ethanol or glucose in the urine, an increase in the 5HTOL to 5HIAA ratio is consistent with the antemortem consumption of ethanol, but not with the postmortem synthesis of ethanol.

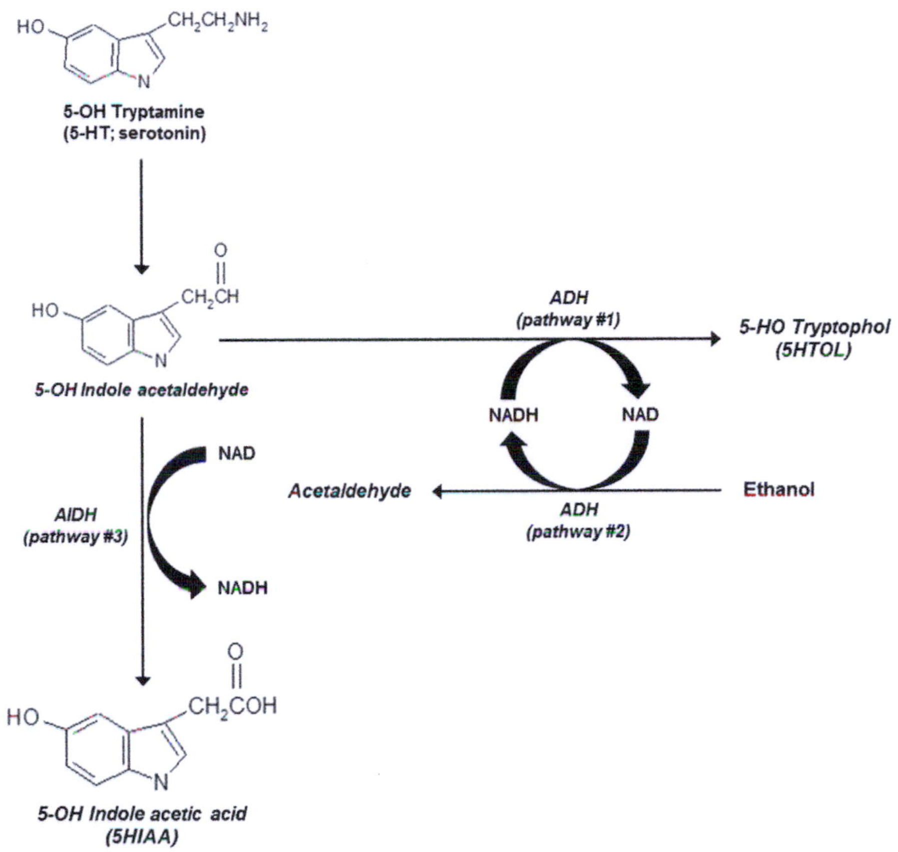

FIGURE 12.1

The effect of ethanol consumption on serotonin metabolism. In the absence of ethanol, serotonin is metabolized to 5-hydroxy indole acetaldehyde and then to either 5HTOL (pathway #1) by aldehyde dehydrogenase (ADH), or to the major end metabolite, 5HIAA (pathway #3), by aldehyde dehydrogenase (AIDH). When ethanol has been ingested, it competes with aldehyde dehydrogenase for the utilization of NAD, thereby decreasing the metabolism of serotonin to 5HIAA via pathway #3. Ethanol also effectively increases the levels of available NADH, thereby enhancing the metabolism of serotonin to 5HTOL via pathway #1. As a result, the ratio of the concentrations of 5HTOL to 5HIAA increases compared to normal values, and an increase in the 5HTOL to 5HIAA ratio is therefore consistent with the antemortem consumption of ethanol.

12.6 WAS THE PRESENCE OF THE DETECTED DRUG DUE TO INTENTIONAL OR UNINTENTIONAL USE?

Although the accurate detection of a drug in samples collected from a subject is generally consistent with the exposure of the subject to the drug, it does not confirm, per se, the conclusion that the drug was used intentionally by the subject. There are numerous circumstances in which the detection of a drug in a subject's body is the result of unintentional or accidental exposure, usually via oral or inhalation routes, or as a result of ante- or postmortem synthesis. Any of these circumstances may result in "innocent" positive results, i.e., results that are analytically accurate, but not the result of intentional use.

Since positive drug results can have serious social and legal consequences and may alter postmortem determination of cause of death, differentiating between intentional and unintentional drug use is an important function of forensic toxicologists. As discussed below, although several approaches to the differentiation of intentional from unintentional exposure to drugs have been proposed, there are problems associated with their use.

12.6.1 UNINTENTIONAL PASSIVE INHALATION

Drugs that can be volatilized, such as marihuana, cocaine, methamphetamine, and phencyclidine, are commonly abused via the inhalation route. However, these drugs may also be inhaled unintentionally or passively from the ambient air by nonsmoking subjects, often referred to as passive inhalers, who are in the vicinity of smokers. As a result of passive inhalation, these drugs are absorbed, distributed, metabolized, and excreted, along with their metabolites, in the same qualitative, but probably not quantitative, manner as the disposition of the drugs in intentional smokers. Consequently, these drugs and/or their metabolites can be detected in samples such as urine and hair collected from the passive inhalers producing the so-called "innocent" positive results. Because the detection of drugs or their metabolites is not proof of intentional exposure, passive inhalation has been used to explain the detection of drugs or their metabolites in samples collected from persons who deny the intentional use. The potential validity of a passive inhalation defense makes the ability to differentiate between passive inhalation and active smoking of a drug a crucial determination.

Often the differentiation between the passive and intentional inhalation of drugs is based upon the findings that the concentrations of drugs and/or their metabolites will be lower in urine, hair, or oral fluid after passive inhalation than after active smoking. Accordingly, cutoff values[2] have been established that are unlikely to be attained as a result of unintentional passive inhalation of these substances consistent with realistic exposure.

As might be expected, the concentration of drugs or metabolites in samples obtained from passive inhalers depends on a number of factors including the amount of drug being smoked, the size and ventilation of the area in which smoking is being conducted, the metabolic and excretion rate in passive inhalers, the period of time

---

[2]In this context, cutoff values are the minimum analyte concentrations consistent with the report of positive results; they may be greater than the limit of detection for the method of analysis.

during which passive inhalation has taken place, and the proximity of passive inhalers to active smokers. Generally, in samples obtained from passive inhalers, it is only under extreme conditions of exposure that urine concentrations of volatile drugs or their metabolites are likely to be detected in concentrations greater than the cutoff values for those analytes. For example, following exposure of a volunteer to the vapor from 200 mg of cocaine freebase in a small room, urine concentrations of cocaine and metabolites less than 50 ng/mL were detected by radioimmunoassay, and benzoylecgonine concentrations less than 15 ng/mL were detected by gas chromatography—mass spectrometry, but no cocaine was detected (Baselt et al., 1991). Therefore, although it is possible that passive inhalation of cocaine could lead to analyte concentrations greater than the cutoff values, the probability of this occurring may require excessive exposure (Cone et al., 1995).

The detection of drugs in hair presents a special problem because a determination of whether the inhalation was intentional or passive is dependent upon whether analytes are located on the exterior or interior of the hair shaft. Following the intentional use of drugs, the drugs and/or their metabolites should be detectable in the interior of hair shafts, whereas following passive exposure the drugs are expected to be adsorbed onto the exterior of the hair shafts. Therefore, removal of drugs adsorbed to the exterior surface of the hair shaft by means of thorough washing of the hair sample (Chapter 9) is essential to ensure that detected drugs are not on the exterior, which is consistent with passive inhalation.

12.6.2 UNINTENTIONAL ORAL EXPOSURE

There are several instances in which the unintentional oral ingestion of a drug leads to the detection of that drug or its metabolite(s) in biological samples. Perhaps the best known example of such an exposure is that of poppy seed ingestion. The consumption of poppy seeds, which contain morphine and codeine, contained in baked goods and other foods, may result in the detection of these opioids in blood, urine, oral fluid, sweat, and hair (Lachenmeier et al., 2010). The claimed ingestion of poppy seeds has gained fame (or notoriety) as the "poppy seed" defense, which is offered most often as an explanation for the presence of morphine in urine (Meadway et al., 1998) or hair (Hill et al., 2005), but possibly also for the presence of codeine (Chang et al., 2012). Whether morphine and codeine will be detected in the urine of a subject following the ingestion of poppy seed-containing foods depends on the consumption of a sufficient number of poppy seeds with a sufficiently high concentration of these drugs.

The validity of the poppy seed defense is enhanced by the detection of thebaine, a naturally occurring compound found in poppy seeds, which is not a metabolite of heroin, morphine, or codeine. The success of the poppy seed defense fails if 6-monoacetylmorphine (6MAM) is detected in the analytical sample since this is a unique metabolite of heroin and is not produced by the metabolism of either morphine or other compounds found in poppy seeds (Musshoff et al., 2013). However, the use of 6MAM as a marker for the use of heroin or the use of thebaine as a marker for or the ingestion of poppy seeds is not without problems because 6MAM has a relatively short half-life in blood (Dubois et al., 2013), and the failure to detect thebaine in urine may be due to variations in the thebaine concentration in poppy seeds as well as the interpersonal rate of thebaine elimination (Meadway et al., 1998).

In many areas of the United States, especially South Florida, much of the currency is contaminated with cocaine (Oyler et al., 1996; Jenkins, 2001; Jourdan et al., 2013). Forensic scientists and law enforcement personnel who handle cocaine samples and bank employees who handle large quantities of currency without gloves and/or respiratory masks may have detectable concentrations of the cocaine metabolite benzoylecgonine in their urine as a result of inhalation or ingestion of cocaine.

The intentional, but generally nonabusive, ingestion of cocaine, by users of cocaine-containing beverages, such as South American "herbal" that contain coca leaf as a mild stimulant (El Sohly et al., 1986; Jackson et al., 1991), may result in the presence of detectable amounts of benzoylecgonine for approximately 1 day in the urine of these users.

Drugs that are prohibited by the International Olympic Committee, or their metabolites, have been detected in the urine of athletes after they ate meat obtained from steroid-treated animals, used nutritional supplements containing ephedrine and other amphetamine-like drugs or used codeine, a permitted drug, that is metabolized to morphine, a prohibited drug (Yonamine et al., 2004).

12.7 WHAT WAS THE SIZE OF THE DOSE?

The determination of the size of the dose used by a subject cannot be determined reliably for most drugs because important parameters such as the duration of drug use, the frequency of drug administrations, the route of administration, and the disposition kinetics are not known. A common exception to this is an estimate of the amount of ethanol consumed, which can be determined by means of the Widmark equation. The Widmark equation is named for the Swedish scientist who developed it and is derived from the equation for the apparent volume of distribution (Appendix A). The equation is

$$A = \frac{(W)\ (R)\ (C + \beta t)}{0.8} \tag{12.1}$$

where

A = volume of ethanol absorbed, expressed in ml of 100% ethanol;
1 oz ≈ 30 mL
W = body weight, expressed in grams; one pound ≈ 454 g
C = blood alcohol (ethanol) concentration, expressed as a decimal; e.g., 100 mg/dL = 0.001%

R = Widmark factor, unitless

β = rate of decline of the blood alcohol concentration (BAC), expressed as a decimal/h

An example of the use of the Widmark equation to estimate the amount of ethanol consumed is presented in Of Interest 12.1.

OF INTEREST 12.1 THE WIDMARK EQUATION

Mr Johnson, who is 6-ft tall and weighed 175 pounds, was involved in an automobile accident at 2:30 a.m. on 9/9/99. At 3:15 a.m. his blood alcohol concentration (BAC) was determined to be 0.11%. Mr Johnson claimed that he had 2 oz of vodka between 12:30 and 1:30 a.m. on 9/9/99. He also stated that he had consumed additional vodka between the time of the accident and the time that the police arrived at the scene. Assuming Mr Johnson's recollection to be correct, how many ounces of 80 proof (40%) vodka did he consume after the accident?

Since this problem requires a determination of the amount of ethanol consumed, Eqn (12.1), the Widmark equation, will be used for its solution.

$$A = \frac{(W)(R)(C + \beta t)}{0.8}$$

W = (body weight in pounds) (454 g/pound) = (175 pounds) (454) = 79,450 g

β = 0.0001–0.00015–0.00020/h, a range of reasonable β values

R = 0.66–0.74–0.80, calculated by means of the R Calculation equations presented below

t = 12:30–3:15 p.m. = 2.75 h

C = 0.0011

Low, average, and high values of A (which represents the amount of ethanol absorbed) are determined by using low values, average values, and high values of both R and β, respectively.

$$A_{low} = \frac{(79450)(0.66)[(0.0011) + (0.0001)(2.75)]}{0.8} \approx 90 \text{ mL } of \text{ 100\% ethanol}$$

$$\approx 7.5 \text{ oz of 40\% vodka}$$

$$A_{ave} = \frac{(79450)(0.74)[(0.0011) + (0.00015)(2.75)]}{0.8} \approx 111 \text{ mL of 100\% ethanol}$$

$$\approx 9.25 \text{ oz of 40\% vodka}$$

$$A_{high} = \frac{(79450)(0.80)[(0.0011) + (0.0002)(2.75)]}{0.8} \approx 131 \text{ mL of 100\% ethanol}$$

$$\approx 11 \text{ oz of 40\% vodka}$$

Mr Johnson consumed a total of approximately 7.5–11 oz (average 9.5 oz) of 49% vodka. Therefore, if Mr Johnson consumed 2 oz of 80 proof vodka prior to the accident, his BAC of 0.11% at 3:15 a.m. is consistent with his having consumed approximately 5.5–7.25–9 oz after the accident.

R Calculation

(Forrest, A.R.W., 1985. The estimation of Widmark's factor. J. Forensic Sci. Soc. 26, 249–252.)

- Body mass index (BMI) = (body weight (BW) in kilograms) ÷ (height in meters)^2

  Mr Johnson's BMI = (pounds/2.2) ÷ (inches/39.37)^2 = (175/3.35) ÷ (62/39.37)^2 = 79.5 ÷ 3.35 = 23.7

Continued

OF INTEREST 12.1 THE WIDMARK EQUATION—cont'd

- Fat as a % of body weight (FBW)
  FBW for men $= (1.340)\ (BMI) - 12.469$
  FBW for women $= (1.371)\ (BMI) - 3.467$
  Mr Johnson's FBW $= (1.34)\ (23.7) - 12.469 = 19.3$
- Total body water (TBW)
  TBW $= [(0.724) \pm (0.034)]\ [(body\ weight) - (body\ weight)\ (FBW)]$
  Mr Johnson's $TBW_{low} = (0.724 - 0.068)\ [79.5 - (79.5)\ (0.193)] = (0.656)\ (79.5 - 15.3) = 42.1$
  Mr Johnson's $TBW_{ave} = (0.724)\ [79.5 - (79.5)\ (0.193)] = (0.724)\ (79.5 - 15.3) = 46.5$
  Mr Johnson's $TBW_{high} = (0.724 + 0.068)\ [79.5 - (79.5)\ (0.193)] = (0.792)\ (79.5 - 15.3) = 50.8$
- R = apparent V_D of ethanol = body ethanol concentration/BAC = TBW/(BW) (0.8)
  Mr Johnson's $R_{low} = 42.1/(79.5)\ (0.8) = 0.66$
  Mr Johnson's $R_{ave} = 46.5/(79.5)\ (0.8) = 0.73$
  Mr Johnson's $R_{high} = 50.8/(79.5)\ (0.8) = 0.80$

12.8 WHAT WAS THE ROUTE OF ADMINISTRATION?

It may be possible to identify the route of administration of a drug by detecting high concentrations of drugs or their metabolites at the site of administration. However, an elevated drug concentration at a specific site is not always indicative of the route of administration. The detection of drugs at injection sites or of undissolved tablets in stomach contents is apparently consistent with intravenous or oral administration, respectively, of these drugs. However, the presence of dissolved drugs in gastric contents may be a consequence of ion trapping following nonoral administration.

12.9 WHAT WAS THE ELAPSED TIME BETWEEN THE LAST DOSE AND SAMPLE COLLECTION?

The time at which a drug was administered cannot be established from the detection or quantitation of a drug in a single sample. The interval between the time that the last dose of a drug was administered and the time that an analytical sample was collected can be determined only as an approximation because the half-life of drugs and their metabolites in various samples varies. In addition, a number of factors that may not be known, including the size and number of doses, the frequency of use, and the detection limit of the analytical method, make an accurate determination of the elapsed time between the last drug dose and the collection of the analytical sample virtually impossible.

Although an accurate estimate of the time that a drug was used may not be possible, it is often possible to establish an estimated chronology of drug use. In many cases, an estimation that the range of the elapsed time between the last use of a drug and death, or the collection of samples, was minutes and not days, or days and not minutes, is an extremely valuable approximation.

Generally, detection periods for drugs in blood range from several minutes to a few hours (for example, for delta-9-tetrahydrocannabinol (Δ9THC)) to days or weeks (for example, for 11-nor-9-carboxy delta-9-tetrahydrocannabinol (THC COOH)). In urine, the approximate detection periods for several drugs of abuse and/or their metabolites can range from hours (for ethanol) to a few days (for morphine, cocaine, amphetamine, phencyclidine (PCP), and/or their metabolites), to weeks (for THC COOH). Drugs may be detected in hair for periods ranging from months to years or decades.

An estimate of the survival period of a subject after the administration of ethanol may be made based on knowledge of its distribution kinetics and a determination of the concentrations in blood and vitreous humor. The time required for ethanol to attain distributional equilibrium is in the order of 0.5—2 h, at which time the ratio of the BAC to the vitreous humor alcohol concentration is approximately 0.8, a ratio essentially the same as a reasonable estimate of the relative water concentrations in the two samples (Kugelberg and Jones, 2007). However, the value of, and the time at which, the equilibrium ratio is attained in a subject are only estimates because they may be influenced by several factors. The time at which the equilibrium ratio is attained is influenced by the rate of absorption of ethanol from the gastrointestinal tract, which in turn may be influenced by factors that either increase the rate of absorption (high ethanol beverage concentrations, carbonation, drugs that increase the rate of gastric emptying, and decreased blood glucose levels) or decrease the rate of absorption (the presence of food in the stomach, carbohydrates such as fructose, drugs that decrease the rate of gastric emptying, and beer with a high carbohydrate concentration) (Jones, 2008). The value of the equilibrium ratio may be influenced by factors, such as the presence of ophthalmic disease, dehydration, or postmortem synthesis of ethanol, that influence the water or ethanol concentration of either sample. Therefore, to account for the possibility that these factors may influence the ratio, it is reasonable to conclude that a postmortem ratio of approximately 1.0 is consistent with the establishment of equilibrium and survival of the decedent for approximately 1—2 h after consumption of the last drink (Felby and Olsen, 1969). For example, a ratio of blood to vitreous humor ethanol concentrations of 0.93 is more consistent with an estimate that the last drink consumed by a subject was likely to have been consumed approximately 2 h, rather than 15 min, prior to death.

12.10 WAS THE SUBJECT A NAÏVE OR A CHRONIC USER?

The differentiation between naïve and chronic use of certain drugs frequently is based upon the ratio of parent drug to metabolite concentration (P:M). Generally, chronic use is associated with a low P:M ratio and acute use is associated with a high P:M ratio. These estimates are based on the assumption that metabolites will accumulate following chronic use if they have a longer half-life than the parent compound. However, alternate causes of high and low P:M values are possible (Druid and Holmgren, 1997):

- a high P:M may be the result of slow metabolism caused by polymorphism of the CYP 2D6 gene

- a low P:M ratio may be the result of acute use following chronic use or post-mortem production of metabolites, as is the case with certain benzodiazepines.[3]

An additional method for the differentiation between acute versus chronic drug use is the demonstration of drug concentration gradients in hair shafts, fingernails, or toenails. Since the approximate rate of growth of head hair is approximately 1 cm/month, and of fingernails is approximately 0.2–0.5 cm/month, the period of use prior to the collection of the samples may be estimated by the presence of drug in specific segments of these samples.

The chronic use of many drugs results in the development of tolerance and/or addiction in the user. In these chronic users, it is likely that the observed symptoms are less pronounced than would be expected based on the determined drug concentration (Section 12.14.1).

12.11 WAS THE PRESENCE OF AN ANALYTE CONSISTENT WITH "OLD" USE OR "NEW" USE?

Occasions arise in which persons are required to submit samples for toxicological analysis to determine whether they have abstained from the use or abuse of drugs. These persons include parolees, drug abusers in drug treatment programs, and divorced parents—all of whom must remain drug-free in order to continue their parole or to preserve custody rights, respectively. For certain drugs, the mere presence of the drug or its unique metabolite(s) in the blood is an indicator of recent use, whereas the presence of the drug or its metabolites in urine may be due to "old use," that is, use that occurred prior to the legal restraint against use was instituted. One drug for which the latter determination is problematic is Δ9THC, a highly lipid soluble molecule that is sequestered in adipose tissue in amounts that are a function of the duration and magnitude of marihuana use. Upon cessation of use, Δ9THC released from its adipose storage sites is metabolized and the metabolites, primarily THC COOH, are excreted into the urine in varying amounts and rates for varying periods of time depending on the amount of drug that had been sequestered. Because of this, the urine concentration of THC COOH fluctuates in consecutive urine samples. As a result of this fluctuation, an increase in the concentration of THC COOH in a urine sample is not sufficient evidence, per se, of recent marihuana use. Methods for differentiating between new and old marihuana use based on an increased ratio of either THC COOH (Huestis and Cone, 1998) or cannabinoids (Manno et al., 1984) to creatinine concentrations in consecutively collected urine samples have been suggested. However, the false-positive and false-negative rates of these methods differ and can be large; they may be influenced by the sensitivity and specificity of the method of analysis used and the presence of conditions in subjects that may alter creatinine levels.

---

[3]Benzodiazepines are a class of anxiolytic (antianxiety) drugs.

12.12 IS THE PRESENCE OR CONCENTRATION OF AN ANALYTE A VIOLATION OF A STATUTE OR REGULATION?

Virtually all countries of the world attempt to minimize the dangers of drug abuse by establishing statutes that provide penalties to operators of automotive vehicles and planes in the presence and/or at specific concentrations of drugs. Countries, or governmental entities within countries, have established legally mandated blood ethanol concentrations presumed to be consistent with the inability to operate motor vehicles in a safe manner, which carry with them specific penalties for violation. In the Unites States, this so-called "legal level" is 0.8% in all states, with the exceptions of commercial drivers for whom the legal level is 0.04% and persons under the age of 21 who are not permitted to have any ethanol in their blood (Centers for Disease Control and Prevention, 2015; Federal Motor Carrier Safety Administration).

12.13 DID THE DRUG OR CHEMICAL CAUSE OR CONTRIBUTE TO AN ADVERSE EVENT?

Determining whether the presence and/or concentrations of specific analytes in ante-mortem or postmortem samples contributed to or caused an adverse effect such as an automobile accident or death is not a simple task. In fact, concluding that there is a correlation between analyte presence and/or concentrations and events is frequently difficult and often impossible. In this section, we will consider attempts to make these correlations and present factors that influence the ability to do so.

12.13.1 CORRELATING EFFECTS WITH ANALYTE CONCENTRATIONS IN BLOOD

The analytical results that are most widely correlated with effects are blood concentrations. The basis for the use of blood concentrations for this purpose is based on two considerations: there is a correlation between the concentrations of analytes in blood and the concentrations of analytes at their target sites, and the database correlating blood concentrations and effects is larger than for any other sample. In other words, blood analyte concentrations are proportional to the analyte concentrations at the target, which in turn are proportional to the quantitative effect produced.

Blood concentrations consistent with therapeutic uses, toxic effects, and lethal effects have been defined as follows (Winek et al., 2001):

- *Therapeutic blood level*: The concentration of drug and/or its active metabolite(s) present in the blood (serum or plasma) following therapeutically effective dosage in humans.

- *Toxic blood level*: The concentration of drug and/or its active metabolite(s) or chemical present in the blood (serum or plasma) that is associated with serious toxic symptoms in humans.
- *Lethal blood level*: The concentration of drug and/or its active metabolite(s) or chemical present in the blood (serum or plasma) that has been reported to cause death, or is so far above-reported therapeutic or toxic concentrations, that one can judge that it might cause death in humans.

There are several blood concentration databases in which drug blood concentrations are correlated with therapeutic use, toxic exposure, or lethality (Table 12.1). Even a cursory review of the correlations reported in these databases reveals the wide range of blood concentrations recorded within and among the three effect levels. Often, these blood concentration ranges are as large as one to two orders of magnitude, and on occasion even greater, because of the manner of data collection: subjects from whom data are collected are of different ages, of different ethnic and national origins, and of both genders; not all samples are collected after the establishment of equilibrium; nonvalidated analytical methods are often used; samples are handled improperly; and samples are stored under varying conditions for varying periods. Because of the great intra- and interdatabase variance, these correlations should be considered to be a first approximation of the blood concentrations that are consistent with effects produced by the drugs—they should not be considered to represent an absolute interpretation, especially when additional available evidence has not been considered.

Of note is the phenomenon of hysteresis, a phenomenon in which the blood concentrations of a drug and the intensity of its effects are out of phase with each other. A diagrammatic representation of counterclockwise hysteresis is presented in Figure 12.2. Counterclockwise hysteresis is observed for the euphoria and increased heart rate caused by Δ9THC for which delay in the establishment of equilibrium between the blood and the target receptor, and a slow production of active metabolites has been proposed as mechanisms for this phenomenon (Cocchetto et al., 1981; Huestis, 2002).

12.13.2 CORRELATING EFFECTS WITH ANALYTE CONCENTRATIONS IN SAMPLES OTHER THAN BLOOD

When blood is not available, analyte concentrations in other samples can be determined with the intent of correlating these concentrations with effects. The basis of making such a correlation is that the effect produced by the analyte is proportional to its concentration at the target site, which is proportional to its concentration in blood, which is proportional to the concentration in the nonblood sample. For example, if, hypothetically, it has been reported that the skeletal muscle to blood ratio of drug X at equilibrium is 1.5:1, then the determination of a 0.21 mg/L drug X concentration in skeletal muscle would be assumed to be 0.14 mg/L in blood, the effect of which can be determined from blood database correlations.

Table 12.1 Sources of Information Regarding Therapeutic, Toxic, and Lethal Blood Concentrations of Various Drugs

Augsburger, M., Donze, N., Menetrey, A., Brossard, C., Sporkert, F., Giroud, C., Mangin, P., 2005. Concentration of drugs in blood of suspected impaired drivers. Forensic Sci. Int. 153(1), 11–15.

Baselt, R.C., Cravey, R.H., 1977. A compendium of therapeutic and toxic concentrations of toxicologically significant drugs in human biofluids. J. Anal. Toxicol. 1(2), 81–103.

Caplan, Y.H., Ottinger, W.E., Crooks, C.R., 1983. Therapeutic and toxic drug concentrations in post mortem blood: a six year study in the state of Maryland. J. Anal. Toxicol. 7(5), 225–230.

Dawson, A.H., Whyte, I.M., 1999. Therapeutic drug monitoring in drug overdose. Br. J. Clin. Pharmacol. 48(3), 278–283.

Druid, H., Holmgren, P., 1997. A compilation of fatal and control concentrations of drugs in postmortem femoral blood. J. Forensic Sci. 42(1), 79–87.

Flanagan, R.J., 1998. Guidelines for the interpretation of analytical toxicology results and unit of measurement conversion factors. Ann. Clin. Biochem. 35 (Pt 2), 261–267.

Jones, A.W., Holmgren, A., 2009. Concentration distributions of the drugs most frequently identified in post-mortem femoral blood representing all causes of death. Med. Sci. Law. 49(4), 257–273.

Jones, A.W., Holmgren, A., Kugelberg, F.C., 2007. Concentrations of scheduled prescription drugs in blood of impaired drivers: considerations for interpreting the results. Ther. Drug Monitor. 29(2), 248–260.

Jonsson, A.K., Soderberg, C., Espnes, K.A., Ahlner, J., Eriksson, A., Reis, M., Druid, H., 2014. Sedative and hypnotic drugs—fatal and non-fatal reference blood concentrations. Forensic Sci. Int. 236, 138–145.

Musshoff, F., Padosch, S., Steinborn, S., Madea, B., 2004. Fatal blood and tissue concentrations of more than 200 drugs. Forensic Sci. Int. 142(2–3), 161–210.

Reis, M., Aamo, T., Ahlner, J., Druid, H., 2007. Reference concentrations of antidepressants. A compilation of postmortem and therapeutic levels. J. Anal. Toxicol. 31(5), 254–264.

Repetto, M.R., Repetto, M., 1997a. Habitual, toxic, and lethal concentrations of 103 drugs of abuse in humans. J. Toxicol. Clin. Toxicol. 35(1), 1–9.

Repetto, M.R., Repetto,M., 1997b. Therapeutic, toxic, and lethal concentrations in human fluids of 90 drugs affecting the cardiovascular and hematopoietic systems. J. Toxicol. Clin. Toxicol. 35(4), 345–351.

Repetto, M.R., Repetto, M., 1999. Concentrations in human fluids: 101 drugs affecting the digestive system and metabolism. J. Toxicol. Clin. Toxicol. 37(1), 1–9.

Schulz, M., Iwersen-Bergmann, S., Andresen, H., Schmoldt, A., 2012. Therapeutic and toxic blood concentrations of nearly 1000 drugs and other xenobiotics. Crit. Care. 16(4), R136.

Stead, A.H., Hook, W., Moffat, A.C., Berry, D., 1983. Therapeutic, toxic and fatal blood concentration ranges of antiepileptic drugs as an aid to the interpretation of analytical data. Hum. Toxicol. 2(1), 135–147.

Winek, C.L., Wahba, W.W., Winek Jr., C.L., Balzer, T.W., 2001. Drug and chemical blood-level data 2001. Forensic Sci. Int. 122(2–3), 107–123.

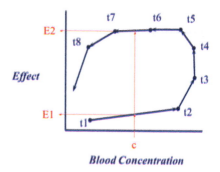

FIGURE 12.2

A hypothetical hysteresis plot.

Perhaps, the drug whose blood concentration is estimated from its concentration in another sample is ethanol. Average ratios between ethanol concentrations in blood and other samples at equilibrium are presented in Table 12.2. Although an average value of 2100:1 is used in the United States as the ratio of ethanol concentration in blood and exhaled alveolar air, there is an extensive intrapersonal variation of this ratio. Also, specific conditions such as an elevated body temperature can alter the results.

Unfortunately, the correlation of effects with analyte concentrations in samples other than blood is usually difficult or impossible to achieve. This attempt at interpretation fails primarily because any proportionality that exists between the concentrations of a drug in blood and other samples exists at equilibrium. However, it is usually the circumstance in both antemortem and postmortem cases that determining whether a drug has attained equilibrium is difficult. However, a method has been used in antemortem cases to estimate the blood ethanol concentration from urine based on establishing that equilibrium is likely to have occurred between these two samples (Of Interest 12.2).

Table 12.2 Approximate Ratios of Ethanol Concentrations in Various Samples to Whole Blood Concentrations at Equilibrium

Plasma or serum	1.15:1
Saliva	1.15:1
Urine	1.3:1
Alveolar air	1:2100
Vitreous humor	1.25:1

OF INTEREST 12.2 ESTIMATING THE BLOOD ETHANOL CONCENTRATION FROM THE ANALYSIS OF A URINE SAMPLE

A method for estimating the blood ethanol concentration (BAC) based upon the ethanol concentration in a urine sample (UAC) at the time of the urine collection is summarized as follows (Haggard et al., 1940):

1. The subject is observed for a minimum of approximately 1½ h to ensure that no ethanol is consumed and also to allow sufficient time for equilibrium between the blood and the urine to be established.

2. At the end of the observation period, the subject is asked to completely empty his/her bladder. Eliminating all of the urine in the bladder eliminates the possibility that ethanol in the bladder was excreted when the BAC was greater or less than it is during the 1½ h observation period. This urine sample is discarded.

3. After the initial urine elimination, the subject is observed for a period of 30 min, again ensuring that the subject does not consume any ethanol. During this period, any ethanol excreted into the bladder is in equilibrium with the BAC at the time of its excretion.

4. At the end of the 30 min observation period, a second urine sample is collected and the UAC in this second urine sample is determined. The ethanol concentration in this urine sample is a time-weighted average of the ethanol excreted during the 30 min observation period.

5. The BAC is determined by dividing the ethanol concentration in the second urine sample by 1.3, an accepted average equilibrium ratio between blood and urine ethanol concentrations.

   Errors in estimating the BAC may be made by use of this method if:

   • the bladder is not emptied entirely, which may be the case in many subjects

   • the average equilibrium ratio between blood and urine ethanol concentrations for the subject is not 1.3, due to variations in the water content of urine resulting from diet, renal function, diuresis caused by ethanol consumption[1] and/or health of the subject

   • the time of the second observation period is greater than 30 min.

   The estimation of the BAC based on urine ethanol concentrations cannot be made as described above in postmortem cases, because the collection of a second urine sample is obviously not possible, and therefore, equilibrium between the BAC and UAC cannot be established. In antemortem cases, the estimation cannot be made if the observation period between the collection of the first and second urine samples is much greater than 30 min because as the second observation increases, the time-weighted average of the UAC deviates to a greater extent from the true BAC, which has been decreasing.

   [1]Diuresis is the increased production of urine. Ethanol causes diuresis by inhibiting the release of the antidiuretic hormone from the posterior lobe of the pituitary gland, thereby decreasing the reabsorption of water from the kidney and diluting the urine.

12.14 FACTORS THAT INFLUENCE THE INTERPRETATION OF ANALYTE CONCENTRATIONS

As discussed in previous chapters, analyte concentrations in samples cannot be interpreted in a vacuum, but must be considered in conjunction with the other relevant evidence in the case being evaluated, since many factors can influence interpretation. Several of the factors that make accurate interpretations difficult and often impossible are explained in the following sections.

12.14.1 TOLERANCE

One of the most important factors that can influence the interpretation of analytical results is the phenomenon of tolerance because many drugs encountered by forensic toxicologists have the potential to cause both tolerance and addiction. Tolerance is described as a state in which, after repeated administration of a drug, a greater than initial dose of the drug is required to produce the desired effect. For example, if an individual takes heroin for extended periods of time, increased doses will be required to achieve the desired effect. Addiction is the phenomenon by which symptoms are produced when a person stops taking a drug. If a heroin addict suddenly stops taking the drug, adverse effects, withdrawal signs, and symptoms will be experienced.

The two types of tolerance, pharmacokinetic tolerance and pharmacodynamic tolerance, are characterized by compensatory mechanisms developed to counteract the effects caused by the repeated and prolonged drug exposure. Pharmacokinetic tolerance describes a state in which the prolonged use of a drug results in a physiological change in one or more of the four basic mechanisms of drug disposition. Pharmacodynamic tolerance refers to the phenomenon by which there is an alteration in the interaction of a drug with its receptor, and/or the effect that is produced by the formation of a drug–receptor complex. These compensatory mechanisms result in a need for greater doses of the drug being necessary to achieve their physiological effect. For example, when an individual becomes tolerant to the effects of ethanol, the rate of ethanol metabolism is increased (dispositional or pharmacokinetic tolerance) and the expression of specific receptors is downregulated (pharmacodynamic tolerance). Because addiction is generally accompanied by tolerance, the adverse effects experienced upon the sudden discontinuation of drug administration are influenced by the specific compensatory mechanisms that have been established in the cell. For this reason, the adverse effects associated with drug withdrawal are always opposite to the effects produced by the drug. The symptoms of withdrawal typically last from 1 week to 10 days—the length of time often required for the compensatory adaptations made by the cell to revert to a normal state.

Because tolerance can develop to both pharmacokinetic and pharmacodynamic events, answers to several of the questions asked in the previous sections of this chapter can be influenced by both the presence of tolerance and the absence or decreased tolerance due to abstinence. Since there are no biomarkers that can be used to determine directly whether a subject is tolerant or addicted to a drug, or the degree of tolerance, conclusions concerning these factors must be made indirectly. Several approaches have been employed in an attempt to determine whether tolerance is present due to active drug use or has diminished due to drug abstinence.

Often, knowledge of a subject's drug use is available from friends of the subject who can provide information about the subject's pattern of drug abuse including duration of use, frequency of daily use, and route of administration, as well as whether there has been any recent abstinence.

Active drug use, e.g., addiction, with the associated pharmacodynamic tolerance, renders addicts less susceptible to the effects of the drug; this may be evident by the absence of the signs and symptoms associated with elevated blood concentrations in nontolerant persons. An example of this are persons who have blood ethanol levels of 0.4% or greater and who are awake and driving (more likely pointing) a car (Jones and Harding, 2013). Blood ethanol concentrations in this range are consistent in non-tolerant persons with severe CNS depression causing coma or death.

In addition to the pharmacodynamic tolerance that can develop to ethanol, pharmacokinetic tolerance to ethanol, which is typified by an increased rate in the decline of the blood ethanol concentration (β) that is two or more times greater than in non-tolerant ethanol users, can develop (Winek and Murphy, 1984; Jones, 1999). This presents a problem in the back-extrapolation of blood ethanol concentrations from the time of the blood collection to the time of interest, or in Widmark calculations, since there is such a potential difference in the rates.

12.14.2 POSTMORTEM REDISTRIBUTION

In the broadest sense, postmortem redistribution (PMR) is the phenomenon by which drugs and chemicals move from one site to another in the body after death. The movement, due to diffusion, is from organs (the so-called "drug reservoirs") in which there are high concentrations of drugs into other fluids and organs.

The extent of PMR that a drug undergoes is influenced by one or more factors, including the following:

- *Apparent volumes of distribution (V_D)*: It has been proposed that the greater the V_D, the more likely it is that PMR will occur and to a greater extent. The basis for this opinion is that drugs with V_D values greater than the total body water are distributed in the nonwater compartments of the body where, due to characteristics such as high lipid solubility or nonspecific protein binding, they are sequestered in organs that become "drug reservoirs." As a result, there is a greater concentration gradient between these sites and adjacent organs and fluids so that PMR is expected to be meaningful when cell contents become more acidic and lyse, releasing these drugs from organs into the blood or adjacent organs (Yarema and Becker, 2005).
- *The postmortem interval, i.e., storage period I*: The extent of the PMR can be influenced by the length and conditions of storage period I.
- *Acidic or basic character of the drugs*: Basic drugs become more ionized under the acidic postmortem condition and are more readily soluble in the aqueous blood compartment (Yarema and Becker, 2005).

The PMR from several major drug reservoirs into other organs and blood is summarized as follows (Ferner, 2008; Pelissier-Alicot et al., 2003; Yarema and Becker, 2005).

- *Stomach*: Drugs that remain unabsorbed in the stomach can be transported via the circulation into the vena cava and the chambers of the heart or diffuse directly into organs in close proximity of the stomach, e.g., left lobe of the liver, left lung, and left ventricle.
- *Lungs*: PDR occurs by diffusion from the pulmonary veins and lobes of the lungs into the right-side chambers of the heart, the inferior vena cava, and peripheral blood.
- *Liver*: Drugs in the liver may be redistributed through the hepatic vein into the right chambers of the heart and the peripheral circulation.
- *Heart*: Several drugs found in high concentrations in the myocardium can enter cardiac blood directly.

The PMR of drugs and chemicals into the blood is of major concern because most interpretations are based on blood drug concentrations. As is apparent, there are several mechanisms by which drugs can be redistributed into heart blood resulting in an increase above the antemortem values. This PMR-mediated increase in antemortem and perimortem analyte concentrations in heart blood can led to erroneous interpretations. For this reason, drug concentrations in blood collected from peripheral blood vessels, such as the femoral vein, rather than in heart blood, are preferred as analytical samples, as they are assumed to be more accurate representations of antemortem blood analyte concentrations (Jones and Pounder, 1987; Prouty and Anderson, 1990; Pounder et al., 1996). However, this assumption may not be valid in all cases because there are conditions that cause PMR into peripheral blood resulting in an increase in antemortem and perimortem analyte concentrations. An example of this is the PMR of fentanyl, a potent opioid, which is a basic drug, has a large volume of distribution and is highly lipophilic—characteristics generally accepted to be consistent with extensive PMR. The postmortem concentration of fentanyl in femoral blood samples has been shown to increase in human and experimental animal samples during storage period I (Olson et al., 2010; Ceelen et al., 2012; Krinsky et al., 2014). The increase in femoral analyte drug concentrations, as illustrated by fentanyl, can occur as a result of several events including:

- the diffusion of analytes from skeletal muscles;
- the improper collection of the femoral sample, e.g., collection by means of a "blind stick" or the collection of a large volume without ligation of the vessel, leading to contamination of femoral blood with blood with a higher concentration from a more central location, such as the iliac vein (Chapter 8);
- continued blood circulation during the perimortem period due to resuscitative efforts or "postmortem circulation" (Of Interest 12.3).

Therefore, although probability and the extent of PMR into femoral blood are lower than into heart blood, PMR is still possible, and therefore the concentrations in femoral veins cannot be assumed to be consistent with antemortem concentrations in all cases, or to represent them more accurately than heart blood concentrations.

> **OF INTEREST 12.3 POSTMORTEM CIRCULATION**
>
> Starting at approximately 24-h postmortem, there is movement of blood in the cadaver. This movement of blood, often referred to as "postmortem circulation," occurs over a postmortem period of several hours in several stages (Fallani, 1961) as presented in Corry (1978) and Prouty and Anderson (1990).
>
> The stages of postmortem blood movement are:
> - a local movement from the right side of the heart into the nearby blood vessels of the neck and chest;
> - a generally retrograde movement of blood from inferior vessels such as the inferior vena cava and abdominal aorta to the superior vessels such as the superior vena cava and the thoracic aorta respectively;
> - movement of blood from the left side of the heart into the peripheral arteries (extensive movement into peripheral veins because of the presence of the valves);
> - movement of blood into the veins due to elevated pressures and advanced putrefaction.
>
> The consequence of the postmortem movement of blood is that the blood collected, at least 24 h after death, may have been in different locations prior to death and as a result may have contributed to the postmortem redistribution of analytes.

The likelihood and extent of PMR of a drug are often determined by the ratio of the concentration in a central (heart) blood sample to that in a peripheral (femoral vein) sample, i.e., the C/P ratio, with higher ratios representing a greater degree of PMR. Generally, this ratio is an indicator of whether PMR has occurred in a specific case. However, the C/P ratio can vary widely due to:

- postmortem events that may occur primarily during storage period I, but also possibly during storage period II before the initial analyses are performed, e.g., incomplete antemortem absorption, continued postmortem metabolism, degree of putrefaction, and analyte degradation or synthesis
- several variables in the studies in which the C/P ratios have been determined, e.g., determination in experimental animals or humans, the route of administration, site and methods of blood sample collection, and methods of analysis.

Because of these factors that cause variation in reported C/P ratios, determining the degree to which PMR has influenced the analytical results is at best challenging and often impossible. Forensic toxicologists should rely on reported C/P ratios as guides to, or indicators of, the possible role of PMR in the interpretation of analytical results, but they should not assume that the C/P ratios of analytes in specific cases are equal to values reported in the literature or observed in previous cases. Examples of the variation in reported C/P ratios are presented in Table 12.3.

In summary, PMR does occur and many factors that influence the likelihood and extent of occurrence have been determined, however, the simultaneous occurrence of several of these factors generate a complexity causing PMR to be "a toxicological nightmare" (Pounder and Jones, 1990).

Table 12.3 C/P Ratios of Selected Drugs[a]

Drug	C/P
Acetaminophen	0.7–2.8
Amitriptyline	0.9–13.9
Codeine	0.7–11.4
Diazepam	0.2–12
Doxepin	1–20
Haloperidol	1.4–10
Morphine	1–5.8
Phenylpropanolamine	0.8–4.6
Salicylate	0.5–3

[a] Dalpe-Scott, M., Degoffe, M., Garbutt, D., Drost, M., 1995. A comparison of drug concentrations in postmortem cardiac and peripheral blood in 320 cases. Can. Soc. Forensic Sci. J. 28, 113–121.

12.14.3 AGE-RELATED PHARMACOKINETICS AND PHARMACODYNAMICS

Several of the events and mechanisms of pharmacokinetics and pharmacodynamics, as well as the manners and rates at which they occur are affected by age.

In the pediatric population, the kinetics of disposition differs meaningfully from those in adults.[4] For example (de Wildt, 2011; Lu and Rosenbaum, 2014):

- the gastric pH is neutral at birth, fluctuating until approximately 2 years of age when it has decreased to the acidic adult values; these fluctuations affect the ionization and absorption of acidic and basic drugs
- the ratio of body water to fat increases from birth during the first year of life, influencing the distribution of drugs depending on their lipo- and hydrophilicity
- the maturation of metabolic enzyme systems varies with type. Phase I cytochrome p450 (CYP) enzymes, such as CYP 2D6 and CYP 3A4, develop at different rates after birth, but all have activities comparable to those of adults at approximately 1–2 years of age. The isoforms of the important 5-diphosphosglucuronic acid glucuronyltransferase phase II family of enzymes responsible for the glucuronidation of many drugs develop at widely varying times after birth. For example, the isoform UGT 2B7 that converts morphine into morphine-6-glucuronide and morphine-3-glucuronide, active and inactive metabolites, respectively, generally has adult activity by 6 months of age, whereas UGT1A6, involved in the metabolism of aspirin and acetaminophen, is not fully active until 10 years of age

---

[4]The FDA has defined four groups within the pediatric population: neonates (birth–1 month), infants (1 month–2 years), developing children (2–12 years), and adolescents (12–16 years) (Lu and Rosenbaum, 2014).

- the renal clearance of drugs is decreased below adult levels in neonates and infants. This increases the half-lives of drugs eliminated by the kidney increasing their duration of action.

Pediatric pharmacokinetics demonstrates the pharmacological adage that the young are not just small adults; they have unique dispositional characteristics that must be considered by forensic toxicologists in the interpretation of analytical results.

The effect of age on the interpretation of analytical results is not as clear in older adults as in the pediatric population. It may be that this is due to the lack of a clear definition of the age at which geriatric studies begin; the age of "older adults" may range over a period of five or more decades and the pharmacokinetic and pharmacodynamic effects seen in older adults often are due to specific comorbidity, e.g., pathologies of the liver and kidneys, that varies widely among the members of this population. For these reasons, it is difficult to make definitive statements concerning the pharmacokinetic and pharmacodynamic changes that occur with advancing age. However, certain trends have been identified in the elderly (McLean and Le Couteur, 2004; Ginsberg et al., 2005; Desoky, 2007):

- the volumes of distribution of water and lipid-soluble drugs are decreased and increased, respectively, due to decreased total body water and increased body fat in older adults;
- older adults have decreased activity of cytochrome p450 enzymes and decreased renal clearance, both of which can increase the half-lives of drugs eliminated by these mechanisms.

The pharmacokinetics and pharmacodynamics in pediatric and geriatric populations can differ meaningfully from those seen in young adults. These differences can influence the interpretation of analytical results, including interpretations regarding the estimation of last use and effects of active metabolites, the differentiation of antimortem use and postmortem production, the differentiation between chronic and acute use, and the interpretation of fluid and tissue drug concentrations, because the databases on which these interpretations are made include little if any data obtained for the pediatric and geriatric populations.

REVIEW QUESTIONS

1. Describe the difference between inductive reasoning and deductive reasoning.
2. Under what conditions might analytical results alone not be sufficient to conclude with "a reasonable scientific probability" whether a drug caused, or contributed to, of the signs and symptoms of a subject?
3. How might the analysis of hair allow for a determination of whether drug exposure was intentional or due to unintentional passive exposure?
4. What is the Widmark equation and for what purpose is it utilized?
5. The analytical results most commonly utilized to correlate analyte concentration to effects are blood drug levels. Why?

APPLICATION QUESTIONS

1. Discuss two types of nonanalytical case-related evidence that might significantly influence a forensic toxicology interpretation.

2. It is generally true that the accurate detection of either exogenous substances or their unique metabolites is a proof of exposure to these substances; however, there are several exceptions to this rule. Describe two scenarios in which exogenous substances or their metabolites might be detected in samples in the absence of intentional exposure.

3. Describe how the analysis of serotonin metabolism may be useful in differentiating between antemortem ethanol consumption and postmortem production of ethanol.

4. Discuss the challenges encountered when attempting to determine when (i.e., how recently) marihuana was used. Describe a strategy that might be beneficial in answering this question. What are some of the strengths and weaknesses of this strategy?

REFERENCES

Albermann, M.E., Musshoff, F., Doberentz, E., Heese, P., Banger, M., Madea, B., 2012. Preliminary investigations on ethyl glucuronide and ethyl sulfate cutoffs for detecting alcohol consumption on the basis of an ingestion experiment and on data from withdrawal treatment. Int. J. Leg. Med. 126 (5), 757–764.

Baranowski, S., Serr, A., Thierauf, A., Weinmann, W., Grosse Perdekamp, M., Wurst, F.M., et al., 2008. In vitro study of bacterial degradation of ethyl glucuronide and ethyl sulphate. Int. J. Legal Med. 122 (5), 389–393.

Baselt, R.C., Yoshikawa, D.M., Chang, J.Y., 1991. Passive inhalation of cocaine. Clin. Chem. 37 (12), 2160–2161.

Beck, O., Helander, A., 2003. 5-hydroxytryptophol as a marker for recent alcohol intake. Addiction (Suppl 2), 63–72.

Boumba, V.A., Ziavrou, K.S., Vougiouklakis, T., 2008. Biochemical pathways generating post-mortem volatile compounds co-detected during forensic ethanol analyses. Forensic Sci. Int. 174 (2–3), 133–151.

Ceelen, L., De Zwart, L., Voets, M., Hillewaert, V., Monbaliu, J., Teuns, G., et al., 2012. Post-mortem redistribution of fentanyl in the rabbit blood. Am. J. Forensic Med. Pathol. 33 (2), 119–123.

Centers for Disease Control and Prevention. Alcohol and Public Health, January 5, 2015. Retrieved from: http://www.cdc.gov/alcohol/faqs.htm.

Chang, J., Wang, M., Appleton, C., 2012. Headache bread—a case of high codeine containing variety of poppy seed. J. Anal. Toxicol. 36 (4), 288.

Cocchetto, D.M., Owens, S.M., Perez-Reyes, M., DiGuiseppi, S., Miller, L.L., 1981. Relationship between plasma delta-9-tetrahydrocannabinol concentration and pharmacologic effects in man. Psychopharmacology 75 (2), 158–164.

Cone, E.J., Yousefnejad, D., Hillsgrove, M.J., Holicky, B., Darwin, W.D., 1995. Passive inhalation of cocaine. J. Anal. Toxicol. 19 (6), 399–411.

Corry, J.E., 1978. Possible sources of ethanol ante- and post-mortem: its relationship to the biochemistry and microbiology of decomposition. J. Appl. Bacteriol. 44, 1−56.

Costantino, A., Digregorio, E.J., Korn, W., Spayd, S., Rieders, F., 2006. The effect of the use of mouthwash on ethylglucuronide concentrations in urine. J. Anal. Toxicol. 30 (9), 659−662.

Druid, H., Holmgren, P., 1997. A compilation of fatal and control concentrations of drugs in postmortem femoral blood. J. Forensic Sci. 42 (1), 79−87.

Dubois, N., Demaret, I., Ansseau, M., Rozet, E., Hubert, P., Charlier, C., 2013. Plasma level monitoring of the major metabolites of diacetylmorphine (heroin) by the "chasing the dragon" route in severe heroin addicts. Acta Clin. Belgica 68 (5), 359−367.

El Desoky, E.S., 2007. Pharmacokinetic and pharmacodynamic crisis in the elderly. Am. J. Ther. 14, 488−498.

El Sohly, M.A., Stanford, D.F., elSohly, H.N., 1986. Coca tea and urinalysis for cocaine metabolites. J. Anal. Toxicol. 10 (6), 256.

Ernst, M.F., Poklis, A., Gantner, G.E., 1982. Evaluation of medicolegal investigators' suspicions and positive toxicology findings in 100 drug deaths. J. Forensic Sci. 27 (1), 61−65.

Fallani, M., 1961. Contributo allo studio della circolazione ematica postmortale. Minerva Me- Dicolegale 81, 108−115.

Felby, S., Olsen, J., 1969. Comparative studies of postmortem ethyl alcohol in vitreous humor, blood, and muscle. J. Forensci Sci. 14 (1), 93−101.

Ferner, R.E., 2008. Post-mortem clinical pharmacology. Br. J. Clin. Pharmacol. 66 (4), 430−443.

Ginsberg, G., Hattis, D., Russ, A., Sonawane, B., 2005. Pharmacokinetic and pharmacodynamic factors that can affect sensitivity to neurotoxic sequelae in elderly individuals. Environ. Health Perspect. 113 (9), 1243−1249.

Haggard, H.W., Greenberg, L.A., Carroll, R.P., Miller, D.P., 1940. The use of ethanol in the chemical test for ethanol. JAMA 115, 1680−1683.

Helander, A., Dahl, H., 2005. Urinary tract infection: a risk factor for false-negative urinary ethyl glucuronide but not ethyl sulfate in the detection of recent alcohol consumption. Clin. Chem. 51 (9), 1728−1730.

Helander, A., Beck, O., Jones, A.W., 1995. Distinguishing ingested ethanol from microbial formation by analysis of urinary 5-hydroxytryptophol and 5-hydroxyindoleacetic acid. J. Forensic Sci. 40 (1), 95−98.

Helander, A., Olsson, I., Dahl, H., 2007. Postcollection synthesis of ethyl glucuronide by bacteria in urine may cause false identification of alcohol consumption. Clin. Chem. 53 (10), 1855−1857.

Hill, V., Cairns, T., Cheng, C.C., Schaffer, M., 2005. Multiple aspects of hair analysis for opiates: methodology, clinical and workplace populations, codeine, and poppy seed ingestion. J. Anal. Toxicol. 29 (7), 696−703.

Hoiseth, G., Yttredal, B., Karinen, R., Gjerde, H., Christophersen, A., 2010. Levels of ethyl glucuronide and ethyl sulfate in oral fluid, blood, and urine after use of mouthwash and ingestion of nonalcoholic wine. J. Anal. Toxicol. 34 (2), 84−88.

Huestis, M.A., Cone, E.J., 1998. Differentiating new marijuana use from residual drug excretion in occasional marijuana users. J. Analyt. Tox. 22 (6), 445−454.

Huestis, M.A., 2002. Cannabis (marihuana)—effects of human behavior and performance. Forensic Sci. Rev. 14, 15−60.

Jackson, G.F., Saady, J.J., Poklis, A., 1991. Urinary excretion of benzoylecgonine following ingestion of health Inca tea. Forensic Sci. Int. 49 (1), 57−64.

Jenkins, A.J., 2001. Drug contamination of US paper currency. Forensic Sci. Int. 121 (3), 189–193.

Jones, A.W., 1999. The drunkest drinking driver in Sweden: blood alcohol concentration 0.545% w/v. J. Stud. Alcohol 60 (3), 400–406.

Jones, A.W., 2008. Biochemical and physiological research on the disposition and fate of ethanol in the body. In: Garriott, J.C. (Ed.), Garriott's Medicolegal Aspects of Alcohol, fifth ed. Lawyers & Judges Publishing Company, Tucson, AZ.

Jones, A.W., Harding, P., 2013. Driving under the influence with blood alcohol concentrations over 0.4 g%. Forensic Sci. Int. 231 (1–3), 349–353.

Jones, G.R., Pounder, D.J., 1987. Site dependence of drug concentrations in postmortem blood—a case study. J. Anal. Toxicol. 11, 186–190.

Jourdan, T.H., Veitenheimer, A.M., Murray, C.K., Wagner, J.R., 2013. The quantitation of cocaine on U.S. currency: survey and significance of the levels of contamination. J. Forensic Sci. 58 (3), 616–624.

Krinsky, C.S., Lathrop, S.L., Zumwalt, R., 2014. An examination of the postmortem redistribution of fentanyl and interlaboratory variability. J. Forensic Sci. 59 (5), 1275–1279.

Kugelberg, F.C., Jones, A.W., 2007. Interpreting results of ethanol analysis in postmortem specimens. Forensic Sci. Int. 165, 10–29.

Lachenmeier, D.W., Sproll, C., Musshoff, F., 2010. Poppy seed foods and opiate drug testing—where are we today? Ther. Drug Monitor 32 (1), 11–18.

Lu, H., Rosenbaum, S., 2014. Developmental pharmacokinetics in pediatric populations. J. Pediatr. Pharmacol. Ther. 19 (4), 262–276.

Manno, J.E., Ferslew, K.E., Manno, B.R., 1984. Urine excretion patterns of cannabinoids and the clinical application of the EMIT dau cannabinoid urine assay for the of substance treatment. In: Agurell, S., Dewey, W.L., Willette, R. (Eds.), The Cannabinoids: Chemical Pharmacologic and Therapeutic Aspects. Academic Press.

McLean, A.J., Le Couteur, D.G., 2004. Aging biology and geriatric clinical pharmacology. Pharmacol. Rev. 56 (2), 163–184.

Meadway, C., George, S., Braithwaite, R., 1998. Opiate concentrations following the ingestion of poppy seed products—evidence for 'the poppy seed defence'. Forensic Sci. Int. 96 (1), 29–38.

Musshoff, F., Brockmann, C., Madea, B., Rosendahl, W., Piombino-Mascali, D., 2013. Ethyl glucuronide findings in hair samples from the mummies of the capuchin catacombs of Palermo. Forensic Sci. Int. 232 (1–3), 213–217.

Olson, K.N., Luckenbill, K., Thompson, J., Middleton, O., Geiselhart, R., Mills, K.M., et al., 2010. Postmortem redistribution of fentanyl in blood. Am. J. Clin. Pathol. 133 (3), 447–453.

Oyler, J., Darwin, W.D., Cone, E.J., 1996. Cocaine contamination of United States paper currency. J. Anal. Toxicol. 20 (4), 213–216.

Paul, R., Elder, L., 2008. Scientific Thinking. The Foundation for Critical Thinking, pp. 21–31.

Pelissier-Alicot, A.L., Gaulier, J.M., Champsaur, P., Marquet, P., 2003. Mechanisms underlying postmortem redistribution of drugs: a review. J. Anal. Toxicol. 27 (8), 533–544.

Pounder, D.J., Jones, G.R., 1990. Post-mortem drug redistribution—a toxicological nightmare. Forensic Sci. Int. 45, 253–263.

Pounder, D.J., Fuke, C., Cox, D.E., Smith, D., Kuroda, N., 1996. Postmortem diffusion of drugs from gastric residue: an experimental study. Am. J. Forensic Med. Pathol. 17 (1), 1–7.

Prouty, R.W., Anderson, W.H., 1990. The forensic science implications of site and temporal influences on postmortem blood-drug concentrations. J. Forensic Sci. 35, 243–270.

Reisfield, G.M., Goldberger, B.A., Crews, B.O., Pesce, A.J., Wilson, G.R., Teitelbaum, S.A., et al., 2011. Ethyl glucuronide, ethyl sulfate, and ethanol in urine after sustained exposure to an ethanol-based hand sanitizer. J. Anal. Toxicol. 35 (2), 85–91.

Rohrig, T.P., Huber, C., Goodson, L., Ross, W., 2006. Detection of ethyl glucuronide in urine following the application of Germ-X. J. Analyt. Tox. 30 (9), 703–704.

Stewart, C., Stolman, A., 1960. The toxicologist and his work. In: Stewart, C., Stolman, A. (Eds.), Toxicology: Mechanisms and Analytical Methods, vol. 1. Academic Press, New York.

Walsham, N.E., Sherwood, R.A., 2012. Ethyl glucuronide. Ann. Clin. Biochem. 42, 110–117.

de Wildt, S.N., 2011. Profound changes in drug metabolism enzymes and possible effects on drug therapy in neonates and children. Expert Opin. Drug Metab. Toxicol. 7 (8), 935–948.

West, R., Crews, B., Mikel, C., Almazan, P., Latyshev, S., Pesce, A., et al., 2009. Anomalous observations of codeine in patients on morphine. Ther. Drug Monit. 31 (6), 776–778.

West, R., West, C., Crews, B., Almazan, P., Latyshev, S., Rosenthal, M., et al., 2011. Anomalous observations of hydrocodone in patients on oxycodone. Clin. Chim. Acta; Int. J. Clin. Chem. 412 (1–2), 29–32.

Winek, C.L., Murphy, K.L., 1984. The rate and kinetic order of ethanol elimination. Forensic Sci. Int. 25 (3), 159–166.

Winek, C.L., Wahba, W.W., Winek Jr., C.L., Balzer, T.W., 2001. Drug and chemical blood-level data 2001. Forensic Sci. Int. 122 (2–3), 107–123.

Yarema, M.C., Becker, C.E., 2005. Key concepts in postmortem drug redistribution. Clin. Toxicol. 43 (4), 235–241.

Yonamine, M., Garcia, P.R., de Moraes Moreau, R.L., 2004. Non-intentional doping in sports. Sports Med. 34 (11), 697–704.

Ziavrou, K., Boumba, V.A., Vougiouklakis, T.G., 2005. Insights into the origin of postmortem ethanol. Int. J. Toxicol. 24 (2), 69–77.

Reports

13

When I use a word, it means just what I choose it to mean — neither more or less.
Humpty Dumpty

Forensic toxicologists prepare two types of reports: laboratory reports and expert reports. The format of these reports differs, but in all cases the contents must be clear, understandable, and accurate. Forensic toxicologists who prepare reports are well advised to adhere to the old adage—"Say what you mean and mean what you say" because these reports will be analyzed and dissected by judges, attorneys, and other experts.

13.1 LABORATORY REPORTS

Following the completion of an experimental analysis, forensic toxicology laboratories will prepare a formal report that outlines the analytical findings. In postmortem forensic toxicology laboratories, this report becomes a component of the autopsy report. There are numerous types of forensic toxicology laboratory reports. There is no "best" type of report and no universally accepted type. Each forensic toxicology laboratory uses a report format that has been determined to be appropriate for its needs and that meets any prevailing regulations or statutes.

13.1.1 THE MINIMUM REPORT

Generally, forensic toxicology laboratory reports are short documents containing a bare minimum of information, e.g., name of the subject, type of the sample analyzed, and qualitative and/or quantitative results. Regardless of the length of laboratory report, it is reasonable to expect that, at a minimum, reports should include the following (SOFT/AAFS, 2006):

- name and identifying code number of the subject. This is of obvious importance for maintenance of a chain of custody;
- identification of the laboratory in which the results were obtained;
- name of the agency that submitted the samples that were analyzed;

Forensic Toxicology. http://dx.doi.org/10.1016/B978-0-12-799967-8.00013-X

- date on which the samples were submitted;
- type of the samples submitted;
- samples that were analyzed;
- date(s) on which the samples were analyzed;
- date on which the report was prepared;
- results; and
- the name of the person who reviewed or certified the results, usually not the person who performed the analysis, but the lab director or staff member responsible for reviewing and certifying the results.

13.1.2 ADDITIONAL INFORMATION

Commonly, additional information pertaining to the samples, methods of analysis, results, and interpretation of the results, which are not included in the list of minimum inclusions in laboratory reports, are also included in the report. Additionally, information pertaining to sample handling, including the site of blood collection (i.e., left heart, right heart, or peripheral vessel) and the type of preservative used, if any, is also included in the laboratory report. The significance of this information has been discussed in Chapter 6. Certain aspects of sample handling are usually not included in reports, including:

- the specific location from which certain samples are collected, e.g., which lobe of the liver or of the lung;
- the volume or weight of the sample;
- the type and size of the container in which the sample was collected and stored; and
- the conditions under which the samples had been stored prior to analysis.

It is not reasonable to expect that a detailed description of the method of analysis is included in the report, and generally no information related to the method of analysis is included in the report. Although the drugs detected, the concentration of each drug detected, and the specific samples in which the drugs were detected are stated in all reports, the raw data on which these results are based such as chromatograms, or mass spectra, are not included in laboratory reports. The omission of a description of the methods of analysis in a report is of some significance, however, because without the knowledge of the type of methods employed, the specificity and sensitivity of the method cannot be determined, and the potential validity of the results (assuming the procedures were conducted properly) cannot be determined.

Any report that will become a component of the official record must be clear and unambiguous. Unfortunately, forensic toxicology laboratory reports often use language that may be confusing and/or misleading. One source of potential confusion is the use of the word "negative." "Negative" means that the concentration of the drug is zero—that no drug is present in the sample. Of course, forensic toxicologists cannot determine that **no** drugs are present; they can only determine that no drugs were detected. Therefore, a more accurate and appropriate way to describe the failure of an analytical protocol to detect specific drugs in the sample is by use of the phrase "not detected." "Not detected" means either the drug was not present in the sample or was present at a concentration lower than the detection limit for the method of analysis utilized (the detection limit for each drug should be stated in the report).

Reports often contain statements such as "No other drugs were detected" or "No volatiles were detected." These and similar statements are not informative and may be confusing. The vagueness of these statements often leads nontoxicologists, e.g., attorneys, police, and insurance investigators, to conclude that **no** other drugs were present in the sample. However, in actuality, such statements in the context of a forensic toxicology laboratory report mean simply that no other drugs, detectable by the methods used, were detected. This confusion can be minimized and possibly eliminated if reports include a list of the specific analytes that are detectable by the methods used, as well as the detection limits of the methods for each of these analytes. Although the list of the specific drugs detectable by a modern method of analysis such as LC/MS/MS would be extensive, comprised of dozens of analytes and/or metabolites, its value exceeds any inconvenience associated with its inclusion in the report.

A phrase that should not be used in laboratory reports is "inconclusive results." This is a phrase that is misleading. If an analysis is performed to determine whether a specific drug is present in a sample, the result of that analysis is either positive or not detected. The word "inconclusive" implies that there is evidence of the presence of the drug. If the results meet the criteria of the limit of detection (LOD), then the result is "positive." If not, then the result is "not detected." There is no analytical circumstance in which the term "inconclusive" should be applied in a laboratory report.

A summary of the pharmacology and/or toxicology of the drugs detected in a sample, as well as the blood and tissue levels that are ***consistent with*** therapeutic, toxic, and lethal effects of the drugs, is often included in a laboratory report. Because it is not practical to present a thorough discussion of the interpretation of the results, this information is generally comprised of a brief summary statement of the available literature on the topic, or simply data derived from a single source. In either instance, these data allow only a first approximation of, or a guide to, the interpretation of the analytical data, as the interpretation should be made in light of the facts of the case, e.g., age, gender, existing pathology, tolerance, and addiction (Chapter 12). Because toxicologists may not be aware of all of the facts and findings of the case, including those that may influence the interpretation, it is often difficult for a comprehensive interpretation to be included in a laboratory report. For this reason, the toxicology findings are only one part of a clinical or postmortem case, and do not stand alone. Any interpretation of these findings must be made by an attending physician or a forensic pathologist.

The results of toxicological analyses performed in clinical toxicology laboratories often are included in a report that presents all the laboratory results obtained for a patient, rather than being presented as a separate document. These reports usually contain therapeutic (often misidentified as "normal") ranges for the drugs detected as well as an H (high) or L (low), as an interpretation of the analytical results. Many clinical toxicology analyses are unconfirmed presumptive tests. When this is the case, the reports contain statements clearly declaring and emphasizing that the toxicology results have not been confirmed, that a chain of custody has not been maintained and that the results are to be used for clinical and not forensic purposes. The failure to confirm the results and to maintain a chain of custody often renders the results inadmissible if there is an attempt to introduce them at trial.

If the case is litigated, an attorney may request the court to issue a subpoena requiring the laboratory to produce specific records pertaining to the analysis on which a laboratory report is based. For example, in a case in which the defendant has been charged with Driving While Intoxicated, based in part on the blood ethanol results reported by a commercial forensic toxicology laboratory, the defense attorney may request the court to issue a subpoena compelling the laboratory to produce specific records of the following information:

- A detailed description of the standard operating procedure for the collection of a forensic blood sample to be analyzed for ethanol.
- The specific procedure followed for the collection of the blood sample, which was analyzed for ethanol, from the defendant.
- A detailed step-by-step description of the method of analysis, standard curves, and mathematical methods used to determine the defendant's blood alcohol (ethanol) concentration (BAC).
- Any records pertaining to the evaluation of the method of analysis, including validation studies and/or control charts.
- Records of the specifications, methods of preparation, and storage of all reagents used generally in the laboratory, and specifically for the analysis conducted on the defendant's blood.
- Log books for the instrument(s) used for the analysis of the defendant's blood for 1 year prior to the analysis of the defendant's blood.
- Identification of potential sources of false-positive and false-negative results that may be obtained through the use of the method of analysis.
- A list of any endogenous or exogenous substances known to interfere with the method of analysis.
- The raw data obtained in the analysis utilized for the BAC determination in the defendant's blood, including data obtained from blanks, controls, and standards.
- The identity of the laboratory technician who performed the analysis of the defendant's blood.
- The results of any internal and external proficiency tests for BAC determinations in which the laboratory participated during the past 2 years.
- Copies of any certifications and/or licenses for BAC determinations held by the laboratory.

Under order of a subpoena, many laboratories, usually large laboratories, provide the so-called litigation packet. This packet is a compilation of the entire record pertaining to the analysis of samples obtained from a person and contains most of the items listed above; additional requested records will have to be produced.

13.2 EXPERT REPORTS

Forensic toxicologists are often called upon to review evidence in both civil and criminal cases and to offer expert opinions on a number of matters within the purview of their expertise. When this occurs, forensic toxicologists may be required to write a report in which they identify the records that they reviewed, including police reports, witness statements, medical records, and laboratory reports; summarize the facts of the case relevant to their opinions; provide a summary of the pharmacology and toxicology of the analytes detected; and state their opinions.

Forensic toxicologists must be extremely careful in the choice of language used in these reports as the reports are meant to assist the trier of fact in understanding the toxicological issues in a legal proceeding. Reports that contain sloppy or confusing language, inaccurate scientific notation, assumption of facts not in evidence, and incorrect interpretation of the scientific literature will be obstacles to the determination of scientific fact and may result in an incorrect determination being made, especially if there are no alternate expert reports available.

Rules for the content of an expert report vary somewhat from state to state, but in general, they contain some or all of the content in the Federal Rules of Civil Procedure (2015), which require that a person who has been identified as a potential witness must prepare and sign a report that contains the following:

- "a complete statement of all opinions the witness will express and the basis and reasons for them;
- the facts or data considered by the witness in forming them;
- any exhibits that will be used to summarize or support them;
- the witness' qualifications, including a list of all publications authored in the previous 10 years;
- a list of all other cases in which, during the previous 4 years, the witness testified as an expert at trial or by deposition; and
- a statement of the compensation to be paid for the study and testimony in the case."

In certain states, expert reports must contain an identification of the evidence reviewed, a summary of the facts, and the opinions of the expert. There is no requirement for an extensive explanation of the basis for the expert's opinions. In other states, not only are the identification of the evidence reviewed, a summary of the facts, and the opinions of the expert required but also a presentation of the scientific basis of the opinion. In these states, the expert's testimony may be limited to the scope of the information presented in the report.

REVIEW QUESTIONS

1. Describe the two main types of reports that forensic toxicologists are responsible for preparing.
2. What minimum components must be included in a laboratory report?
3. What components are typically included in an expert report?
4. List the components that the Federal Rules of Civil Procedure dictate that a potential witness must include in a written report.
5. Who is responsible for preparing a laboratory report and/or an expert report?

APPLICATION QUESTIONS

1. Discuss two types of additional information that are commonly included in a laboratory report. Why is the inclusion of this additional information valuable? Are there any circumstances under which the inclusion of additional information might be detrimental to the report?
2. Discuss the differences in meaning between the terms "negative" and "not detected," in the context of a forensic toxicology laboratory report. Why is "not detected" considered to be more precise and accurate language?
3. Describe the purpose of an expert report. What factors must a forensic toxicologist take into consideration when preparing an expert report? What kind of language would you, as a forensic toxicologist, use in an expert report—would you consider your audience when making language and/or content choices for your report—why or why not?
4. Discuss why forensic toxicology laboratory reports often serve as only one component of a clinical or postmortem case. Why do they not often function as stand-alone documents?

REFERENCES

Fed. R. Civ. R. 26(a)(2)(b), (2015).

SOFT/AAFS, 2006. Forensic Toxicology Laboratory Guidelines. From: http://www.soft-tox.org/files/Guidelines_2006_Final.pdf (retrieved 03.11.12).

Testifying

Facts are stubborn things; and whatever may be our wishes, our inclinations, or the dictates of our passion, they cannot alter the state of facts and evidence.
John Adams, 1770

It is of the utmost importance that the chemical analysis in cases of suspected poisoning should be entrusted to a competent chemist capable not only of conducting it with system and accuracy but also of meeting the numerous objections that may at the subsequent trial be brought against his evidence.
F. Thornton and M. Stillé, 1855

There are a series of events, ranging from the practical to the legal, that occur as a result of going to court. This section is not, and should not be considered to be, a legal treatise. It is a summary of the opinions of the authors, who are not attorneys, and is based on experience and should be construed as just that.

14.1 PRELIMINARIES

14.1.1 GETTING TO THE COURTHOUSE

Forensic toxicologists scheduled or under subpoena to testify as expert witnesses must arrive at the courthouse on time. They do not want the same fate to befall them as befell Raspail in the LaFarge matter or to be held in contempt if they are under subpoena. Since traffic is a problem in major metropolitan areas, extra time should be allowed for unforeseen occurrences that will increase travel time. Generally, judges are not sympathetic about excuses from late-arriving experts; they may respond to tardiness by reminding the expert that they, and probably everyone else in the courtroom, were able to get to court on time. Allow yourself plenty of travel time.

14.1.2 WAITING TO TESTIFY

After arrival at the courthouse, experts should expect to wait, often for prolonged periods, before they are called to the stand. Experts must remember that—"The

Forensic Toxicology. http://dx.doi.org/10.1016/B978-0-12-799967-8.00014-1

wheels of justice turn slowly, but exceedingly fine." Therefore, they should be prepared to occupy themselves with appropriate diversions, e.g., books, newspapers, crossword puzzles, for what may be hours of waiting.

While waiting, experts should not enter the courtroom unless they have been told to do so by the attorney who will call them. In many cases, the judge will allow experts to sit in the courtroom to hear the testimony of others, especially if that testimony is relevant to, or is the foundation of, the expert's opinion.

14.1.3 ENTERING THE COURTROOM

When experts are called to the stand and they enter the courtroom, virtually everyone in the courtroom will look at them. This is a classic example of having only one chance to make a first impression. Therefore, as experts walk to the stand, it is to be expected that some jurors will formulate an opinion of them based on their overall appearance, including the manner of dress, posture, and gait, and any other physical or behavioral signs that can be detected. Before experts take the oath, some jurors will have formulated an opinion about whether they should trust and believe the testimony they are about to hear.

14.1.4 BEING SWORN IN

Before taking the stand, experts will be sworn in. They will swear or affirm that they will tell the truth, the whole truth, and nothing but the truth. This is a very high standard. Experts must tell truth and nothing but the truth. In other words, do not lie. Telling the whole truth is another matter. It is often not possible or desirable for an expert to tell the whole truth (see below).

14.1.5 VOIR DIRE

After being sworn in, experts undergo *voir dire* by the attorneys who called them. This is the procedure by which attorneys elicit information concerning the qualifications of their experts in order to convince the judge that they are qualified and competent to testify as expert witness and thus provide opinion testimony in the area of their expertise. The experts will be asked to discuss their education, their professional experience, the professional organizations to which they belong, their record of research (articles published and presentations made), any certifications or licenses that they hold, and the number of times and the courts in which they have testified. Opposing attorneys then may stipulate to their expertise and offer no objection to the expert's acceptance as an expert witness, and generally, they will be accepted. Alternatively, the opposing attorney may question them further, if not to have their testimony excused then to limit their testimony to more specific areas of their expertise or to point out deficiencies in their qualifications to the jury to demonstrate that they may not be as "expert" as was suggested. No matter how many organizations experts belong to, they may be asked about three or four that they do not belong to. No matter how many publications they have, they will be asked about a journal in which they have not published.

There are no absolute requirements other than whether the experts know more about the topic than the lay person: "Similarly, the expert is viewed, not in a narrow sense, but as a person qualified by 'knowledge, skill, experience, training, or education' (Federal court)." Judges will evaluate the overall qualifications of experts.

14.2 QUALIFICATION OF THE EXPERT WITNESS

Outside of the courtroom, it was once joked that an expert was someone from out of town who had slides (today the expert would have a PowerPoint). However, this definition does not meet the standards of the law.

The Federal Rules of Evidence (2015), Rule 702, identify an expert as follows:

A witness who is qualified as an expert by knowledge, skill, experience, training, or education may testify in the form of an opinion or otherwise if:

(a) the expert's scientific, technical, or other specialized knowledge will help the trier of fact to understand the evidence or to determine a fact in issue;

(b) the testimony is based on sufficient facts or data;

(c) the testimony is the product of reliable principles and methods; and

(d) the expert has reliably applied the principles and methods to the facts of the case.

There are several criteria used to determine whether a proposed expert possesses the requisite qualifications, including education, training, experience, research publications, memberships in professional organizations, prior testimony as an expert, and board certification. These qualifications are elicited on *voir dire*,[1] the process by which the proposed expects answer questions pertaining to these aspects of their qualifications, following which the judge determines whether a proposed witness is qualified to testify as an expert in a specific area.

Is a forensic toxicologist with an MS degree, 20 years of experience, and 15 publications the equivalent of one with a PhD, 5 years of experience and 6 publications? It depends. The trial judge makes a decision as to whether the toxicologist will be allowed to testify as an expert witness based on his understanding of the expert's qualifications as they apply to the scientific issues at hand. This process of *voir dire* by which experts are identified and qualified by the court to provide opinion testimony is not always efficient (Of Interest 14.1).

Generally, if the judge decides to allow expert testimony from a witness, he will describe for the jury the role of the expert, explaining that the expert may be allowed

---

[1]*Voir dire* is derived from French and is translated loosely as "to speak the truth."

OF INTEREST 14.1 AN EXPERT?

The occasional failure of the *voir dire* process is illustrated by a case in which the issue was whether a man was of sound mind when he changed his will a few days before his death to leave a significant amount of his estate to his second wife. As might be expected, the first wife and her children were upset and brought suit claiming that the will was changed while the man was hospitalized and under the influence of drugs included in his treatment, and, therefore, was not of sound mind to change his will. The plaintiffs retained, as an expert, a scientist who analyzed samples for pesticide content for the federal government. The expert had never taken a toxicology course, nor did he have any degrees in toxicology or a related disciplines or any forensic experience. The sum total of his "expertise" was the detection of pesticides—experience that had no relevance to the toxicology issue in this case. In spite of his shortcomings, the judge accepted him as an expert in the field of toxicology and allowed him to render an opinion as to whether the decedent had been under the influence of medication when he altered his will.

---

to provide opinion as well as factual testimony. In addition, the judge will tell the jurors that even though the witness is an expert, they can afford as much weight to the testimony as they see fit and can accept or reject the testimony of the expert (Of Interest 14.2).

OF INTEREST 14.2 THE CSI EFFECT

A jury's knowledge of science is often meager and based not on education, but rather on personal experience, rumors, and myth. Forensic scientists who fail to explain the differences between science and fiction may fail to convince the jury of their competence and reliability and may not be able to gain the trust of jurors. The problem of science versus popular beliefs was recognized early in the history of forensic toxicology by Christison who was of the opinion that expert testimony was "… an interaction between expert and popular knowledge" (Burney, 2006, p. 53). In 2002, Time magazine coined the phrase "CSI effect" to explain a jury's inaccurate understanding and unrealistic expectations of the limitations (or lack thereof) of the forensic sciences (Cole, 2015). This theory proposes that jurors have been unable to understand that the CSI stable of television dramas and other programs of the same ilk are not real and that some or much of what they present is science fiction. Since then, this view of a jury's expectations has been advanced in part by attorneys who argue that the popularity of these programs has made the selection of a knowledgeable jury with reasonable expectations of what forensic science is able to achieve much more difficult. Studies have shown that the CSI effect may not be due entirely to the television viewing habits of the public, but is rather more accurately described as a "tech effect," the product of rapidly developing technological advances in the everyday lives of jurors, e.g., laptop computers and cell phones in the size of cigarette packs with computer capabilities (Shelton, 2012). If there are heightened and unrealistic expectations of the capabilities of science, regardless of their genesis, experts including forensic toxicologists must respond.

An example of the personal experience and opinions of jurors overriding scientific testimony occurred in the 1990 trial of D.C. Mayor Marion Barry who was arrested and charged with 14 counts related to possession and use of cocaine (Walsh and Gellman, 1990, p. A1). The testimony of an FBI analyst that the substance in a plastic bag found in Barry's possession was crack cocaine was not challenged or disputed by the defense. However, during jury deliberations, two jurors disagreed with the testimony because the substance that was shown to the jury did not look like crack to them—it was the wrong color and looked like sugar! Barry was convicted on one of the 14 counts.

14.3 ADMISSIBILITY OF SCIENTIFIC TESTIMONY

Even after being qualified, the testimony of expert witnesses is limited. There have been several landmark cases in which the type of evidence that may be rendered by experts has been delineated. Interestingly, all but one of these cases has involved toxicology issues.

14.3.1 FRYE V. UNITED STATES (FRYE V. UNITED STATES, 1923)

In 1921, James Frye was arrested and tried for the murder of a physician in Washington, DC. At trial the defendant sought to have the results of the so-called "systolic blood pressure deception test" (a crude precursor to the polygraph) introduced to support his claim of innocence. The trial refused and Frye was convicted (see the article by Starrs (1882) for a thorough discussion of this case). He appealed to the Court of Appeals of the District of Columbia which affirmed the trail court's decision and stated:

> *Just when a scientific principle or discovery crosses the line between the experimental and demonstrable stages is difficult to define. Somewhere in this twilight zone the evidential force of the principle must be recognized, and while courts will go a long way in admitting expert testimony deduced from a well-recognized scientific principle or discovery, the thing from which the deduction is made must be sufficiently established to have gained **general acceptance in the particular field in which it belongs**. (Emphasis added)*

This decision of the appellate court, which came to be known as the Frye rule, was the widely held standard of the admissibility of scientific evidence for decades, largely until the Daubert decision.

14.3.2 PEOPLE V. WILLIAMS (PEOPLE V. WILLIAMS, 1958)

Iverson Williams was convicted of the use of narcotics in part on the basis of the results of the Nalline test that was administered to him. The administration of the narcotic antagonist Nalline to a person who had used a narcotic recently would result in a measurable dilation of that person's pupil due to the reversal of the narcotic effect of papillary constriction. Williams appealed his conviction on the basis that the admission of the results of the Nalline constituted prejudicial error. Although the court concluded that the Nalline test had not attained "general acceptance by the medical profession as a whole," the appellate court affirmed the use of the test. The 1958 decision stated:

> *All of the medical testimony points to the reliability of the test. It has been generally accepted by those who would be expected to be familiar with its use. In this age of specialization, more should not be required.*

The court's opinion narrowed the Frye standard so that general acceptance by experts within a field was sufficient for admissibility.

14.3.3 COPPOLINO V. STATE (COPPOLINO V. STATE, 1970)

Carl Coppolino, a physician, was convicted of the murder of his wife by injecting her with the muscle relaxant drug succinylcholine. The toxicological testimony presented at trial was based on the detection of the metabolites of this drug in greater than normal concentrations in the decedent's body. Coppolino appealed the decision and argued that the method used for the detection of the metabolites was a novel test that had been developed for this case and did not meet the acceptance standards of either the Frye or Williams cases. The decision of the Florida Supreme Court stated:

> *The tests by which the medical examiner sought to determine whether the death was caused by succinylcholine chloride were novel and devised specifically for this case. This does not render the evidence inadmissible. Society need not tolerate homicide until there develops a body of medical knowledge about some particular lethal agent. The expert witnesses were examined and cross-examined at great length and the jury could either believe or doubt the prosecution's testimony as it chose.*

14.3.4 DAUBERT V. MERRELL DOW PHARMACEUTICALS, INC. (DAUBERT V. MERRELL DOW PHARMACEUTICALS, 1993)

Jason Daubert and Eric Schuller brought suit against Merrell alleging that their limb reduction birth defects were caused by the antinausea drug Bendectin that their mothers had taken while pregnant. An expert for the plaintiffs testified that an epidemiological study he had conducted demonstrated that Bendectin caused limb reduction defects. The US District Court ruled that this was merely a reanalysis of previously published human data and that it was not demonstrated the teratogenicity of Bendectin. Plaintiffs appealed to the United States Court of Appeals for the Ninth Circuit which ruled that

> *… the reanalysis of epidemiological studies is generally accepted by the scientific community only when it is subjected to verification and scrutiny by others in the field. Plaintiffs' reanalyses do not comply with this standard; they were unpublished, not subjected to the normal peer review process, and generated solely for litigation.*

The US Supreme Court granted certiorari in 1992 and delivered an opinion in which it held that the Federal Rules of Evidence and not Frye v. United States "occupy the field."

> *Faced with a proffer of expert scientific testimony under Rule 702, the trial judge, pursuant to Rule 1049(a), must make a preliminary assessment of whether the testimony's underlying reasoning or methodology is scientifically valid and properly can be applied to the facts at issue. Many considerations will bear on the inquiry, including whether the theory or technique in question can be (and has been) tested, whether it has been subjected to peer review and publication, its known or potential error rate, and the existence and maintenance of standards*

controlling its operation, and whether it has attracted widespread acceptance within a relevant scientific community. The inquiry is a flexible one, and its focus must be solely on principles and methodology, not on the conclusions that they generate.

The Court in recognizing that this ruling might limit the admission of valid scientific testimony opined that "… the rules are not designed to seek cosmic understanding but, rather, to resolve legal disputes."

In summary, the Court held that "good science" was the test of admissibility. The burden that this placed on trial judges was expressed by Judge Kozinski of the Ninth Circuit (Kaufman, 2001).

We judges are largely untrained in science and certainly no match for any of the witnesses whose testimony we are reviewing.

Our responsibility, then, unless we badly misread the Supreme Court's opinion, is to resolve disputes among well-credentialed scientists about matters squarely within their expertise, in areas where there is no scientific consensus as to what is and what not is "good science," and occasionally to reject such expert testimony because it was not "derived by the scientific method."

Mindful of our position in the hierarchy of the federal judiciary, we take a deep breath and proceed with this heady task.

14.4 EXPERT TESTIMONY

Expert witnesses are in unique positions because they have one foot in the laboratory and one foot in the courtroom, these are different worlds—entirely different worlds. The role of expert witnesses is to aid the trier of fact by providing or explaining evidence in areas that are outside of the purview of the lay person. Experts should never act as advocates for either the prosecution or defense. Their roles are those of impartial scientists whose only function is to provide honest information and opinions to the trier of fact. Guilt or innocence is not their professional concern. However, when they enter a courtroom, experts find themselves in an adversarial system in which their testimony will be carefully examined by an advocate who wishes to minimize the impact of this testimony by eliciting its shortcomings through intense cross-examination (Burney, 2002).

When forensic toxicologists testify as expert witnesses, they are permitted to present both factual and opinion testimony. Allowing experts to provide opinion testimony dates to the eighteenth century (Of Interest 14.3). As scientists, expert witnesses have been educated and trained in the methods of scientific inquiry and have been held to the relatively high standards of proof of scientific inquiry. Forensic scientists, with that background, enter a courtroom in which, generally, they are the only scientists present and in which the standards differ from those in the scientific community. Therefore, they will be presenting scientific information to nonscientists

---

OF INTEREST 14.3 HISTORY OF EXPERT WITNESS TESTIMONY

Until the late eighteenth century in England, persons who possessed special knowledge, education, and skills in their particular science or art traditionally appeared in court only at the request of the Court, either as part of the jury or as advisors to the Court. These individuals were not designated or defined as experts or differentiated in any way from lay witnesses, and could testify as to their opinions only if based on their direct knowledge of the facts. A person with expert knowledge would most likely have to be found in the area in which the case was filed in order to qualify to testify.

In 1782, the case of **Folkes v. Chadd**, known as the "Wells Harbor" case, changed the legal status of expert witnesses and laid the foundation for rules governing expert evidence. Expert witnesses no longer served as jurors or Court advisors as they had in the past, but now appeared as partisan witnesses called by parties in support of their case. The issue in the Wells Harbor case concerned the cause of decay of the harbor serving the city of Wells. In question was whether the decay was due to a slow, natural process or the result of the erection of embankments by plaintiffs on surrounding land which allegedly prevented the entry of water and the ability of ships to navigate to the harbor. In allowing civil engineering experts to testify in behalf of the parties, the Court held that "professional men, when examined on the subject of their art or science are of necessity allowed to state their opinion."

It has been suggested that the true issue in this case was the legal status of Newtonian (natural) philosophers. Some believed that only those experts who believed in natural law and were familiar with the particular facts in question should be permitted to testify, but the Wells Harbor Court believed that all kinds of science should be heard in court where the experts could give unbiased opinions subject to cross-examination. This case was said to be "a junction where the expanding late eighteenth-century cultures of law and science finally crossed paths."

Tal Golan, 2004. Laws of Men and Laws of Nature, Harvard University Press, Cambridge, pp. 44–50.

---

in a nonscientific setting. There are differences between legal facts and scientific facts. A legal fact is the evidence that has been introduced and accepted in a case and, at least for that case, is a virtual absolute. However, scientists know there are few, if any, absolute facts and whereas there are many scientific theories, there are few scientific laws. They know that most theories have been altered as additional knowledge is gained. Courts are aware of these limitations and generally have established standards of expert testimony which allow scientific experts to present opinions that they hold with a "reasonable scientific certainty" or "a reasonable scientific probability." These standards have different meanings in the law and in science.

Usually, factual testimony consists of what experts have done, e.g., analyses conducted, files reviewed, etc. Their opinions are the interpretations and conclusions they have been able to draw from the facts, e.g., the concentration of drug X detected in the blood of the defendant is consistent with physical impairment. The direct examination of a forensic toxicologist by a prosecutor might include the following questions and answers, which elicit information concerning the blood ethanol concentration (BAC) (facts) and the interpretation of that concentration (opinion).

Q: Did you have occasion to analyze a blood sample collected from the defendant?
A: Yes.

Q: What are the results of that analysis?

A: I determined that the blood contained ethanol in a concentration of 0.23%.

Q: Do you have an opinion as to the effect of that blood ethanol concentration?

A: Yes.

Q: What is that opinion?

A: It is my opinion that this blood concentration of ethanol is consistent with physical impairment, alteration of behavior, and impairment of judgment.

It is not unusual that experts in forensic toxicology present differing opinions based on their interpretations of the same evidence (Chapters 12 and 13). This results in a "battle of the experts" in which the casualties are the jurors, judges, and the parties in the case all of whom are challenged to determine which opinion is accurate in areas in which they have no competence and which apparently is sufficiently complex that the experts cannot agree. This is ironic since the reason that the experts are allowed to testify and to provide opinion testimony is to provide information to assist the trier of fact in understanding the evidence. There are two primary reasons that experts disagree. First, it is possible that because the evidence is limited or conflicting the judgment of the experts differs as to the significance or meaning of the evidence. For example, one of the experts may assign greater value to the results of blood concentrations and the other to the signs and symptoms of the subject. This difference of opinion may be due to the complexity of the case or to the incompetence of one or both of the experts. In either case, the differences are based on honest (albeit possibly incompetent) opinions.

Unfortunately, the second reason for opposing opinions is an unpleasant truth: there are forensic scientists who knowingly provide expert opinions that are slanted or undeniably false. The obvious reason that these experts lie is that they have been paid to do so. The most important quality that expert witnesses must possess is honesty—they must provide honest and unbiased testimony. They must tell the truth. "The one-eyed man is king in the land of the blind" often pertains to experts in a courtroom since often they are the only persons in the courtroom who understand what the testimony means. Therefore, the presentation of biased or false testimony is often unchallenged (unless the opposing side has an expert of its own) and is virtually sanctified as a result of the witness providing such testimony having been designated as an expert by the judge.

14.4.1 BE PREPARED

There is no substitute for preparation—prepare, prepare, prepare! Experts must be well prepared for each and every court appearance and should master the material about which they are to testify. They should never assume that any appearance will be "routine," but rather must be prepared to discuss the evidence they received and analyzed, the scientific principles behind the tests they conducted, the procedures of the tests they conducted, the conclusions, and the basis for them. Furthermore, experts should be prepared to defend their conclusions/opinions and to discuss reasons that they rejected other possible conclusions and opinions. Prior to trial, experts should review their proposed testimony, develop a line of questions that they would ask if they were the opposing attorney, and prepare answers to them.

Experts never should assume that the attorneys who will cross-examine them are not as knowledgeable as they are since the attorney may have been briefed by scientists who are as knowledgeable as the experts.

14.4.2 DEVELOP A LINE OF QUESTIONING PRIOR TO TRIAL

Forensic toxicologists must discuss several aspects of their testimony with the attorneys who will call them as witnesses. The discussion should include the specific testimony that the expert is willing to provide as well as the strengths and weaknesses of the testimony. Often, attorneys are not familiar with the specialties of their experts and, therefore, it is therefore essential that the experts explain to the attorneys both the reasoning by which they formulated their opinions as well as the extent to which these opinions can be extended. Experts should assist the attorney in formulating the questions that should be asked on direct examination. A coherent line of questioning that presents both the foundation for the expert opinions, as well as the opinions, in a clear, logical, and easy-to-follow manner should be formulated. Often the questions for direct examination, as well as the anticipated answers, are written. This written "script" not only allows the attorney to ask the appropriate questions in the appropriate order, but also prepares the expert for the specific questions to be asked. Further, the "script" alerts the attorney if the answer given by the expert is not what was agreed upon. In addition, experts should anticipate questions that might be asked by the opposing attorney during the cross-examination and should provide questions that can be asked on redirect to counter those questions.

14.5 THE DOS AND DON'TS OF EXPERT TESTIFYING

What follows is a summary of some of the most important aspects of providing effective expert testimony.

14.5.1 TELL THE TRUTH

The cardinal responsibility of an expert witness is to tell the truth. An expert must tell the truth if the jury is to be aided in making a decision. In addition, experts have taken an oath to tell the truth, the whole truth, and nothing but the truth, and a violation of that oath by not telling the truth can lead to a prosecution for perjury. It should not be difficult to tell the truth and nothing but the truth, although as discussed above it is a problem for some exerts.

However, telling the *whole* truth can be difficult if not impossible. For example, how can a forensic toxicologist tell the whole truth in response to the following question: "Will you please explain the metabolism of ethanol?" Books have been written on this topic. Experts cannot and are not expected to tell "the whole truth" by reciting the entire scientific body of knowledge or everything that they know about the metabolism of ethanol. Therefore, there are aspects of the metabolism of ethanol that should be omitted, not only for brevity but also in the interest of clarity since too many minutiae may confuse the jurors and prevent them from extracting the salient information relevant to their decision-making. Therefore, an abbreviated answer must be given. However, the abbreviated answer must contain the information that is needed by the jury in order to understand the issue adequately and to render a decision. What should be omitted? It is easier to determine what should not be omitted. It is essential that information of a probative value is not omitted, i.e., aspects of this topic that are relevant and important, so that the trier of fact can adequately understand the testimony and draw valid conclusions. Expert witnesses must not eliminate anything from their testimony simply because it does not agree with their opinions, nor can they eliminate that information because it may buttress opposing opinions. Nothing of probative value, *i.e.*, nothing that will aid the trier of fact in the decision-making process should be omitted.

Nobody knows everything (although there are experts who apparently believe that they do). All experts will be asked questions that they are unable to answer. They should admit this shortcoming without hesitation or embarrassment. Experts who attempt to answer a question if they are uncertain of the correct answer are digging holes for themselves; the holes will get deeper and deeper as the attorney recognizes the situation and continues the line of questioning on this topic. "I don't know" is a perfectly acceptable answer and has the added advantage of limiting any further questioning on that specific topic. Of course, an excess of "I don't know" answers may call purported expertise into question. In many cases, experts may feel that they should be able to provide an answer to a question, but are unable to do so because they have forgotten the correct answer to the specific question asked. What can be an effective admission of ignorance was the answer used by an expert in psychiatry who was once asked a question in the area of his expertise that he could not answer. He responded, "That's a very good question and I should be able to answer it and at one time I would have been able to answer it, but I have forgotten that information. It's not something which I use frequently or on which I rely." He felt that his answer resonated well with the jury because it was honest and the jury concluded that not only was he a competent expert, but also an honest expert. We all have learned more than we can remember and we should admit it when we have forgotten something that we should know or once knew.

In addition to questions with the field of expertise of expert witnesses, questions of a personal nature that may be embarrassing to answer often are asked. Such questions may include, "How much are you being paid?" "What was your grade in forensic toxicology?" These questions should be answered forthrightly and without evasion, hesitation, or attempts at obfuscation. If your grade was a B−, say so; do not say that it was about a B. "About" is a red flag which will only bring out the shark in many attorneys who will then ask a number of additional questions until you finally admit that it was a B−.

Also, experts should correct errors as soon as they recognize them by simply stating: "I was wrong what I should have said was …"

14.5.2 DO WHAT THE JUDGE SAYS

Do what the judge says. Do everything the judge says. Do not argue with a judge. In all cases and under all circumstances, experts must do what the judge says. Always respond to a judge's instructions courteously—"Yes, your honor." Failure to do so may result in unpleasant consequences, possibly including the failure to make it home for dinner!

An expert who was testifying in federal court was asked by opposing counsel whether he knew what shock was. He answered that he had an opinion, but not an expert opinion since he did not think that it was within the purview of his expertise as a forensic toxicologist. After a bench conference, the judge asked the expert whether he did have an opinion of the definition of shock. The expert responded as he had before and was told by the judge to answer the question—and he did. On another occasion, a defense attorney stood and objected to a question posed by the prosecutor. The judge overruled the objection. The defense attorney apparently taken aback by the judge's ruling remained standing and in a moment of disbelief said, "Wait a minute your honor." The judge responded by saying: "I have ruled on your objection and the court will not wait—sit down." The defense attorney realizing the error and potential consequences of his misdirected enthusiasm sat down.

Do what the judge says.

14.5.3 BE PROFESSIONAL

Most jurors have never seen a scientist. Their concept of a scientist may be based on the actor, in a white lab coat, on a television ad who explains the "science" behind the effectiveness of an antacid. Although their vision may be misguided, the jurors may have in their mind's eye an idea of what a scientist looks like. The vision includes a certain manner of dress, speech, language, and general deportment—how the experts sit in the witness chair, their tone of voice, their dress, etc. Both male and female expert witnesses would be well advised to dress in a professional manner and demonstrate a neat and well-groomed personal appearance. When experts are called to the courtroom to testify, they will walk from the door of the courtroom to the witness stand. During the minute or so that it takes to reach the witness stand, jurors will be watching and evaluating the experts' appearance and deportment and may have already formed an opinion as to whether they want to listen to what the expert has to say.

Jurors will respond to information other than the testimony itself in making their decision as to whether to believe the expert (Rosenthal, 1983).

Communications to jurors entail not only primary *content—the subject matter of the testimony—designated as the* message, *but also* secondary *content emanating from the witnesses as sources, from peripheral aspects of the message itself, and from the environment of the trial—designated as the* para message.

The general implication is that when confronted with complex or confusing testimony, expert or otherwise, jurors will shift their focus to observable characteristics of the sources of information, or to other ancillary elements of the situation, and will be guided in their response by information and inferences derived from such data.

A witness from Stanford University was extremely articulate, his hair was short and trim, he wore glasses and a brown business suit, and presented himself in a very conservative and positive way. What struck me about the jury's response to the witness was the universal perception that he was "a real scientist." "Some of the others looked like hippies." "This guy was real scientist … I could tell," were typical comments.

Under no circumstance, even if their integrity or competence is impugned, should experts, lose their self-control, lose their tempers, raise their voices above normal volume, get into a shouting match, respond in kind to snide or sarcastic questions, or act impolitely in manner or speech.

14.5.4 ATTEMPT TO EDUCATE THE JURY

Experts are in the courtroom to assist the trier of fact in understanding scientific or technical evidence that is beyond their knowledge or experience. The most efficient method of achieving this goal is to educate the trier of fact. The expert is not in court to impress the jury, but rather to present and explain scientific evidence in such a manner that it is understandable by the jurors and judge, the majority of who do not understand the language or principles of science. Therefore, this is a teaching role for experts and a learning experience for the jury. To accomplish this, the evidence must be presented using language and concepts appropriate for a nonscientific population. This is to be done without "talking down" to, but rather by "talking to," the jury. Experts are present to inform the judge and jury and should do so in their terms.

The expert must be prepared to present definitions of scientific terms in a manner consistent with conversational English. For example, a definition of scientific words or phrases should be 25 words or less, should not contain scientific or technical terms of art, and should be understood by a person with the scientific knowledge of a seventh grader. For example, a forensic toxicologist may be asked to define alcohol dehydrogenase. One potential answer might be "ADH is an NAD-requiring enzyme that metabolizes ethanol into its oxidation product acetaldehyde." This answer is correct, but probably is unintelligible to most jury members simply because it contains several words that are not common to a lay person, i.e., NAD, enzyme, metabolizes, oxidation, and acetaldehyde. A better answer might be, "Alcohol dehydrogenase, also known as ADH, controls the breakdown of ethanol in the body into another substance." Of course, experts should be prepared to expand this definition and discuss the concepts in greater detail if asked to do so, but whenever possible explanations should be made in the language of the jury. It is a good idea for forensic toxicologists to prepare "boilerplate" definitions of terms and phrases that they will be asked to define on a regular basis in court, e.g., forensic toxicology, central nervous system, drug. They should practice these definitions with friends and relatives who do not have a science background until they have developed definitions that are accurate and understandable. Experts not only have the duty to present information that is probative and accurate, but also they must do so in a manner that is understood by the jurors. It is important to remember that the trier of fact will find it difficult to accept the testimony of an expert if the testimony has not been understood.

Frequently in a jury trial, it is a good idea to provide a few minutes what might be called "foundational testimony" in which experts present the concepts that are the foundation for their subsequent testimony. For example, experts in forensic toxicology frequently testify in cases involving ethanol, and the foundational testimony in these cases might include an overview of the basic toxicology of ethanol. The few minutes required to do this improves the testimony in several ways. First, experts are provided with an opportunity to briefly discuss the foundation of their subsequent testimony so that the jury will better understand the basis for the conclusions they have drawn. This provides the members of the jury and the judge with an opportunity to evaluate the experts' competence to provide expert opinions on which they should rely. For example, if experts are to testify as to the interpretation of a BAC, they might first provide a discussion of the disposition of ethanol in the human body and an explanation of why the BAC can be correlated with the effects produced by ethanol. Generally, one or more members of the jury will find this information to be informative and interesting since it is likely that they, or someone they know, drink ethanol and it might be of reasonable interest to know what happens after ethanol is consumed! Second, not only will the jurors have an opportunity to determine whether experts have the requisite expertise, but also whether they can explain the scientific material to them in a manner that they will understand. Experts who cannot explain their disciplines and opinions in language that is accessible to jurors are not of much value. Third, during this "lecture" on the pharmacology and toxicology of ethanol, experts are afforded an opportunity to observe how their testimony is being received and to identify those jurors who are interested and paying attention. Not all jurors are interested in what experts have to say and often they wish to be elsewhere. However, generally one or more of the jurors will be interested in the testimony as evidenced by them looking at the experts, taking notes, nodding in agreement as the experts speak, and occasionally even sitting on the edges of their seats. These are the jurors to whom experts should direct their evidentiary testimony on the specific issues in the case, in the anticipation that these jurors will attempt to understand the testimony and perhaps may be able to explain it to other jurors during the juror deliberation.

A portion of such "foundational testimony" in an ethanol case is presented below.

Q: Dr _____, what is ethanol?

A: Ethanol is the chemical that is a member of a class of chemicals known as alcohols. Ethanol is the alcohol found in all alcoholic beverages.

Q: Dr _____, would you explain to the jury how the body handles ethanol when a person drinks an alcoholic beverage?

A: Certainly. When a person drinks ethanol in any form, the ethanol goes to the stomach and then to the small intestine. From these organs the ethanol is transferred into the circulatory system that is the blood supply of the body. Virtually all of the ethanol that is consumed enters the circulatory system from the stomach and small intestine.

After the ethanol enters the circulatory system, it is transported in the blood throughout the body to all of the organs of the body such as the brain, the liver, and the kidneys.

As the ethanol is circulating throughout the body, it is being changed to other chemicals. This process of changing ethanol to other chemicals is known as metabolism and occurs mainly in the liver. The chemicals into which ethanol is changed cannot produce the same effects as ethanol. Therefore, the metabolism of ethanol is a method by which the body terminates the action of ethanol. The small percent of ethanol that is not metabolized is excreted from the body by the kidneys.

Q: Would you please describe what effects ethanol has on the brain?

A: Yes. Ethanol exerts an inhibitory or depressant effect on the central nervous system or CNS, which includes the brain and the spinal cord. This inhibitory or depressant effect causes the brain to function at a level lower than it would normally function in the absence of ethanol. In other words ethanol prevents the brain from working in a normal manner. When the brain is exposed to ethanol, the ethanol inhibits the normal action of the brain, causing the brain to function in an abnormal manner. As the amount or concentration of ethanol in the blood increases, the effect of ethanol in the brain also increases and the inhibition of normal brain activity also increases. Therefore, the blood concentration of ethanol is related to the inhibition of normal brain activity.

Q: Based on what you have said, would I be correct in concluding that if the BAC is known, the relative extent of the effect on the brain can be determined?

A: Yes.

Q: Have studies been conducted in which the BAC of persons has been correlated with their physical and behavioral actions.

A: Yes.

Q: Doctor you have mentioned that ethanol is a CNS depressant. What does it do to the brain?

A: Ethanol has several adverse effects on the brain that may be observed. These include impairment of physical ability, alteration of behavior, impairment of judgment, and diminished attention to divided tasks.

Q: Doctor could you elaborate on these effects?

A: Certainly. The impairment of physical activity is consistent with a loss of visual acuity, diminished physical coordination, and an increase in reaction time, that is, it would take longer to react to a stimulus or an event. For example, it would take longer to apply the brakes in an emergency.

The alteration of behavior may be manifest in a variety of ways. Some persons become very silly, others become aggressive, and still others become morose. Although the alteration may vary from person to person, the behavior while under the influence of ethanol is not normal.

By impaired judgment, I mean that a person under the influence of ethanol is not able to process information in a normal manner and take appropriate action. The classic example is that a person who has been drinking all night thinks that he is able to drive a car. Diminished attention to divided tasks refers to the inability to apply appropriate attention to each of several tasks simultaneously. A good example is that a person who is under the influence of ethanol may concentrate on steering the car and keeping a tight grip on the steering wheel, but pay little attention to the speed of the car.

14.5.5 ANSWER THE QUESTION

The role of experts is to aid the trier of fact by answering questions. The role of attorneys is to elicit the information that they think is relevant by asking questions. Therefore, experts **should answer questions that are asked** and not questions that they think have been asked or that they think should have been asked. Students and new forensic scientists often have difficulty in doing this; they have a tendency to add additional information that extends beyond the scope of the question.

In order to answer a question, experts must wait until they have heard and understood the entire question. Some experts have a tendency to answer the question before it has been asked completely because they think that they know what the question will be. This is a dangerous practice since it may confuse the jury if the answer is not responsive to the question that was to be asked. On the old TV show "Name That Tune," contestants were rewarded if they could identify the name of a song after having heard just a few notes. However, in the courtroom there is no reward for attempting to answer a question before the question has been asked in its entirety.

After the question has been asked, experts must ensure that they have understood the question; if they do not understand the question, they should ask for clarification. There are several ways of asking for clarification, including the simplest and most direct: "I'm sorry I don't understand the question, would you please repeat it or rephrase it for me?" Experts should not ask for clarification by providing one or more possible interpretations of the answer: "Do you mean …"; "I'm not sure that I understand the question, but I think you mean …" Attorneys should be allowed to clarify the question that they wish to ask.

Of course, experts must be certain that they do not attempt to answer any question based on the materials, e.g., text books, journal articles, theories, and their own testimony in prior cases, with which they are unfamiliar or that they have forgotten. They should ask to see—May I see the material from which you are reading (which you are quoting)?—and they should review the materials e.g., books, articles, text book chapters, or a transcript of an expert's prior testimony in another case, about which the attorney is asking questions.

Once the question has been asked and understood, experts should take a few seconds to organize their thoughts before answering. This is to ensure that their answer is accurate and presented in a logical, easy-to-follow manner and that their brains and mouths are synchronized. These few seconds may seem like an eternity since the attorneys, the judge, the jury, and the gallery are awaiting an answer. However, this interval is vital since it will minimize the likelihood of incorrect answers and increase the likelihood of coherent, organized, reasoned, and deliberate answers. Remember, extra points are not awarded for speed.

When the answer is given it should be in a measured volume and pace. The jury must hear and understand the answer. Experts should speak slower than their normal conversational speed since their answer may contain terms and concepts with which the jury is unfamiliar and it will take them some time to process what they have heard. The jury members are not scientists but rather lay persons who are unfamiliar with the subject matter.

The answer to the question should answer the question—nothing more. For example, the correct answer to the question, "Do you have an opinion as to the effects that are consistent with a 0.23% BAC?" is "Yes or No," as opposed to "Yes, it is consistent with impairment of behavior, judgment, and physical coordination." The question asked was "**Do you** have an opinion?" **not what is your opinion**. If attorneys wish additional information, they will ask—they are not bashful.

After answering a question, experts must wait for the next question; they should not feel a need to fill a quiet void in the courtroom. They have done their immediate job; they have answered the question asked. The ball is now in the attorney's court to ask the next question and fill the void.

Experts must be careful not to attempt to answer questions outside of their area of expertise. For example, a forensic toxicologist may be asked if the death of a person in whom a drug was detected was caused by that drug. Questions such as this that are directed at the cause of death are outside of the purview of the forensic toxicologist. "I'm sorry but that is outside of my area of expertise" is a reasonable response to such questions. The forensic toxicologist may decide to offer the further opinion that the concentration of the drug was consistent with a lethal concentration, an entirely appropriate opinion for forensic toxicologists, but they must never opine as to the cause of death.

14.5.6 USE PROPER LANGUAGE

Experts must minimize some of the bad habits of everyday speech, e.g., "Uh-Uh" and "You know." These utterances are attempts to keep the mouth at the same speed as the thought process of the brain. Speaking slowly will help to eliminate these annoying expressions, which if not eliminated become the focal point of the testimony. No slang, technical terms or terms of art should be used unless they have been fully defined or explained. The lay jurors are not familiar with and will not understand such language.

Vague language should not be used, e.g., "… or something like that," "… there may be better examples," "… I think that it does," "… I saw what I thought was a peak on the chromatogram." This language is confusing to the jurors who cannot judge the import of such weak statements. The expert should testify to a reasonable scientific probability and do so with confidence and clarity.

Experts must be able to pronounce, spell, and define all scientific and technical words and phrases properly. The expertise of expert witnesses who use words and phrases that they cannot pronounce, spell, or define is rightfully suspect, and jurors may lose confidence in the validity of the testimony being offered. For the forensic toxicologist, this includes several scientific words and phrases that they routinely will be asked to define and spell such as toxicologist, alcohol dehydrogenase, acetyl-cholinesterase, and glucuronide.

At all times experts should use words carefully. As has been said many times, "words have meaning, they have consequences."

14.5.7 BEWARE OF "TRICK" QUESTIONS

Experts must listen very carefully to the questions asked in order to avoid falling for an artfully phrased question designed to confuse or trick them. Experts must remember the adage that "the devil is in the details." There may be a trap, a catch, or a trick in the way that a question is phrased. The question may be formulated to confuse, embarrass, or divert the expert from the testimony at hand. Beware of the details.

Some examples of these types of questions are presented below, along with reasonable responses.

Loaded Questions

Q: "Have you ever made a mistake?"

A: "Probably. But I have no reason to believe that I did so in this case. I followed accepted methods of analysis that have been evaluated and found to be reliable in our laboratory."

Questions that Cannot Be Answered

Q: "Answer this question yes or no."

A: "I know that because you want a thorough and clear answer to that question, I can't answer it with a simple yes or no answer."

Questions with Faulty Premises

Q: "Let me ask you to assume ..." (The assumptions are irrational.)

A: "I'm sorry but your assumptions are irrational and I can't give you an answer based on irrational assumptions."

Questions Based on Past Lab Performance

Q: "Is your laboratory still making the type of errors it made in the _____ case?"

A: "That case has been thoroughly reviewed as have many others like it. It was the only error of its type that was made. In the 5 years since that case no such error has been made."

Questions Not Based on Acceptable Standard of Proof

Q: "Is it possible that the defendant was sober and not impaired as you have testified?"

A: "Although it is not theoretically impossible that the defendant was sober, it is my opinion with a reasonable scientific certainty that the defendant's blood ethanol concentration was consistent with impairment."

Intentionally Confusing Questions

Q: "You're not telling the jury that the defendant hadn't been smoking any marihuana, are you, or aren't you?"

A: "It is my opinion with a reasonable scientific probability that the defendant had smoked marihuana prior to a sample being collected from him."

REVIEW QUESTIONS

1. Define and describe the process of *voir dire*.
2. The cardinal responsibility of an expert witness is to tell the truth. However, it is often difficult for an expert to tell "the whole truth." Why?
3. Discuss the ways in which the role of an expert witness is similar to the role of a teacher.
4. If you, as a forensic toxicologist, are called upon by a defense attorney to testify on behalf of his client, is it your responsibility to act as an advocate for the client? Why or why not?
5. Imagine that you are called upon to testify as an expert witness in a case. How would you prepare for your testimony? What type of information would you need to gather and/or analyze? What documents would you collect? With whom would you speak prior to the court date?

APPLICATION QUESTIONS

1. Although judges have the ultimate responsibility for evaluating the overall qualifications of an expert witness, there are several criteria that are utilized to determine whether a proposed expert possesses the requisite qualifications to serve in an expert witness capacity. Describe the criteria that generally must be met by a forensic toxicologist in order to be deemed "qualified" to testify as an expert.

2. Describe one landmark court case in which the ruling of the case helped to delineate the types of evidence that may be rendered by expert witnesses.
3. Describe the major differences between scientific testimony and expert testimony.
4. In their function as expert witnesses, forensic toxicologists must often work closely with the attorney who has called them. Describe the types of interactions that you, as a forensic toxicologist, might have with an attorney. What are your responsibilities when interacting with an attorney? What information or advice should you provide to the attorney with whom you are interacting?

REFERENCES

Burney, I.A., 2002. Testing testimony: toxicology and the law of evidence in early nineteenth-century England. Stud. Hist. Phil. Sci. 33, 289–314.

Burney, I.A., 2006. Poison, Detection and the Victorian Imagination. Manchester University Press, New York.

Cole, S.A., 2015. A surfeit of science: the "CSI effect" and the media appropriation of the public understanding of science. Public Understanding Sci. (Bristol, England) 24 (2), 130–146.

Coppolino v. State: 223 so.2d 68 (Fla. Dist. Ct. App. 1968, App. Dismissed, 234 so.2d 120 (Fla. 1969), Cert. Denied, 399 U.S. 927 (1970).

Daubert v. Merrell Dow Pharmaceuticals; 951 F,2d 1128 (1991), 61 LW 4805, (1993).

Fed R. Evid. 702(a)(b)(c)(d); (2015).

Frye v. United States: 293 F. 1013 (D.C. Cir. 1923), (1923).

Kaufman, H.H., 2001. The expert witness. Neither Frye nor Daubert solved the problem: what can be done? [Electronic version]. Sci. Justice: J. For. Sci. Soc. 41 (1), 7–20.

People v. Williams; 331P.2d 251, 164 Cal. App.2d Supp. 1958, (1958).

Rosenthal, P., 1983. Nature of jury response to the expert witness. J. For. Sci. 28, 528–531.

Shelton, D.E., 2012. Forensic Science Evidence: Can the Law Keep up with Science? LFB Scholarly Publishing, El Paso.

Starrs, J.E., 1882. A still-life watercolor: frye v united states. J. For. Sci. 27, 684–694.

Walsh, E., Gellman, B., August 23, 1990. Chasm Divided Jurors in Barry Drug Trial. The Washington Post, pp. A01.

Principles of Pharmacokinetics

A familiarity with the fundamentals of pharmacokinetics is essential for the modern forensic toxicologist. Drug disposition is the term used to describe the four major events that occur after the administration of a drug or exposure to a chemical—absorption, distribution, metabolism, and excretion. The rate at which these four events of drug disposition occur is known as pharmacokinetics. This chapter will present the basic principles of pharmacokinetics that are relevant to the forensic toxicologist.

A.1 INTRODUCTION

The effect of a drug can be defined as local or systemic. A local reaction is one that takes place at the specific site of application, such as the gastrointestinal tract (GIT) in the case of oral administration or the epithelial layer in the case of topical application. Systemic effects are effects that are produced at a site other than the site of application. For example, the oral administration of an analgesic agent, which effectively applies the drug to the GIT, may have an effect on a distant location such as the brain. Forensic toxicologists generally are interested in drugs that elicit systemic effects, rather than local effects.

Drug disposition is a term that is used to describe the four major events that occur after a drug has been administered; these events include absorption, distribution, metabolism, and excretion. In order for a drug to produce a systemic effect it must enter the circulatory system; that is, it must undergo the process of absorption.[1] A drug that is absorbed into the circulatory system is then transported to other sites throughout the body, leaves the circulatory system, and enters organs and tissues; this is the process of distribution. Following distribution, a drug may remain as an unmodified free drug, or it may be modified through one of more chemical reactions during the process of metabolism. Finally, the drug and/or its metabolites will reenter the circulatory system and will be eliminated from the body by various mechanisms of excretion. An understanding of the mechanisms of these four dispositional events is of the utmost importance to forensic toxicologists.

---

[1]This is true for all routes of administration other than those by which the drug is introduced directly into the circulatory system, e.g., intravenous administration by which the drug is introduced directly through a vein into the circulatory system.

A.2 ACID—BASE CHEMISTRY

Many drugs are weak acids or weak bases and can therefore exist in both nonionized and ionized forms at the physiological pH values in various locations in the body. Because nonionized forms of drugs are more likely to diffuse across cellular membranes, it is important to understand the effect that pH has on the ratio of the ionized to the nonionized forms, as this will influence the disposition of the drug.

According to the Arrhenius theory of acids and bases, acids are substances that dissociate in aqueous solutions to produce hydrogen ions, whereas bases are substances that dissociate in aqueous solutions to produce hydroxyl ions. The Bronsted—Lowry acid—base definition specifies that acids are proton donors and bases are proton acceptors.

The equilibrium dissociation constant, K_a, for an acid or a base is a quantitative measure of the amount of dissociation in aqueous solutions. For weak acids, the ionization is represented as

$$AH \overset{K_a}{\rightleftharpoons} A^- + H^+$$

and for weak bases, the ionization reaction is represented as

$$BH^+ \overset{K_a}{\rightleftharpoons} B + H^+$$

Due to the many orders of magnitude that are spanned by dissociation constants for various substances, a logarithmic measure of the constant is commonly used, in which the pK_a for an acid or a base is equal to the negative log of the equilibrium dissociation constant of the acid:

$$pK_a = -\log_{10}K_a$$

The difference between a weak acid and a strong acid is the degree of ionization in water; strong acids undergo significantly more ionization in water than do weak acids, so it follows that the dissociation constants for strong acids in water are relatively high and the dissociation constants for weak acids in water are relatively low. For example, the weak acid, acetylsalicylic acid, has a K_a of approximately 3×10^{-4} and a pK_a of approximately 3.5; an acidic drug with a pKa lower than 3.5 would be considered a stronger acid than acetylsalicylic acid. Conversely, strong bases have higher pK_a values than do weak bases. Many drugs of interest to forensic toxicologists are weak bases that have pK_a values between 7 and 10. It is important to note, however, that a pK_a value alone does not indicate if a substance is an acid or a base; this determination is based upon the chemical structure of the compound.

The Henderson—Hasselbalch equation allows for the degree of ionization of acids and bases to be determined at various pH values. The Henderson—Hasselbalch equation for an acid is expressed as

$$pK_a = pH + \log_{10}\frac{[AH]}{[A^-]}$$

and the Henderson—Hasselbalch equation for a base is expressed as

$$pK_a = pH + \log_{10} \frac{[BH^+]}{[B]}$$

As an example, if acetylsalicylic acid, which has a pK_a of approximately 3.5, is placed in a buffered solution with a pH of 7, the Henderson—Hasselbalch equation predicts that the dissociated conjugate base will predominate. For acids, for every unit the pH of the solution is greater than the pK_a value of the acid, 10 times more of the acid will be ionized as compared to unionized; for every unit the pH of the solution is lower the pK_a value of the acid, 10 times more of the acid will be unionized as compared to ionized. Conversely, for bases, if the pH of the solution is greater than the pK_a of the base the majority of the base will be unionized, and if the pH of the solution is lower than pKa of the base the majority of the base will be ionized. The Henderson—Hasselbalch equation is exceedingly useful for forensic toxicologists because it allows for the prediction of the degree of ionization of drugs in various body compartments, which possess characteristic pH values. This information is important for the determination of the movement of a drug throughout the body as the absorption of a drug is influenced by its ionization state. It is important to note that *the Henderson—Hasselbalch equation is an equilibrium equation* and applies only when a state of equilibrium is present.

A.3 TRANSMEMBRANE MOVEMENT

As a drug is distributed throughout the body it must cross semipermeable cellular membranes, which are comprised of phospholipid bilayers with both integral and peripheral proteins attached, as described by the fluid mosaic model. A subset of integral membrane proteins includes transmembrane proteins, which belong to several functional classes including receptor proteins and transport proteins. Plasma membranes are fluid structures with dynamic and changing microenvironments.

Although there are several mechanisms by which a drug may transverse a semipermeable membrane, the most common mechanism of transport is diffusion. Diffusion is a form of passive transport by which substances move across a membrane from a region of high concentration to a region of lower concentration. Generally only small, uncharged, lipid-soluble drugs may cross cellular membranes via diffusion. The rate at which a drug crosses a cell membrane is directly proportional to the concentration gradient of the drug across the membrane, the surface area of the membrane, and the partition coefficient of the drug, and is inversely proportional to the distance the drug has to travel across the membrane.

The partition coefficient of a drug is expressed as the solubility of the drug in an organic solvent divided by the solubility of the drug in water:

$$\text{Partition coefficient} = \frac{\text{Solubility of drug in organic solvent}}{\text{Solubility of drug in water}}$$

As the partition coefficient increases, the rate at which a drug crosses a cell membrane also increases. The partition coefficient of a drug can be estimated by adding water, an organic solvent, and the drug of interest to a container such as a separatory funnel, mixing thoroughly, allowing the layers to separate and then determining the concentration of the drug in both the water phase and organic phase. Substances have different partition coefficients in different organic solvents; so to determine the movement of a drug throughout the body, it is necessary to know what the partition coefficient of the drug is in a cellular membrane; it has been found that the partition coefficient for a drug in the cell membrane is approximately equal to what the coefficient is for the drug in olive oil. Because the unionized forms of drugs are more lipid soluble than the ionized forms, it predicted that the ionized form would predominate in the water phase and the unionized form of the drug would predominate in the organic phase of a separation.

In addition to simple diffusion, drugs may also be transported across cellular membranes through facilitated diffusion mediated either by channel proteins or carrier proteins. Both types of facilitated diffusion are passive processes in which transmembrane proteins facilitate the movement of substances down their concentration gradients from a region of high concentration to a region of low concentration. Drugs may also be transported across cell membranes up their concentration gradients via active transport. Active transport is mediated by transmembrane transport proteins that utilize energy from the hydrolysis of the high-energy bonds in ATP to move substances from an area of low concentration to an area of high concentration. Active transport is responsible for only a minority of the movement of drugs into and out of cells. Finally, drugs may be moved into cells via endocytosis and/or out of cells via exocytosis.

A.4 ABSORPTION

The first event of drug disposition is absorption, the process by which drugs enter the circulatory system. Unless a drug is administered directly into the circulatory system, it must be able to cross cellular membranes in order to be absorbed into the circulatory system.

The pathway by which drugs enter the circulation is influenced by several factors including the route of administration, the lipid solubility of the drug, the pK_a of the drug, and the pH of the physiological fluid in which it is located, which vary in different body compartments. For example, the approximate pH values in the stomach, the small intestine, and the blood are 2, 7, and 7.4, respectively. In order for a drug to move throughout the body by diffusion, for example, from the stomach or small intestine into the circulatory system and then the cells, the drug must be in a nonionized form. Therefore, the rate of diffusion of a drug throughout the body is dependent upon the pH of the body compartment, the relative degree of ionization of the drug, and the partition coefficient of the drug.

Although there are several routes by which drugs may be administered, those of foremost interest to forensic toxicologists include the oral, intravenous, and inhalational routes.

A.4.1 ORAL ADMINISTRATION

Oral administration is one of the most common routes of drug administration and results in the passage of the drug through the GIT. Although dependent upon the acid—base chemistry of the drug, in general, the absorption of orally administered drugs occurs primarily in the stomach and small intestine. When absorbed from the GIT, drugs enter the surrounding capillaries, which drain into the portal vein, which carries blood to the liver where the hepatic vein empties into the inferior vena cava and ultimately into the heart. Orally administered drugs may be metabolized in the stomach or liver before they enter the systemic circulation, this is known as first-pass metabolism. Before reaching the heart, orally administered drugs reside in a state of localized circulation between the GIT and the liver, termed enterohepatic circulation.

The oral availability of a drug is therefore dependent upon both its stability in the GIT as well as its ability to be absorbed from this compartment. For example, drugs that are proteins, such as insulin, may be degraded in the low pH of the stomach. Highly lipid-soluble drugs, such as Δ9-tetrahydrocannabinol, do not dissolve well in aqueous solutions, and therefore cannot be absorbed well from the GIT. Drug formulations often take these factors into consideration and are designed to regulate the rate of dissolution, and thus the rate of absorption, of a drug in the GIT. To elicit a physiological effect, orally administered drugs must first dissolve and be absorbed before finally traversing through enterohepatic circulation to enter systemic circulation to be transported to a target site; the onset of action of oral administration is thus often relatively slow as compared to intravenous or inhalational drug administration.

A.4.2 INTRAVENOUS ADMINISTRATION

Absorption is not necessary following intravenous administration because the drug is introduced directly into systemic circulation. However, in order for a drug to be administered intravenously, it must be prepared in soluble form because undissolved materials cannot be injected into a vein. After intravenous injection, drugs are carried through the venous system to the vena cava and ultimately the heart, so the rate at which a drug enters systemic circulation is much greater than following oral administration. The amount of drug that reaches a target site per unit of time influences not only the degree of effect that is elicited but also the type of effect. Therefore, a drug that is administered via intravenous administration has the potential to elicit both quantitatively and qualitatively different effects than would be achieved via oral administration. A potential disadvantage of intravenous drug administration is a relatively short duration of action as compared to oral administration, due to the rapid peak and decline of drug concentrations in the blood.

A.4.3 INHALATIONAL ADMINISTRATION

Only drugs that can be volatilized without being destroyed by the volatilization process can be administered via inhalation. The volatilization of a substance is achieved by heating, and most drugs that can be volatilized are in the freebase, or nonionic form. When a drug is inhaled, the site of entry into the body is the lungs, which are comprised of many alveoli that have a rich capillary system, resulting in a rapid and extensive absorption of volatilized drugs. Drugs thus absorbed enter the systemic circulation quickly and are carried to target sites rapidly and in high concentration. For these reasons, the onset of action, duration of action, and effects elicited from inhalational administration are generally similar to intravenous administration, with the added benefit of increased safety, especially in the case of shared needles among drug abusers.

A.5 DISTRIBUTION

After a drug is absorbed into systemic circulation it can be distributed throughout the body to various cells and tissues. Drug disposition is influenced by many factors, including the lipid solubility of the drug, its ionization state, its size, and pH. As discussed previously, drugs that are small, uncharged, and highly lipid soluble more freely cross cell membranes and are therefore more readily distributed out of capillaries and into tissue. An additional factor that modulates the transport of drugs out of the circulation and into target cells and tissue is plasma protein binding. When a drug enters the circulatory system it has the potential to interact with various plasma proteins including the most abundant protein found in blood plasma, albumin. The binding of drugs to plasma proteins is considered nonspecific binding because it does not trigger the initiation of signal transduction, and thus does not elicit any physiological effects. In the blood, equilibrium is established between free, unbound drug, and protein-bound drug. Owing to the large molecular weight of most proteins, protein—drug complex is too large to diffuse freely across capillary membranes and thus only free drug can be distributed out of the circulation to target sites to elicit physiological effects. However, because of the dynamic nature of the equilibrium within the capillaries, as free drug leaves circulation the equilibrium shifts and drug is released from its protein-binding site and becomes free drug capable of being distributed. Therefore, highly protein-bound drugs generally have a delayed onset of action, but also an extended duration of action as compared to drugs that are not highly protein bound.

Because each albumin protein has multiple binding sites, more than one drug molecule can bind to albumin simultaneously. For this reason, if multiple drugs are administered concurrently and both undergo significant protein binding in the plasma, the two drugs will compete for binding to the available plasma albumin. This competition may be manifested as an increase in the relative amount of free drug(s) available for distribution, due to a decreased level of protein binding resulting from binding site saturation. For example, anticoagulants are highly protein-bound drugs, and if used in conjunction with other protein-bound drugs, the amount of free anticoagulant available to reach the target site increases and may result in bleeding. Forensic toxicologists must therefore be cognizant of the fact that the effects of drugs are due to the distribution of the free drug to target sites and that the effects of protein-bound drugs can be influenced by their concurrent administration with other drugs that bind highly to plasma proteins.

A.5.1 VOLUME OF DISTRIBUTION

The apparent volume of distribution of a drug, V_D, is a theoretical measure of the volume of fluid a drug must be distributed into to result in the measured plasma concentration of free drug. The apparent volume of distribution of a drug is represented as

$$V_D = \frac{Q}{C}$$

where

Q = the dose of drug administered (mg)
C = the concentration of free drug in the blood plasma (mg/L) at the time of administration

The V_D of a drug can be determined experimentally by administering a known dose (Q) of drug to a laboratory animal, collecting blood samples at various time points following administration and measuring the concentration (C) of free drug in the plasma at each time point. To calculate V_D accurately, the dose of a drug and the plasma concentration of free drug must be considered at the same time point. When performing this experimental protocol, the dose of the drug is known at time zero (the time of administration), but the plasma concentration cannot be measured at time zero. Therefore, it is necessary to measure the free drug concentration in plasma samples over multiple time points, generate a plot of plasma concentration versus time, and extrapolate from the plot a theoretical free drug plasma concentration at time zero. The hypothetical plasma concentration at time zero represents the amount of free drug that would be found in the plasma if all of the administered drugs entered into the systemic circulation instantaneously. As an example, if 1000 mg of a drug is administered at time zero, and the theoretical plasma concentration at time zero is determined to be 20 mg/L by this process, the V_D of the drug is 50 L. In this manner, apparent volumes of distribution have been calculated experimentally for most drugs of interest to forensic toxicologists, and these values are of practical use for the determination of the compartments into which drugs are distributed following absorption. During the process of distribution, drugs leave the blood plasma, enter the interstitial fluid, and ultimately may be transported into cells. The V_D value for a drug of interest can therefore be utilized to determine the body compartment(s) into which the drug is distributed. If the V_D of a drug is 3 L or less, it can be concluded that the drug is poorly distributed and remains predominantly in the blood compartment; if the V_D is between 12 and 18 L (the sum of the volumes of the blood plasma and interstitial fluid), it can be concluded that the drug is distributed to the interstitial fluid, and if the V_D of a drug is between 40 and 50 L, it must be concluded that the drug is highly distributed and can be found in the blood, the interstitial fluid and the intracellular fluid.

Interestingly, the V_D for some drugs may be calculated to be greater than the sum total of the volumes of all three aqueous compartments in the body. For example, if 1000 mg of drug is administered at time zero, and the theoretical plasma concentration at time zero is determined to be 1 mg/L, the V_D of the drug is equal to 1000 L. Because the total volume of the aqueous compartments of the body is between 40 and 50 L, the drug must be distributed somewhere in addition to the aqueous compartments. This scenario is most often observed for highly lipid-soluble drugs, which are distributed readily into the fat, or drugs that are highly protein bound in tissues, resulting in inflated apparent volumes of distribution. Drugs that possess high partition coefficients are highly lipid soluble and have elevated apparent volumes of distribution are often stored in fat; these drugs may redistribute out of fat and back into circulation postmortem. This process is called postmortem redistribution and is important to forensic toxicologists because it may result in artificially elevated free drug concentrations in the plasma in locations surrounding the area in which the drug was stored (Chapter 12). Certain highly distributed drugs may also be sequestered in the liver and heart via protein binding, but the bonds binding the drug to protein may break postmortem resulting in the release of free drug back into circulation. Postmortem redistribution may result in local plasma drug concentrations that are two to five times greater than the systemic blood concentrations during life. Thus, it is preferable for blood to be collected from regions that are located at a distance from the heart, the liver, and other organs that are potential sites of protein-bound drug sequestration; blood collected from these sites is less likely to be significantly affected by postmortem redistribution. The apparent volume of distribution of a drug is therefore directly proportional to the partition coefficient of the drug, which is proportional to the degree of postmortem redistribution. Highly water-soluble, nonprotein-bound drugs generally undergo minimal postmortem redistribution.

A.5.2 ENTEROHEPATIC CIRCULATION

The enterohepatic circulation is a process by which drugs cycle between the GIT and the liver, inhibiting the rate at which the drugs are distributed to other areas of the body. Portions of orally administered drugs are absorbed from the GIT, primarily from the stomach and small intestine, into the capillaries of the GIT, which empty into the portal vein; unabsorbed drug will be excreted in the feces. The drugs are transported via the portal vein to the liver. From the liver, drugs enter the hepatic vein, through which they are transported to the heart, enter the systemic circulation, and transported to its target site. Alternately, a portion of the drug that enters the liver may be acted upon by the enzyme, glucuronyl transferase to form drug-glucuronide metabolites. Several classes of drugs may form glucuronides, including those that possess phenolic hydroxyl groups, carboxylic acids, or amines. After formation, drug-glucuronides are excreted from the liver into the bile, which is stored in the gallbladder. When bile is emptied into the small intestine, the glucuronide metabolites it contains are hydrolyzed by the enzyme β-glucuronidase to the free, nonglucuronide, version of the drug; the free drug can be reabsorbed and the cycle begins anew (Figure A.1).

Depending upon the physical characteristics of a drug, it may cycle through the enterohepatic circulation for extended periods of time, with a portion of the free drug being excreted in feces, and a portion entering the systemic circulation with each cycle. Drugs that enter the enterohepatic circulation have increased half-lives when administered orally as opposed to alternate routes of administration.

A.5.3 DISTRIBUTION INTO THE CENTRAL NERVOUS SYSTEM

The mechanisms of drug distribution into the central nervous system, the brain, and the spinal cord are of great importance to forensic toxicologists because the brain is a target organ for virtually all drugs of abuse. The brain is of central importance to virtually all physiological functions, so it is a very highly protected organ. In order

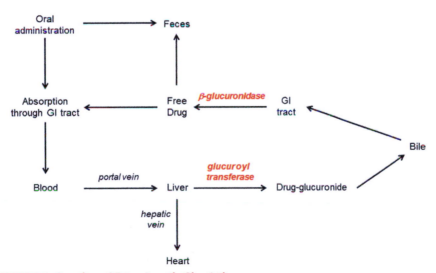

FIGURE A.1 Overview of Enterohepatic Circulation

Distribution through enterohepatic circulation results in a drug continually cycling between the gastrointestinal tract and liver. Some percentage of an orally administered drug may be excreted in feces, some of the drug will be absorbed into the capillaries to enter the blood, and some may be transported to the liver where it may enter systemic circulation or be acted upon by glucuronyl transferase.

for a drug to reach the neurons, it must transverse the blood—brain barrier (BBB) or the blood—cerebral spinal fluid barrier (BCSF) barrier. The BBB and the BCSF are anatomical and chemical barriers that prevent the unregulated passage of substances from the circulatory system into the neurons. The BBB, which is arguably the most restrictive barrier to entry into the brain, comprises both physical and metabolic factors that function to limit the entry of substances into the central nervous system. The foundation of the BBB is the intrinsic anatomy of the capillary endothelial cells in the brain. In many regions of the body the endothelial cells lining capillary walls contain gap junctions, which are small channels through which low molecular weight molecules can pass freely, regardless of their ionization state or lipid solubility. The endothelial cells lining brain capillaries, however, are joined together by tight junctions and do not contain gap junctions (or contain these junctions to a significantly diminished extent), thereby effectively prohibiting the free passage of many substances. Additionally, approximately 85% of brain capillaries are closely associated with astrocyte processes which provide an additional layer of cellular membranes that must be crossed by a drug in order to enter the neurons. Due to this distinct anatomy of the brain, only drugs that are largely nonionized, highly lipid soluble, and small in size may readily diffuse out of the circulatory system and cross the BBB; drugs that do not possess these characteristics cannot easily diffuse across the BBB.

In addition to the physical component of the BBB, the cytoplasm and organelles of the BBB endothelial cells contain enzymes that can metabolize certain drugs, thereby preventing the active free drug from entering the neurons. The third component of the BBB is a system of pumps located on either the abluminal or luminal membranes of neurons that can actively pump drugs out of the cells, thus ensuring that the concentration of drug in or around the cells will remain low. The three components of the BBB—the physical membranes, the metabolic enzymes, and the active pumps—combine to make it exceedingly difficult to target drugs to the brain.

The second major barrier to drug distribution into the central nervous system is the BCSF barrier. The BCSF is formed by the choroid plexi of the four ventricles of the brain, which are regions of tightly associated capillaries. As blood travels through the choroid plexi, its movement is slowed and the pressure within the plexi forces fluid out of the capillaries. The fluid that is forced out of circulation at the choroid plexi is a protein-free filtrate of blood that, upon entering the central nervous system, becomes cerebral spinal fluid. Cerebral spinal fluid bathes the brain and the spinal cord and makes contact with ependymal cells, which are cells that line the ventricles of the brain. Drugs that exit the circulation at the choroid plexi therefore come into contact first with the cerebral spinal fluid, and then with the ependymal cells lining of the ventricles. Because the ependymal cells are not joined together by tight junctions as the capillary endothelial cells in the brain are, drugs can more readily transverse this barrier to enter the neurons. Thus, although the BCSF forms a barrier against the entry of substances into the neurons, it does not provide as effective a barrier as the BBB does.

In order for a drug to be distributed into the central nervous system it must circumvent the anatomical and metabolic barriers of either the BBB or BCSF. Drugs that are not highly protein bound, largely nonionized, highly lipid soluble, and small in size may successfully diffuse out of the circulation. However, drugs that do not possess these physical and chemical characteristics do not readily enter the central nervous system unless they are administered in high doses, or are transported in via carrier proteins. To be transported efficiently by a carrier protein, drugs must have structures that are structurally similar to the endogenous ligand of the transport molecule. A major class of carrier protein in the central nervous system is composed of transmembrane proteins that transport amino acids into the neurons, so certain drugs that resemble amino acids are distributed to the central nervous system via this mechanism of carrier protein transport.

A.6 METABOLISM

The third event in drug disposition is metabolism, which can be defined as the biochemical modification of drugs, also referred to as the parent drugs, generally by enzymatic systems. The end products of a metabolic reaction, the metabolites, may elicit greater effects than the parent drug, lesser effects, or different effects, depending upon the nature of the parent drug. There are many aspects of drug metabolism that are of interest to forensic toxicologists, including, but not limited to:

1. *The mechanisms of metabolism of a drug of interest*: There are two major mechanisms of drug metabolism, enzymatic metabolism and nonenzymatic metabolism. Some drugs can be metabolized both enzymatically and non-enzymatically, whereas others undergo only enzymatic or nonenzymatic mechanisms of metabolism. A familiarity with the mechanism(s) of drug metabolism is useful as a means of anticipating or describing potential drug metabolites.

2. *The chemical structure of the metabolites formed*: It is useful to have an understanding of the metabolites produced from a parent. Care must be taken when utilizing experimental laboratory animals to investigate the enzymatic metabolism of drugs, as different species sometimes possess different enzymes, resulting in species-specific metabolite formation.

3. *Which metabolites are major metabolites and which are minor metabolites?* Often, the metabolism of a parent drug produces several different metabolites. The major metabolites are defined as the metabolites that are produced in the greatest percentage, and the minor metabolites are produced to a lesser extent. It is sometimes important to be able to predict the percentage of an administered drug will be converted into each metabolite. There are several factors that can influence which metabolites will be produced as the major metabolites and which will be the minor metabolites; these factors include individual genetic

differences resulting in differential enzyme expression, and elevated drug dose resulting in the saturation of enzymatic pathways.

4. *What factors influence the rate and extent of the metabolism of a drug?* Both the rate of drug metabolism, described as the half-life of conversion from parent drug to metabolites, and the extent of metabolism (defined as the percentage of parent drug that is converted to metabolites) may be influenced by many factors, including genetics, gender, race, age, ethnicity, and diet. The specific factors influencing the rate and extent of a metabolic reaction are dependent upon both the identity of the parent drug and the metabolic pathway employed.

5. *Which metabolites can elicit a physiological effect?* The physiological effects elicited by drug metabolites vary widely and are dependent upon the identity of the parent drug and the metabolic pathways involved in metabolite production. Certain drug metabolites elicit no effect because the structure of the parent drug has been altered to such an extent that the metabolites can no longer be distributed to the target molecule and/or can no longer interact with the target molecule. Some metabolites, however, produce quantitatively and qualitatively similar effects as the parent drug, and some metabolites produce different physiological effects entirely.

6. *The kinetics of metabolism:* The rate at which metabolism occurs influences several pharmacological characteristics of a drug, including the half-life and duration of action.

7. *The location of metabolism:* Although drug metabolism may occur in many different body compartments or organs, enzymatic metabolism is dependent upon the presence of both enzymes and cofactors. Therefore, the most common locations for enzymatic metabolism are organs that contain high concentrations of these factors; the liver is the major site of metabolic enzymes and cofactors and is thus the major site of drug metabolism.

8. *Does an analytical method of choice differentiate between a parent drug and its metabolites?* It is of the utmost importance to forensic toxicologists to know if the analytical method of choice in a toxicological analysis is capable of differentiating between a parent drug and its metabolites. This is especially true when the parent drug and its metabolites elicit either qualitatively or quantitatively different physiological effects, or when information about the timing of drug administration or the kinetics of metabolism is desired.

A.6.1 PHASE I AND PHASE II METABOLIC REACTIONS

Metabolic reactions can be divided into two major classes: phase I, or nonsynthetic, reactions and phase II, or synthetic (conjugation), reactions. The chemical structure of a parent drug influences how it will be metabolized. Drugs may progress through a phase I metabolic reaction followed by a phase II reaction, they may be metabolized by a phase I reaction only, or they may proceed directly to a phase II reaction. Phase I reactions include oxidation, reduction, and hydrolysis reactions; oxidations are the most common of these. Phase II reactions include glucuronidation, glycine conjugation, acetylation, and mercapturic acid synthesis reactions, with glucuronidations being the most common phase II reaction. The metabolites produced by both phase I and phase II reactions are typically more water soluble and less lipid soluble than their parent drug. However, a greater percentage of metabolites produced by phase I reactions have some physiological activity as compared to phase II metabolites; this is largely because phase I metabolites remain approximately the same size as the drugs from which they are derived, whereas phase II metabolites can be significantly larger than their parent drug, which may result in steric hindrance preventing the metabolite from reaching its target molecule. Table A.1 provides a comparison of the major characteristics of phase I and phase II metabolic reactions and Table A.2 provides an overview of the locations of selected metabolic enzymes.

A.6.2 PHASE I OXIDATION REACTIONS

Oxidation reactions, the most common type of phase I reaction, are largely controlled by two classes of enzymes: the flavin monooxygenase (FMO) family and the cytochrome p450 family. The FMO and cytochrome p450 enzymes are microsomal (associated with the endoplasmic reticulum) oxidation peroxidation systems that require NADPH and molecular oxygen to function. The mammalian FMO gene family encodes for enzymes that oxidize nucleophilic heteroatoms present in drugs, including nitrogen, sulfur, and phosphorous atoms. Cytochrome p450

Table A.1 Major Characteristics of Phase I and Phase II Metabolic Reactions

Phase I	Phase II
Types of Reactions	
Wide variety, determined by functional group include:	Wide variety, determined by functional group include:
Oxidation	Glucuronidation
Reduction	Glycine conjugation
Hydrolysis	Mercapturic acid synthesis
Characteristics of Metabolites	
Generally less lipid and more water soluble	Generally less lipid and more water soluble
Activity may be greater, less, or different than parent compound	Generally less active than parent compound
Reactions Catalyzed by Nonmicrosomal Enzymes	
Most hydrolyses	Glycine conjugation
Some reductions	Mercapturic acid synthesis
Reactions Catalyzed by Microsomal Enzymes	
Most oxidations	Glucuronidation
Most reductions	Some conjugations
Some hydrolyses	

Metabolic reactions can be divided into two major classes: phase I (nonsynthetic) reactions and phase II (synthetic/conjugation) reactions.

Table A.2 Locations of Phase I and Phase II Metabolic Enzymes

Enzyme	Location
Alcohol dehydrogenase	Cytosol
Aldehyde dehydrogenase	Cytosol, mitochondria
Cytochrome p450	Endoplasmic reticulum
Flavin monooxygenase	Endoplasmic reticulum
Glucuronyl transferase	Endoplasmic reticulum
Glutathione-S-transferase	Cytosol, endoplasmic reticulum

The enzymes involved in catalyzing phase I and phase II metabolic reactions may be located in various cellular compartments, including the cytosol, endoplasmic reticulum, and/or mitochondria.

enzymes are heme proteins that oxidize many of the same drugs as FMOs, but do not generally produce the same metabolites. There are several families, and subfamilies, of cytochrome p450 enzymes, generally designated by CYP followed by an alphanumeric description, for example, CYP2D6. Notably, there are significant individual differences in the expression of cytochrome p450 enzymes; these differences are due to genetic polymorphisms in the genes encoding for the proteins. Although the cytochrome p450 enzymes are ubiquitous, they are found in the highest concentration in the liver. This enzyme family is arguably the most important phase I enzymatic system due to the large number of drugs the enzymes metabolize. Table A.3 provides an overview of selected cytochrome p450 enzymes and examples of the drugs they metabolize.

Cytochrome systems are sometimes called mixed function oxidase systems, and the basic reaction catalyzed by these enzymatic systems is the reaction of oxygen (O_2) with a drug (RH) in the presence of the cofactor NADPH to form an alcohol (ROH), water and $NADP^+$.

$$RH + O_2 + NADPH + H^+ \rightarrow ROH + H_2O + NADP^+$$

In some metabolic pathways, the alcohol produced is the end product, whereas in other pathways catalyzed by cytochromes the alcohol is an unstable intermediary that

Table A.3 Overview of Drugs Metabolized by Cytochrome p450 Enzymes

CYP1A2	CYP2C9	CYP2C19	CYP2E1	CYP2D6	CYP3A4
Acetaminophen	Ibuprofen	Diazepam	Acetaminophen	Amphetamine	Acetaminophen
Caffeine	Phenobarbital	Imipramine	Caffeine	Codeine	Amitriptyline
Haloperidol	Tamoxifen	Phenobarbital	Ethanol	Desipramine	Citalopram
Propanalol	Tetrahydrocannabinol	Phenytoin	Theophylline	Lidocaine	Diazepam
				Metoprolol	Erythromycin
				Oxycodone	Imipramine
					Methadone
					Warfarin

The cytochrome p450 family of mixed function oxidase systems is arguably the most important class of phase I metabolic enzymes due to the large number of drugs metabolized by the enzymes.

will spontaneously produce another product. Each cytochrome p450 subtype possesses specificity with regard to the drug(s) it can metabolize; this specificity is determined by how well the enzyme can bind to specific drugs. Most cytochrome p450 enzymes can, however, metabolize multiple drugs, potentially resulting in competition between drugs for enzyme-binding sites. Additionally, multiple cytochrome p450 subtypes may metabolize the same drug. CYP3A4, which is found in the liver, small intestine, and stomach, is an especially important subtype as it can metabolize approximately 50% of all clinically utilized drugs. The reactions catalyzed by cytochrome p450 enzymes are diverse and include, among others, aliphatic oxidation, aromatic oxidation, N-dealkylation, O-dealkylation, S-dealkylation, N-oxidation, S-oxidation, P-oxidation, epoxide formation, oxidative deamination, oxidative desulfuration, and oxidative dehalogenation reactions.

A third class of enzymes that catalyze phase I oxidation reactions is the dehydrogenase family, nonmicrosomal enzymes, which includes alcohol dehydrogenase (a cytosolic enzyme) and aldehyde dehydrogenase (a mitochondrial enzyme). The dehydrogenases are of particular importance to forensic toxicologists because of their role in the metabolism of ethanol; alcohol dehydrogenase converts alcohols to aldehydes, for example, ethanol to acetaldehyde, and aldehyde dehydrogenase converts aldehydes to acids, for example, acetaldehyde to acetic acid. The activity of both enzymes is reversible.

A.6.3 PHASE II REACTIONS

The most common type of phase II reaction is glucuronide synthesis, a reaction in which glucuronic acid is transferred to a drug substrate by a glucuronyl transferase to form a drug-glucuronide. Many drugs can be metabolized to form glucuronides, with the glucuronide product generally being more water soluble, larger, more highly ionized, less active, and less toxic than the parent drug.[2] Glucuronidation occurs primarily in the liver, although glucuronyl transferases can be found in most major body organs including the GIT where glucuronide synthesis reactions play a major role in enterohepatic circulation. The rate and extent of glucuronide synthesis reactions is influenced by gender, age, liver function, and glucuronyl transferase activity.

Mercapturic synthesis reactions, which are a major pathway for the detoxification of electrophiles, including those produced as a result of cytochrome p450 oxidation reactions, are a second common phase II reaction. Mercapturic acid synthesis reactions are catalyzed by the family of glutathione-S-transferases (GSTs), which are found in the liver, intestines, kidneys, adrenal gland, and testes, and which catalyze the conjugation of the reduced form of the naturally occurring nucleophile, glutathione, to electrophilic substrates. This activity results in the production of metabolites known as

---

[2]Although most glucuronides are inactive there are certain notable exceptions. Morphine can be metabolized to morphine-3-glucuronide, morphine-6-glucuronide, and morphine-3,6-glucuronide, of which, one, morphine-6-glucuronide is an active metabolite.

mercapturic acids that generally have increased water solubility and decreased toxicity compared to their parent drug. GST expression is controlled by the GST gene family, with genetic variability resulting in variable expression of specific GST subtypes within the population. Interestingly, a deficiency in certain GST subtypes is suspected to be associated with increased susceptibilities to various forms of cancer, possibly due to the diminished ability of GST to detoxify potentially mutagenic electrophiles.

A.7 EXCRETION

Excretion, the process by which the body eliminates a drug and/or its metabolites, is the fourth and final event of drug disposition. Drugs or their metabolites theoretically can be excreted in any substance that leaves the body, including urine, feces, saliva, air, or hair. Although the mechanism of excretion of a drug is influenced by the physical and chemical characteristics of the compound, that is, volatile compounds may be excreted in exhaled air; drugs that are not absorbed well and/or enter enterohepatic circulation may be excreted in feces, the major mechanism of excretion for most drugs and their metabolites is renal excretion, with the vehicle of excretion being the urine.

A.7.1 RENAL EXCRETION

The kidneys receive about 25% of the total cardiac output of blood and filter approximately 175—190 L of plasma water each day, resulting in the formation of between 1 and 2 L of urine daily. Each kidney is supplied with blood by a renal artery and drained by a renal vein; urine exits each kidney through a duct called the ureter and drains into a common urinary bladder before being expelled through the urethra. The mammalian kidney has two distinct regions: the outer renal cortex and the inner renal medulla. Each kidney contains approximately 1 million nephrons, which are the functional units of the kidneys. A nephron consists of a single long tubule and a tightly woven ball of capillaries called the glomerulus; a capsule-shaped membranous structure called Bowman's capsule surrounds and receives filtrate from the glomerulus. When blood enters the glomerulus, the osmotic pressure increases and small, nonprotein molecules are forced out of circulation and into the interior of the Bowman's capsule. Drugs that can be filtered through the glomerulus are generally small, nonprotein bound, unionized, and highly lipid soluble. From the Bowman's capsule, the filtrate passes through three distinct regions of the nephron, the proximal tubule, the loop of Henle, and the distal tubule. Fluid from several nephrons flows into a collecting duct, which leads to the renal pelvis, which is drained by the ureter. The proximal and distal tubules in the nephrons play an important role in osmoregulation and in the excretion of drugs; as filtrate travels through the tubules it becomes increasingly concentrated such that the urine is much more concentrated than the body fluids. In the proximal tubules, the passive reabsorption of water, salts, and other small molecules and the active secretion of drugs and/or

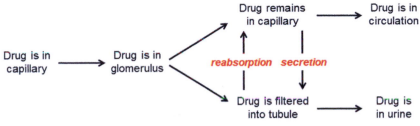

FIGURE A.2 Pathway of Renal Excretion

The major mechanism of excretion for most drugs and their metabolites is renal excretion, with the vehicle of excretion being the urine. As a drug or metabolite travels through the tubules it can be reabsorbed from the proximal tubule back into the capillaries to reenter systemic circulation or secreted in the filtrate.

metabolites can occur. As a drug or metabolite travels through the tubules it can be reabsorbed from the proximal tubule back into the capillaries to reenter systemic circulation; alternately, it can be secreted in the filtrate from the capillaries. Approximately 80% of water and NaCl is reabsorbed in the proximal tubules, resulting in a decrease in the total volume of the filtrate and an increase in the drug concentration in the tubule, thereby necessitating the active secretion of the compounds. The reabsorption of water continues in the distal tubules under the influence of the antidiuretic hormone; the reabsorption of water further concentrates the drugs and/or metabolites in the filtrate so that passive reabsorption may occur.

The secretion of hydronium ions into the distal tubule from the capillaries causes an acidification of the urine, thus influencing drug reabsorption. As the urine pH decreases, the ionization of weak acids decreases leasing to an increase in reabsorption and a decrease in the rate of urinary excretion. Conversely, the acidification of the urine in the distal tubules results in an increased ionization of weak bases, leading to a decreased reabsorption and an increase in the rate of urinary excretion. Figure A.2 illustrates the pathway of renal excretion.

A.7.2 CLEARANCE AND ELIMINATION KINETICS

The analysis of renal clearance and elimination kinetics provides important information about kidney function. The glomerular filtration rate, which is defined as the amount of blood filtered by the glomerulus per minute, can be estimated by measuring the clearance of inulin, a polymeric carbohydrate that is filtered at the glomerulus and neither reabsorbed nor secreted. The glomerular filtration rate of inulin resulting from normal kidney function is approximately 130 mL/min. Creatinine clearance may also be used as a measure of glomerular filtration rate as it is relatively easy to measure in blood and urine, is neither reabsorbed or metabolized by the kidneys, and is only minimally secreted; the glomerular filtration rate of creatinine is comparable to the rate of clearance of inulin in normally functioning kidneys. If the glomerular filtration rate is known, then the renal clearance, which is the volume of blood plasma cleared of a drug in 1 min, can be calculated. Real clearance is expressed as

$$\text{Renal Clearance} = \frac{\text{Filtration Rate} + \text{Secretion Rate} - \text{Reabsorption Rate}}{\text{Plasma Concentration}}$$

It is important to note that the renal clearance volume is a theoretical value because no defined volume of blood is cleared entirely of drug in the kidneys. The clearance of a drug may be calculated as follows:

$$C_r = \frac{U \times V}{P}$$

where C_r is equal to the clearance of the drug from the blood plasma (mL/min), U is the concentration of drug in 1 mL of urine over a period of time, V is the number of milliliters of urine formed in the period of time, and P is the concentration of free drug in 1 mL of plasma at midpoint in the period of time. The maximum renal clearance volume in humans is approximately 650 mL/min, which corresponds to the complete tubular secretion of drug; the minimum renal clearance is 0 mL/min, which corresponds to the complete reabsorption of drug. The renal clearance rate alone provides no information about the extent to which the plasma concentration of drug has been decreased as a result of urinary excretion. However, if the renal clearance rate is known, the renal elimination rate (the half-life of drug elimination by the kidneys) may be determined. The half-life of renal clearance ($t_{1/2}$) may be calculated as

$$t_{1/2} = \frac{V_D}{\text{Renal Clearance Rate}}$$

where V_D is the volume of distribution for the drug of interest. Highly water-soluble drugs, which possess low volumes of distribution, are therefore excreted in urine very rapidly. Conversely, highly lipid-soluble drugs, which possess high volumes of distribution, are excreted more slowly by the kidneys. The extended half-life of renal clearance for lipid-soluble drugs is generally due to the distribution into, and gradual release of the drugs from fat, rather than an impaired excretion of the drugs by the kidneys. The analysis of the clearance and elimination kinetics of renal drug excretion is important to forensic toxicologists because it provides some insight into how long a drug can reasonably be predicted to stay in the urine, and therefore, for what duration of time the drug should be detectable in urine.

A.7.3 ALTERNATE ROUTES OF EXCRETION

Although renal excretion is the primary mechanism of drug excretion, drugs are also excreted via biliary clearance, pulmonary excretion, and salivary excretion. The liver secretes between 0.25 and 1 L of bile per day and drugs that are administered orally, and/or enter enterohepatic circulation may be subject to biliary clearance as described previously. Anions, cations, and unionized compounds can all enter the bile, but the optimal molecular weight for biliary excretion is approximately 300—500 Da. It is notable that transport into the bile cannot be considered excretion in the classical sense, as some percentage of the drug will be recycled into systemic circulation.

Salivary excretion is relevant only for drugs that are nonprotein bound in the plasma because protein-bound drugs cannot enter the saliva. As is the case with biliary excretion, some percentage of the drug in saliva will be recycled due to swallowing and reabsorption from the GIT. Interestingly, for many drugs the concentration of drug in saliva is similar to the concentration of free drug in the blood plasma, thus making this excretion a potential vehicle for drug screening.

Pulmonary excretion is a less common mechanism of excretion that is relevant only for volatile compounds, notably ethanol for which the detection in exhaled air is an important tool of law enforcement as a means of estimating the blood ethanol concentration.

A.8 CONCLUSION

Forensic toxicologists must possess a working knowledge of the mechanisms and kinetics of the four major events in drug disposition—absorption, distribution, metabolism, and excretion—in order to make accurate determinations of the qualitative and quantitative effects elicited by drug administration, the duration of action of drugs of interest, and the appropriate timing and method of drug detection and analysis. This understanding is crucial to the interpretation of analytical results.

SUGGESTED READING

Brunton, L., Chabner, B., Knollman, B., 2011. Goodman and Gilman's the Pharmacological Basis of Therapeutics. McGraw-Hill, Columbus.

Golan, D.E., Tashjian, A.H., Armstrong, E.J., Armstrong, A.W., 2012. Principles of Pharmacology: The Pathophysiologic Basis of Drug Therapy. Lippincott Williams and Wilkins, Philadelphia.

Harrold, M.W., Zavod, R.M., 2013. Basic Concepts in Medicinal Chemistry. American Society of Health-Systems Pharmacists, Inc., Bethesda.

Hilal-Dandan, R., Brunton, L.L., 2014. Goodman and Gilman's Manual of Pharmacology and Therapeutics. McGraw-Hill, New York.

Katzung, B.G., Trevor, A.J., 2015. Basic and Clinical Pharmacology. McGraw-Hill, Columbus.

Klaassen, C.D. (Ed.), 2001. Casarett & Doull's Toxicology: The Basic Science of Poisons. McGraw-Hill, New York.

LaDu, B.N., Mandel, H.G., Way, E.L., 1971. Fundamentals of Drug Metabolism and Disposition. The Williams and Wilkins Company, Baltimore, MD.

Lemke, T.L., Williams, D.A., Roche, V.F., Zito, S.W., 2013. Foye's Principles of Medicinal Chemistry. Lippincott Williams and Wilkins, Philadelphia.

Patrick, G.L., 2015. An Introduction to Medicinal Chemistry. Oxford University Press, Oxford.

Rang, H.P., Ritter, J.M., Flower, R.J., Henderson, G., 2015. Rang and Dale's Pharmacology. Elsevier.

Stringer, J.L., 2011. Basic Concepts in Pharmacology: What You Need to Know for Each Drug Class. McGraw-Hill, Columbus.

Wecker, L., Crespos, L., Dunaway, G., Faingold, C., Watts, S., 2009. Brody's Human Pharmacology. Mosby, St. Louis.

Whalen, K., 2015. Pharmacology. Wolters Kluwer, Philadelphia.

Principles of Pharmacodynamics

B

Pharmacodynamics refers to the study of the effects a drug has on the body and the mechanisms by which those effects are produced. Included in this study is the examination of the various factors that influence drug effects. This chapter will present the basic principles of pharmacodynamics that are relevant to the forensic toxicologist.

B.1 DRUG EFFECTS

In order for a drug (or its metabolites) to elicit a physiological effect, it must interact with a target molecule, which in many cases is a receptor protein, and initiate the process of signal transduction. The effects of a drug can be characterized as therapeutic effects, side effects, or toxic effects. The therapeutic effects of a drug are defined as the specific, desired effects of drug administration. For example, a physician may prescribe a narcotic to relieve pain; the relief of pain is the therapeutic effect. The dose of a drug that is anticipated to produce the desired effects, for instance, the relief of pain, without resulting in significant adverse or undesired effects, is called the therapeutic or effective dose. Side effects are defined as all of the effects that are produced by a therapeutic dose of a drug and that are not the desired therapeutic effects. For instance, if an opioid is prescribed for the relief of pain, the therapeutic dose may achieve the desired effect of analgesia, but it may also result in the side effect of constipation. If, however, an opioid is prescribed to treat diarrhea, constipation would be the therapeutic effect and pain relief would become a side effect. It is therefore important to note that the therapeutic effects and the side effects of a drug are dependent upon the purpose of drug administration. Whereas side effects are produced at the therapeutic dose of a drug, toxic effects occur only when doses greater than the normal therapeutic dose of a drug are administered. If a therapeutic dose of aspirin is administered, the side effect of an upset stomach may result. However, if a dose exceeding the therapeutic dose of aspirin is administered, tinnitus may occur. Because tinnitus occurs only as the result of the administration of a greater than therapeutic dose of aspirin, and not as a result of the administration of a normal, therapeutic dose of the drug, it is considered to be a toxic effect rather than a side effect. The occurrence of toxic effects indicates that a dose exceeding the normal therapeutic dose has been taken. It is therefore evident that the dose of a drug influences the effects elicited by drug administration (i.e., a therapeutic dose elicits therapeutic effects, whereas an elevated dose may produce toxic effects). As Paracelsus famously proclaimed, "the dose makes the poison."

Although there are many different ways to describe the dose of a drug, the most straightforward definition of a dose is simply the amount of drug that is administered. As described previously, the therapeutic or effective dose of a drug produces the specific, desired effects, whereas a toxic dose produces toxic effects. There are several factors to take into consideration, however, when determining an effective dose of a drug. First, the route of drug administration influences the magnitude and specificity of response elicited, and therefore influences the dose required to achieve the therapeutic effects. Second, a specific dose and route of administration of a drug may affect different individuals differently. The therapeutic dose of a drug must therefore be calculated carefully with the goal of determining the dose of the drug that elicits the desired effects in a meaningful percentage of a population when administered by a specific route of administration. When calculating a therapeutic dose for a drug, there are two criteria that must be met as emphasized by the Federal Drug Administration: at the therapeutic dose for the specified route of administration, the drug must be efficacious and it must be safe. In order to determine at what dose (or range of doses) a drug is efficacious and safe for a significant percentage of the population, dose–response studies must be performed.

To perform a dose–response study, varying doses of a drug are administered to a population of individuals (or laboratory animals) and the dose of drug administered is plotted against the effect elicited by the drug. The specific effect measured is dictated by the identity of the drug and its target molecules. As is illustrated in Figure B.1, most drugs exhibit a threshold effect, which describes the phenomenon in which at low doses very little effect is observed, as the dose is increased, a

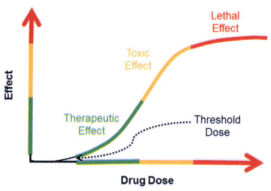

FIGURE B.1 Dose–Response Curve

The dose of drug administered is plotted against the effect elicited by the drug. Most drugs exhibit a threshold effect, in which as the dose is increased, a favorable effect is produced, at more elevated doses an adverse effect is elicited, and finally lethality is induced. The threshold dose is the dose at which the desired effect of the drug is first observed.

favorable effect is produced, at more elevated doses an adverse effect is elicited, and finally the effect elicited by drug administration levels off as lethality is induced. A threshold dose is defined as the dose at which the desired effect of the drug is first observed. Most drugs of interest to forensic toxicologists and most drugs used therapeutically have a threshold dose—a dose below which no effect is observed. In a variation of this most simple dose—response curve, the log dose of drug administered can be plotted against the cumulative response to the drug within a population, where the "response" is defined as either the therapeutic effect or the lethal effect. Figure B.2 illustrates the percentage of a population in which the desired effect, or a lethal effect, is achieved as a function of the log dose of drug administered. A pharmacological characteristic known as the effective dose 50 (ED_{50}) is defined as the dose at which 50% of the population experiences the desired effect (a single drug may have several different ED_{50} values depending upon which desired effect is being measured). The lethal dose 50 (LD_{50}) is defined as the dose at which the drug is lethal to 50% of the population. Traditionally, the toxicity of a drug was represented as the therapeutic index, which is calculated as the LD_{50}/ED_{50} of the drug. Drugs with higher therapeutic indices have superior safety profiles as compared to drugs with lower therapeutic indices. Although the therapeutic index provides valuable information about the safety profile of a drug, an alternate measure of toxicity called the margin of safety can provide a more accurate representation of the potential risks associated with drug administration. The margin of safety is calculated as the LD1/ED99, where the LD1 is the dose that elicits lethality in 1% of the population, and the ED99 is the dose that elicits the therapeutic effect in 99% of the population. In other words, the margin of safety assumes that it is preferable for a drug to elicit a therapeutic effect in 99% of a population, while inducing a lethal effect in only 1% of the population. It is important to note that two drugs may have the same therapeutic index, but very different margins of safety. In such a case, it would

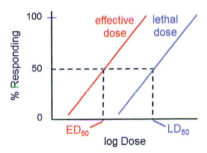

FIGURE B.2 Determination of ED_{50} and LD_{50}

The log dose of drug administered is plotted against the cumulative response to the drug within a population, where the "response" is defined as either the therapeutic effect or the lethal effect. The effective dose 50 (ED_{50}) is the dose at which 50% of the population experiences the desired effect, and the lethal dose 50 (LD_{50}) is the dose at which the drug is lethal to 50% of the population.

be preferable to use the drug with the higher margin of safety, as this indicates that there is very little overlap between the doses that elicit a therapeutic effect and the doses that elicit a lethal effect. There is, however, sometimes a trade-off between efficacy and safety, and there are circumstances in which an individual might be willing to accept a greater risk of toxicity in order to obtain a therapeutic effect.

An interesting phenomenon called hormesis can occasionally be observed if the dose–response curve of a drug is examined carefully. Hormesis is the phenomenon in which relatively low doses of a drug elicit beneficial effects that are not achieved by higher doses of the drug. For instance, ethanol, which can elicit toxic or undesired effects at higher doses, has been shown to increase life span in some individuals who are exposed to low doses of ethanol for prolonged periods of time. The hormesis effect results in a dose–response curve that is described as a J curve. Frequently, when drug efficacy is being evaluated, the effects of very low doses are not investigated thoroughly and the phenomenon of hormesis is overlooked.

B.2 SPECIFIC AND NONSPECIFIC DRUGS

The effects elicited by drugs can be broadly characterized as specific or nonspecific. The effects of certain drugs are inherently linked to their molecular structure; such drugs are called structurally specific drugs. Structurally specific drugs exhibit structure–activity relationships, that is, the structures of drugs are correlated with the effects that they produce. The effects of structurally specific drugs are mediated by binding to a specific target molecule or receptor. For this reason, drugs that are structurally similar often produce similar effects because they can bind to the same target molecules via a lock and key fit—the drug is the key and the receptor or target molecule is the lock. For example, morphine and codeine are structurally similar drugs and both can bind to specific morphine receptors and elicit qualitatively similar effects. Specific drugs may demonstrate major modifications in effect as a result of slight modifications of structure. For example, if the structure of morphine is modified slightly, the analgesic effects elicited from administration may be greatly reduced or greatly enhanced.

Drugs that produce effects due to their physical properties are called structurally nonspecific drugs. A physical property in this context is a property that can be determined without destroying the chemical, for instance, lipid solubility. Physical properties are often not a function of structure and drugs that are structurally similar may vary widely in regards to physical properties. For example, general anesthetics may have varying molecular structures, but they all share the physical characteristic of high lipid solubility, which facilitates their entry into neuronal plasma membranes where their disruption of membrane structure is thought to contribute to their central nervous system depressant effects. Therefore, it is both possible for structurally dissimilar drugs to produce similar effects (due to common physical characteristics) and for structurally similar drugs to produce dissimilar effects (due to the goodness of fit to the target molecule and their varying physical properties).

Generally, structurally nonspecific drugs are less potent than structurally specific drugs, meaning that greater doses of nonspecific drugs must be administered to achieve the desired physiological effect. This phenomenon is at least partly explained by the Ferguson Principle, which was developed to explain the depressant activity of structurally unrelated drugs and which introduced the concept of relative saturation. The Ferguson Principle for nonvolatile drugs states that

$$a = \frac{S_t}{S_0}$$

where a is the relative saturation of the drug, S_t is the molar concentration required to produce a biological effect, and S_0 is the molar solubility of the drug. The same principle applies to volatile drugs, but in place of drug concentrations, partial pressures of drugs are utilized. The Ferguson Principle for volatile drugs is expressed as

$$a = \frac{P_t}{P_0}$$

where a is the relative saturation of the drug, P_t is the partial pressure of the drug in solution or in a gaseous mixture, and P_0 is the vapor pressure of the pure drug. In general, the relative saturation values for structurally specific drugs are less than or equal to 0.1, whereas the relative saturation values of structurally nonspecific drugs are between 0.1 and 1, indicating that significantly greater amounts of nonspecific drugs must be administered in order to achieve the biological effect.

B.3 TARGET MOLECULES

Because there are many more molecules in the human body than there are molecules in a dose of drug, if the drug molecules were to react indiscriminately and equally with all of the body molecules, only a very small percentage of the molecules would be targeted and any physiological effect would likely be negligible. It is therefore necessary that drug molecules react with specific molecules, which are distributed in a heterogeneous manner throughout the body. Furthermore, because different drugs produce different physiological effects, it follows that the varying effects produced by drugs are the result of interactions with different target molecules.

The receptor theory is based upon the principle that structurally specific drugs interact with a small number of molecules, called target molecules, which are distributed with characteristic and varying density among the cells and tissues of the body. The molecular structure of a specific drug determines the target molecule(s) with which the drug will interact. The target molecules with which drugs must interact in order to elicit their specific effects are called receptors. The term receptor can be used to describe any target molecule with which a drug reacts, although most receptors are proteins.

In order for a drug to elicit a physiological effect, two general events must occur: (1) the drug must bind to a target molecule to form a drug–receptor (DR) complex;

and (2) the binding of a drug to a target molecule must stimulate or inhibit the activity of the target molecule and/or must initiate signal transduction. Drugs that alter the activity of target molecules and/or trigger the initiation of signal transduction pathways upon DR complex formation are called agonists. Drugs that bind to target molecules but do not alter the activity of the molecules or stimulate signal transduction are known as antagonists. Drugs that can alter the activity of target molecules and/or trigger the initiation of signal transduction pathways upon DR complex formation, but do so to a lesser extent than agonists are known as partial agonists, and drugs that bind to receptors and cause physiological effects that are the reverse of the effects produced by agonist binding are called reverse agonists.

Carbon monoxide (CO) is an example of a ligand that causes a direct effect when it binds to its target molecule, hemoglobin (Hb). As a result of the binding of CO to Hb, the ability of Hb to function normally is decreased, that is, Hb cannot transport oxygen normally because some of its oxygen binding sites have been occupied by CO. Morphine is an example of a drug that initiates signal transduction when it binds to its receptor; the formation of a DR complex and the resulting signal transduction produces several effects including analgesia and euphoria.

Drug receptors have four defining characteristics:

1. *Specificity*: In order to be defined as a receptor, a target molecule must exhibit specificity of binding, wherein a specific drug or drugs of related structures can bind to the molecule and elicit an effect whereas drugs with dissimilar structures cannot.
2. *Saturability*: Drug receptors are expressed in finite numbers and thus, by definition, it is possible to saturate them with drugs, which as a result of their structures, bind to the receptors specifically.
3. *High-affinity binding*: Receptors are characterized by a high affinity for their drugs and therefore it is possible to saturate them with low drug concentrations.
4. *Reversibility*: Structurally specific drugs interact with their receptors via the formation of chemical bonds and these interactions generally are reversible. However, certain drugs form covalent bonds with their receptors forming essentially permanent, nonreversible DR complexes.

B.4 RECEPTOR THEORIES

Several theories have been developed to describe the ways in which drugs interact with their target receptors. Although the commonly considered receptor theories all have limitations and shortcomings, each provides some insight into the mechanisms by which drugs bind to their specific receptors to elicit a biological effect. Three receptor theories—the occupancy theory, the rate theory, and the two-state theory—will be described. Taken together, the principles of the three theories provide a foundation upon which the activity of agonists and antagonists may be considered.

B.4.1 OCCUPANCY THEORY

The occupancy theory, one of the initial receptor theories developed, is based upon several assumptions:

1. *The law of mass action is applicable to reversible DR interactions*: The law of mass action states that the rate of a homogeneous chemical reaction at a constant temperature is proportional to the product of the concentrations of the reactants. As applied to DR interactions, this law assumes that the greater the concentrations of drug and receptor, the greater the formation of DR complex.

2. *All receptors for a specific drug are identical and equally accessible to the drug*: The assumption that all receptors for a given drug are identical and equally accessible to the drug is inaccurate for several reasons. First, many drugs can bind to several different receptors, that are by definition, not identical. Second, receptors are distributed in a heterogeneous manner in the body, and due to the specific distribution, metabolism, and excretion of drugs following administration, not all receptors are equally accessible to the drug.

3. *The effective concentration of a drug is not significantly reduced by DR complex formation*: In general, the number of molecules of drug in a dose is significantly greater than the number of receptors to which the drug binds. Therefore, even after receptor saturation, the concentration of free, unbound drug is significantly larger than the concentration of bound drug, and is not significantly different than the initial concentration of drug.

4. *The intensity of a pharmacological effect is proportional to the percentage of receptors occupied*: This assumption is based upon the principle that the formation of a DR complex initiates signal transduction, resulting in a biological effect. However, this assumption does not account for several factors including antagonists, receptor desensitization, and cooperativity. First, the assumption dose not account for the lack of activity of antagonists, which, upon binding to a target molecule, elicit no pharmacological effect regardless of the number of receptors that are occupied. The stability with which a drug binds to a target molecule is called affinity, and the ability of a DR to initiate signal transduction is called intrinsic activity. Agonists, partial agonists, and antagonists all may bind to their target molecules with low or high affinity, but only agonists form DR complexes with high intrinsic activity, whereas partial agonists form DR complexes with moderate intrinsic activity, and antagonists form DR complexes with no intrinsic activity. Second, the assumption does not account for the phenomenon of receptor desensitization, in which increasing doses of a drug are needed to produce a given effect, may also be an exception to the assumption that the intensity of a pharmacological effect is directly proportional to the percentage of receptors occupied. Receptor desensitization may be caused by several factors, including a decreasing ability of an agonist to stimulate signal transduction (decreasing intrinsic activity) after prolonged drug administration, receptor downregulation in response to prolonged drug exposure, and/or decreased binding affinity after prolonged drug exposure. Finally, the

assumption dose not account for cooperativity, a phenomenon in which the affinity of a drug for its receptor is influenced by the prior binding of some other receptor drug. In positive cooperativity, the prior binding of another drug to a receptor increases the affinity of a drug for the receptor. In negative cooperativity, the prior binding of a drug decreases the affinity of a drug for its receptor.

5. *The maximum pharmacological effect is produced when all of the drug receptors are occupied*: Although accurate for some DR complexes in certain conditions, there are instances in which the maximum drug effect is produced without all receptors being occupied. Systems in which there are more receptors present than are needed to produce the maximum effect are described as having spare receptors. In these instances, some of the receptors may be blocked or destroyed without reducing the maximum drug effect.

Although several of the assumptions upon which the occupancy theory is based are not accurate in all situations, the theory, nonetheless, serves as a valuable model of DR interactions. Based upon the foundational assumptions of the occupancy theory, if a tissue sample containing a total number of receptors (N_{total}) specific for a drug (D) is exposed to a drug at a concentration of x_A and allowed to reach equilibrium, a specific number of the receptors (N_A) will be occupied, and the number of unoccupied receptors can be represented as $N_{total} - N_A$. Generally, the number of drug molecules administered in the sample significantly exceeds the total number of receptors (N_{total}) so that the formation of the DR complex does not significantly reduce the effective concentration of drug (x_A). In such a situation, the intensity of the pharmacological effect will be proportional to the number of receptors occupied by the drug, with the maximum effect produced when all of the receptors are occupied. The reaction can be expressed as

$$
\begin{array}{ccccc}
\text{D} & + & \text{R} & \underset{K_2}{\overset{K_1}{\rightleftharpoons}} & \text{DR} \\
\text{drug} & & \text{free receptor} & & \text{drug} - \text{receptor complex} \\
(x_A) & & (N_{total} - N_A) & & (N_A)
\end{array}
$$

When the law of mass action is applied to this reaction, the dissociation constant (k_D) for the DR complex can be defined as

$$ k_D = \frac{k_2}{k_1} = \frac{[D][R]}{[DR]} \tag{B.1} $$

This equation resembles the Langmuir adsorption isotherm equation, and a plot of the relationship between drug concentration and receptor occupancy generates a characteristic rectangular parabola curve. The k_D for a DR complex is characteristic of the specific drug and receptor, and is a measure of the affinity of the drug for the receptor as well as the stability of the DR complex. According to the occupancy theory, k_D is equal to the concentration of drug resulting in 50% receptor occupancy at equilibrium. The higher the affinity of a drug for its receptor, the lower the k_D value. Conversely, the lower the affinity of a drug for its receptor, the higher the k_D value.

Saturation curves can be utilized to further illustrate the occupancy theory of DR interactions. An equation established to describe enzymatic reactions states that

$$v = \frac{V_{max}[S]}{[S] + k_M} \qquad (B.2)$$

where v is equal to the velocity of the reaction, V_{max} is the maximum reaction velocity, [S] is equal to the substrate concentration, and k_M is the Michaelis–Menton constant, which is equal to the substrate concentration at which the velocity of the reaction is one half of the maximum velocity. Based upon this equation, an analogous equation can be derived and applied to the reversible interactions between drug and receptor

$$E = \frac{E_M[D]}{[D] + k_D} \qquad (B.3)$$

where

  E = the pharmacological effect
  E_M = the maximum effect
  [D] = the free drug concentration
  k_D = the dissociation constant of the reaction.

The application of this equation to a DR complex, in which the effect has been determined, allows for the generation of a plot of drug concentration versus effect, which produces a characteristic hyperbolic curve. Because k_D is analogous to k_M, [D] is analogous to [S], and E_M is analogous to V_{max}, it follows that since it has been established that k_M is equal to [S] at ½ V_{max}, k_D must be equal to [D] at ½ E_M. In other words, k_D is the drug concentration at which half of the maximum effect is achieved (Figure B.3). A Lineweaver–Burke plot is a method by which to convert the hyperbolic saturation curve into a linear plot from which the value of k_D can more easily be extrapolated. Rather than plotting drug concentration versus effect, Lineweaver–Burke equations plot the reciprocals of these values: 1/drug concentration versus 1/effect. In such a curve, the y-intercept is equal to $1/E_M$ and the x-intercept is equal to $-1/k_D$ (Figure B.4). Lineweaver–Burke plots are commonly used to investigate the characteristics of DR interactions, including the influence of competitive and noncompetitive antagonists on DR complex formation.

B.4.2 RECEPTOR ANTAGONISM AND THE OCCUPANCY THEORY

There are two major classes of receptor antagonists: competitive antagonists and noncompetitive antagonists. The effects of antagonists on agonist activity can be measured experimentally and analyzed via Lineweaver–Burke plots. Competitive antagonists are so named because they compete with agonists for receptor binding. The effects of a competitive antagonist can be reversed by increasing the concentration of the agonist because the antagonist–receptor interactions are reversible. If a dose–response curve of effect as a function of agonist concentration (expressed on a

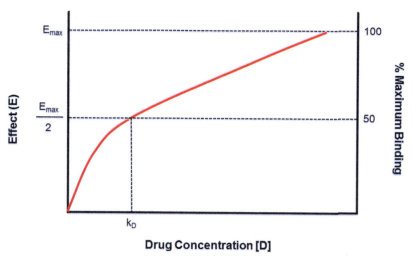

FIGURE B.3 Dose—Effect Curve

The generation of a plot of drug concentration versus effect produces a characteristic hyperbolic curve. The dissociation constant of the reaction, k_D, is equal to the drug concentration at which half of the maximum effect is achieved.

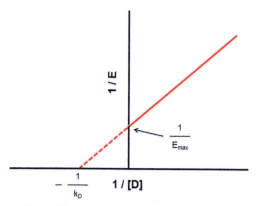

FIGURE B.4 Lineweaver—Burke Plot

Lineweaver—Burke plots are transformations of the typical dose—effect curve in which the reciprocals of drug concentration (1/[D]) and effect (1/E) are plotted. In the resulting linear plot, the y-intercept is equal to the reciprocal of the maximum effect ($1/E_{max}$) and the x-intercept is equal to the negative reciprocal of the dissociation constant of the reaction ($-1/k_D$).

log scale) is plotted, a characteristic sigmoidal curve will be generated in which increasing doses of agonist result in increasing biological effect until a maximum effect is achieved. According to the receptor occupancy theory, the maximum response corresponds with receptor saturation. The addition of a low concentration of competitive antagonist to the assay or sample causes a parallel right shift in the sigmoidal curve but has no effect on the maximum effect of agonist treatment; the addition of a higher concentration of competitive antagonist causes a more pronounced right shift in the dose—response curve, also with no effect on maximum effect (Figure B.5). The characteristic right shift in a dose—response curve observed after cotreatment with a competitive antagonist is due to the competition between the antagonist and the agonist for receptor binding. The inhibitory effect of a competitive antagonist can be overcome by increasing the concentration of the agonist because, as described in the law of mass action, the greater the concentration of the reacting agonist, the greater the probability of receptor binding, and the increasing concentrations of agonist will eventually outcompete the antagonist for receptor binding. In the presence of a competitive antagonist, the dose of drug needed to achieve a desired effect is therefore increased, but the maximum effect is unchanged. The transformation of a standard dose—response curve to a Lineweaver—Burke plot, in which the reciprocals of drug concentration and effect are plotted, allows for the direct investigation of the effects of a competitive antagonist on the E_M and k_D of agonist—receptor interactions. As described previously, the y-intercept of a Lineweaver—Burke plot is equal to $1/E_M$ and the x-intercept is equal to $-1/k_D$. The presence of a competitive antagonist does not alter the

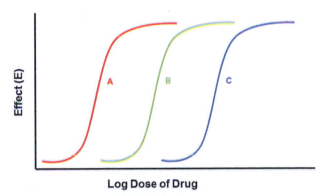

FIGURE B.5 Effects of Competitive Antagonists

When a dose—response curve of effect as a function of agonist concentration (expressed on a log scale) is plotted, a characteristic sigmoidal curve will be generated (A). The addition of a low concentration of competitive antagonist causes a parallel right shift in the sigmoidal curve but has no effect on the maximum effect of agonist treatment (B); the addition of a higher concentration of competitive antagonist causes a more pronounced right shift in the dose—response curve, also with no effect on maximum effect (C).

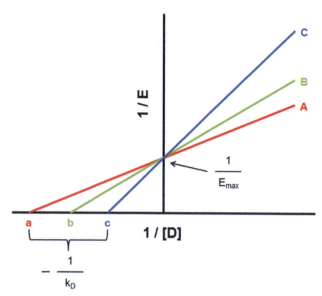

FIGURE B.6 Lineweaver–Burke Analysis of Competitive Antagonist Effects

The transformation of a standard dose–response curve to a Lineweaver–Burke plot, in which the reciprocals of drug concentration and effect are plotted, allows for the direct investigation of the effects of a competitive antagonist on the maximum effect and dissociation constant of agonist–receptor interactions. The y-intercept of a Lineweaver–Burke plot is equal to $1/E_{max}$ and the x-intercept is equal to $-1/k_D$. The presence of a low concentration (B) or high concentration (C) of competitive antagonist does not alter the y-intercept of a Lineweaver–Burke plot of agonist alone (A), which is to be expected as the E_{max} of the reaction is not affected. The presence of a competitive antagonist does cause a dose-dependent rightward shift in the x-intercept, corresponding with an increase in the k_D of the reaction; agonist alone has the lowest k_D (a), the addition of a low concentration of antagonist results in an increase in k_D (b), and the addition of a higher concentration of competitive antagonist results in an even higher k_D (c).

y-intercept of a Lineweaver–Burke plot, which is to be expected as the E_M of the reaction is not affected, but it does cause a right shift in the x-intercept, corresponding with an increase in the k_D of the reaction (Figure B.6). The elevated k_D value characteristically caused by a competitive antagonist is indicative of a decreased stability of the agonist–receptor complex. The decreased stability is, in a sense, an artificial change that is due to the competition from the antagonist making it more difficult for the agonist–receptor complex to form; competitive antagonists change the apparent affinity of an agonist for its receptor by requiring higher concentrations of agonist to produce a given effect. The hallmark characteristics of competitive antagonists, therefore, are their ability to induce parallel right shifts in agonist dose–response curves and to cause increases in the k_D values of agonist–receptor interactions.

Similar to competitive antagonists, noncompetitive antagonists compete with agonists for receptor binding, but noncompetitive antagonists bind covalently and essentially irreversibly to the receptor, whereas competitive antagonists bind reversibly. The irreversible binding of a noncompetitive antagonist to receptor modifies the receptor in such a way as to make it unavailable for agonist binding; the influence of a noncompetitive antagonist can therefore not be reversed by increasing agonist concentration. Because the presence of a noncompetitive antagonist effectively reduces the number of functional receptors available for agonist binding, the maximum effect elicited by agonist treatment is also reduced. The receptors that are not bound by noncompetitive receptor remain unchanged, however, and the affinity of agonist binding to available receptor is unaltered. The effect of a noncompetitive antagonist on agonist—receptor interactions is represented by a nonparallel displacement of the agonist dose—response curve, with a reduced maximum effect plateau (Figure B.7). The altered dose—response curves indicate that in the presence of a noncompetitive antagonist, the dose of agonist needed to achieve a desired effect is increased, but increasing agonist concentration cannot elicit the same maximum effect as is achieved in the absence of the noncompetitive antagonist. Notably, in systems with spare receptors, the presence of a low concentration of a noncompetitive antagonist will result in a parallel right shift in the agonist dose—response curve with no effect on E_M (similar to the shift caused by a competitive antagonist). The transformation of a standard dose—response curve to a Lineweaver—Burke plot demonstrates that the presence of a noncompetitive antagonist results in a decreased E_M (as is represented by an increased y-intercept value) and an unaltered k_D (as is represented by an unchanged x-intercept) (Figure B.8). The constant k_D values of

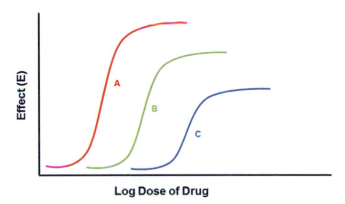

FIGURE B.7 Effects of Noncompetitive Antagonists

When a dose—response curve of effect as a function of agonist concentration (expressed on a log scale) is plotted, a characteristic sigmoidal curve will be generated (A). The addition of a low concentration of a noncompetitive antagonist causes a nonparallel displacement of the dose—response curve with a reduced maximum effect (B); the addition of a higher concentration of a noncompetitive antagonist amplifies this response (C).

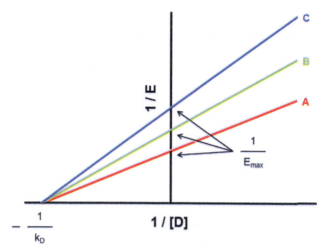

FIGURE B.8 Lineweaver—Burke Analysis of Noncompetitive Antagonist Effects

The transformation of a standard dose—response curve to a Lineweaver—Burke plot demonstrates that as compared to agonist alone (A) the presence of a low concentration (B) or high concentration (C) of noncompetitive antagonist results in a decreased E_{max} (as is represented by an increased y-intercept value) and an unaltered k_D (as is represented by an unchanged x-intercept).

agonist—receptor interactions in the presence of noncompetitive antagonists underscore the fact that the stability of the agonist—receptor complex is unaltered. The hallmark characteristics of noncompetitive antagonists, therefore, are their ability to induce nonparallel displacements in agonist dose—response curves and to cause decreases in the E_M values of agonists—receptor reactions.

B.4.3 RATE THEORY

Because the occupancy theory has certain limitations and is not accepted in its totality, a second theory, the rate theory, was developed to provide an alternative theory of DR interactions. The rate theory, similar to the occupancy theory, states that a drug will bind to its receptors in an equilibrium reaction with a characteristic rate constant for association (k_1) and a characteristic rate constant for dissociation (k_2). The rate theory proposes that the intrinsic activity of a drug, its ability to cause an effect, is a function of the rate at which the DR complex is formed and is proportional to the k_1 and k_2 values of the binding reaction. Based upon this supposition, an agonist is a molecule that has high k_1 and high k_2 values, as the rapid association and dissociation of DR complexes would allow for a high number of complexes to be formed per unit of time, resulting in the production of significant pharmacological effects. Conversely, according to the rate theory an antagonist is a molecule that may have a low, moderate, or high k_1 value for DR association, but must have a low k_2 value. The relatively stable and irreversible DR complexes represented by elevated rates of association compared with low rates of dissociation would limit the number of complexes formed per unit of time and result in limited pharmacological effects. The rate theory, therefore, proposes that the effects produced by a drug are dependent solely upon the rate at which it forms DR complexes. A limitation of this model is that it does not explain the mechanism by which signal transduction is initiated upon DR complex formation, but it assumes that the binding of a drug to its receptor will initiate signal transduction that will persist even after the drug has dissociated from the receptor.

B.4.4 TWO-STATE THEORY

The two-state theory of receptors differs from the occupancy theory and the rate theory in that it proposes that receptors exist in two conformations, an active state called the relaxed, or R, state and an inactive state called the tense, or T, state; these two states are in equilibrium with each other. When activated by ligands, the relaxed state of receptors produces a biological effect whereas the tense state produces no effect. The two-state theory asserts that drugs have different binding affinities for the relaxed and tense states of their specific receptor, and as such, they bind preferentially to the percentage of receptors that are in the state for which they have the greater affinity. The theory further proposes that the binding of a drug to its receptor stabilizes the receptor in either its existing relaxed or tense form. In this manner, drugs do not activate or block the activation of receptors per se, they merely stabilize the receptors in the form in which they already exist. According to the principles of the two-state theory, it follows that agonists are molecules that possess almost complete preferential affinity for the active, R state of their receptors; formation of agonist—receptor complexes thus stabilize the relaxed conformation of the receptor and result in sustained biological activity. Partial agonists are molecules that have significantly greater preferential affinity for the relaxed state as compared to the tense state, but also bind with meaningful affinity to the inactive T state, thus producing quantitatively reduced biological effects compared to full agonists. Antagonists bind with relatively equal affinity to both the relaxed and tense conformations of their specific receptors, thus stabilizing the existing equilibrium and resulting in no measurable effects. Finally, inverse agonists possess almost complete preferential affinity for the tense state of their receptor, thereby producing effects that are opposite to those produced by agonists, which stabilize the relaxed form of the receptor. The two-state theory, therefore, is based upon the principle that drugs do not bind equally to any form of their receptor, but rather, they bind with preferential affinity to a specific conformation of the receptor, resulting in the stabilization of that existing form. Similar to the occupancy theory and the rate theory, the two-state theory provides some valuable insight into DR interactions, but it does not in and of itself provide a complete and accurate representation of drug and/or receptor activity.

B.5 TRANSDUCTION SYSTEMS

To cause a biological effect, the binding of a drug to its receptor must initiate signal transduction. Signal transduction, broadly defined, is the process by which an extracellular signal, that is, the binding of a drug to its membrane receptor, is transmitted across the plasma membrane to intracellular components of signaling pathways, to cause a biochemical change within the cell. The manner in which signals are transmitted is dependent upon the identity and characteristics of the membrane receptor involved. Although there are many different types of cellular membrane receptors, four types are of the most relevance to forensic toxicologists: enzyme-linked receptors, ion channels, intracellular receptors, and G protein-coupled receptors (GPCRs).

B.5.1 ENZYME-LINKED RECEPTORS

Although different types of receptors transmit signals in different ways, a common mechanism of signal transduction is through the activation of enzymatic activity upon drug binding. The enzymes most commonly associated with receptor activation are protein kinases, which are enzymes that trigger the covalent attachment of a phosphate group to a protein through the process of protein phosphorylation. In animals, kinases can phosphorylate proteins on three amino acids: tyrosine, serine, and threonine; most of the kinases associated with receptor activity are tyrosine protein kinases. Phosphorylation is an important and ubiquitous biological on–off switch, by which the addition of a phosphate group generally has an activating effect on the modified protein and the removal of the phosphate (dephosphorylation) elicits a deactivating effect. A defining characteristic of phosphorylation, therefore, is that it is reversible. In one common type of receptor, the cytoplasmic portion of the receptor contains intrinsic kinase activity. In a second common type of receptor, the receptor itself has no kinase activity but its cytoplasmic tail is noncovalently bound to cytoplasmic protein kinases called receptor-associated protein kinases, which may be either constitutively bound to receptor or may associate only after drug binding. For both types of receptors, the kinases (either bound to or a part of the receptors) are normally inactive but drug binding to the extracellular region of the receptor causes kinase activation. A common mechanism of activation is via clustering wherein drug binding to kinase-associated receptors causes receptor dimerization, which draws the intracellular kinases associated with each individual receptor together. The clustering of the kinases results in enzyme activation, and the kinases then phosphorylate the receptor tails, other proteins associated with the receptor or even each other. This initial phosphorylation event initiates a cascade of intracellular signaling events in which a series of proteins interact with each other and pass on the signal that originated in the extracellular space. The removal of phosphate groups by protein phosphatase enzymes often serves to turn off signaling pathways by returning proteins to their original, inactive forms.

B.5.2 ION CHANNELS

Ion channels are transmembrane receptors that exist in either open or closed conformations. When open, ion channels facilitate the passage of specific ions across the plasma membrane and into the interior of a cell, and when closed, ion passage is prevented. The function of ion channels is important in maintaining the ion balance within a cell which is important for cellular function. In some cases, ion channels are constitutively open, but a type of ion channel opens in response to a change in transmembrane potential (voltage-gated channels) or in response to drug binding (drug-gated channels). In the context of drug action, the ion channels of the greatest relevance are drug-gated channels. Most commonly, drugs bind to the extracellular regions of ion channels, causing the transmembrane opening to change in some way so as to allow specific ions to pass through. Occasionally, a drug may bind to a site on the interior of the channel, effectively blocking the passage of ions. Direct drug-gated ion channels are channels in which drug binding alone is sufficient to regulate ion transport through the channel, whereas indirect drug-gated ion channels are those in which drug binding to some other target molecule results in the formation of a molecule (typically a second messenger) that will bind to the ion channel to trigger channel opening. In the case of indirect drug-gated ion channels, therefore, drugs do not bind directly to the channel, but rather modulate channel activity indirectly by binding to some other target receptor, often a GPCR, which transduces a signal to ultimately result in channel activation. Because direct drug-gated channels respond to drug directly they function more rapidly than indirect drug-gated channels, which require an initial reaction to occur before the channel can be activated; for this reason direct drug-gated ion channels are sometimes referred to as fast opening channels, whereas indirect drug-gated channels are referred to as slow opening channels.

B.5.3 INTRACELLULAR RECEPTORS

The majority of receptors are expressed on the cell surface, but some receptors are found in the intracellular space. Intracellular receptors generally elicit effects by either directly or indirectly regulating gene expression, often by modulating the activity of transcription factors. Drugs for intracellular receptors must possess high lipid solubility in order to passively move across the plasma membrane to interact with their specific target molecule(s). The steroid superfamily of receptors is the most common and broadly expressed class of intracellular receptors. In their resting state, steroid receptors are found in the cytoplasm in complex with molecular chaperones such as heat shock proteins. The binding of a naturally occurring glucocorticoid, or a pharmacological derivative of the glucocorticoid family, called corticosteroids, to its specific receptor triggers the displacement of the chaperone protein, which exposes a nuclear localization signal and the DNA binding region of the receptor. The activated DR complex can then enter the nucleus and regulate gene transcription either by binding to specific DNA sequences in the promoters of steroid-responsive genes, or by interacting with specific transcription factors such as NF-κB, and activating or inhibiting their activity.

B.5.4 G PROTEIN-COUPLED RECEPTORS

GPCRs are arguably the receptor class of the greatest interest and importance to forensic toxicologists because approximately 50% of all therapeutically used drugs exert their effects by binding to GPCRs. More than 50 different GPCRs have been characterized, all of which consist of a single polypeptide chain containing seven transmembrane α-helical domains, with an extracellular amino terminus and an intracellular carboxy terminus. GPCRs interact with a class of proteins called G proteins via coupling with the third cytoplasmic loop of the receptors. G proteins, so named because of their interaction with the guanine nucleotides, GTP and GDP, consist of three subunits, the α, β, and γ subunits. In the resting state, G proteins exist as αβγ trimers, with the βγ dimer associated with the cytoplasmic side of the plasma membrane and the α subunit bound to GDP. Drug binding to the extracellular region of a GPCR triggers a conformational change in the cytoplasmic domain of the receptor, facilitating a high-affinity binding to the G protein αβγ trimer. The association of the αβγ trimer with the GPCR triggers the displacement of GDP by GTP on the α subunit, which in turn causes dissociation of the βγ dimer from the α subunit. The active, GTP-bound α subunit diffuses away from the GPCR to interact with a target molecule or molecules. The α subunit possesses intrinsic GTPase activity, and signaling is terminated when the α subunit hydrolyzes the bound GTP to GDP and the resulting GDP-bound α subunit dissociates from its target molecule and associates once again with the βγ dimer. There are three major types of G proteins, G_s, G_i, and G_q, with the three subtypes differentiated by the differing structures of their α subunits. The two major target effector systems of GPCR signaling are the adenylyl cyclase system and the phospholipase C system. The biological effects elicited by a GPCR drug are dependent upon the effector system activated by DR complex formation, which in turn is dependent upon the type of G protein coupled to the specific target receptor.

B.5.5 ADENYLYL CYCLASE SYSTEM

The enzymatic activity of adenylyl cyclase is stimulated by GTP-bound G_s and inhibited by GTP-bound G_i. When activated, adenylyl cyclase catalyzes the conversion of adenosine triphosphate (ATP) to $3'$-$5'$-cyclic adenosine monophosphate (cAMP), and pyrophosphate. Cyclic AMP is a second messenger that plays an integral role in the regulation of multiple cellular processes, including cell metabolism, cell differentiation, ion channel activity, and cell division. The effects of many drugs are facilitated by the modulation of intracellular cAMP levels. Importantly, intracellular cAMP levels are regulated not only via the activation of inhibition of adenylyl cyclase activity but also via the regulation of phosphodiesterase activity; phosphodiesterases are enzymes responsible for the hydrolysis of cAMP. The cellular effects of cAMP are facilitated in large part by the activation of cAMP-dependent protein kinases, namely protein kinase A (PKA). In its resting form, PKA exists as a tetramer comprises two catalytic domains and two regulatory domains; before activation the regulatory domains block catalytic activity. Cyclic AMP activates PKA by binding to specific sites with the regulatory domains and triggering the dissociation of the regulatory and catalytic domains of the kinase. Activated cAMP-dependent kinases, such as PKA, phosphorylate and activate a variety of substrates including the cyclic AMP response element-binding protein (CREB), lipase, glycogen synthase, phosphorylase kinase, myosin-light-chain-kinase, and voltage-gated calcium channels. The biological effects of G_s activation by drug-GPCR complex formation are therefore quite varied, ranging from increased glycogen breakdown to increased force of muscle contraction.

B.5.6 PHOSPHOLIPASE C SYSTEM

The catalytic activity of phospholipase C (PLC) is activated by GTP-bound G_q. Activated PLC-γ catalyzes the breakdown of the membrane lipid phosphatidylinositol 3,4-bisphosphate into two products: the membrane lipid diacylglycerol (DAG) and the soluble second messenger inositol 1,4,5-triphosphate (IP3). DAG remains bound to the plasma membrane where it can shuttle laterally through the phospholipid bilayer, whereas IP3 diffuses away from the membrane into the cytosol; IP3 may be further phosphorylated to form inositol tetrakisphosphate. The activation of PLC by G_q and the resulting production of DAG and IP3 elicits a variety of biological effects. Many effects of IP3 are facilitated by its diffusion away from the plasma membrane and binding to IP3 receptors on the membrane of the endoplasmic reticulum. IP3 receptors are calcium channels, and IP3 binding opens the channels and triggers the release of Ca^{2+} from the endoplasmic reticulum into the cytosol. The depletion of Ca^{2+} stores in the endoplasmic reticulum in turn triggers the opening of Ca^{2+} channels in the plasma membrane, called CRAC channels (calcium release-activated calcium channels), which allows Ca^{2+} to enter the cell from the extracellular fluid. The cumulative effect of IP3 receptor activation and CRAC channel activation is the elevation of Ca^{2+} concentration in the cytosol, which can elicit several biological effects including transcription factor activation. Although DAG remains bound to the membrane, it serves an important role by recruiting of a variety of proteins including GTP exchange factors, which may be involved in MAP kinase signaling pathways, and various protein kinases, including protein kinase C. The proteins recruited by DAG play a role in mediating signal transduction pathways that regulate a variety of cellular processes.

SUGGESTED READING

Brunton, L., Chabner, B., Knollman, B., 2011. Goodman and Gilman's the Pharmacological Basis of Therapeutics. McGraw-Hill, Columbus.

Golan, D.E., Tashjian, A.H., Armstrong, E.J., Armstrong, A.W., 2012. Principles of Pharmacology: The Pathophysiologic Basis of Drug Therapy. Lippincott Williams and Wilkins, Philadelphia.

Harrold, M.W., Zavod, R.M., 2013. Basic Concepts in Medicinal Chemistry. American Society of Health-Systems Pharmacists, Inc., Bethesda.

Hilal-Dandan, R., Brunton, L.L., 2014. Goodman and Gilman's Manual of Pharmacology and Therapeutics. McGraw-Hill, New York.

Katzung, B.G., Trevor, A.J., 2015. Basic and Clinical Pharmacology. McGraw-Hill, Columbus.

LaDu, B.N., Mandel, H.G., Way, E.L., 1971. Fundamentals of Drug Metabolism and Disposition. The Williams and Wilkins Company, Baltimore, MD.

Lemke, T.L., Williams, D.A., Roche, V.F., Zito, S.W., 2013. Foye's Principles of Medicinal Chemistry. Lippincott Williams and Wilkins, Philadelphia.

Patrick, G.L., 2015. An Introduction to Medicinal Chemistry. Oxford University Press, Oxford.

Rang, H.P., Ritter, J.M., Flower, R.J., Henderson, G., 2015. Rang and Dale's Pharmacology. Elsevier.

Stringer, J.L., 2011. Basic Concepts in Pharmacology: What You Need to Know for Each Drug Class. McGraw-Hill, Columbus.

Wecker, L., Crespos, L., Dunaway, G., Faingold, C., Watts, S., 2009. Brody's Human Pharmacology. Mosby, St. Louis.

Whalen, K., 2015. Pharmacology. Wolters Kluwer, Philadelphia.

Immunoassays

C.1 INTRODUCTION

Pluripotent hematopoietic stem cells found in the bone marrow give rise to all blood cells, including the red blood cells, platelets, and white blood cells. The white blood cells, also called leukocytes, form the basis of mammalian immune systems. Hematopoietic stem cells differentiate into two other cell types of more limited developmental potential—the common lymphoid progenitor cells and the common myeloid progenitor cells. Common myeloid progenitor cells differentiate to form most of the cells involved in innate immunity, and common lymphoid progenitor cells give rise to the cells of the adaptive immune system, including T and B lymphocytes. Adaptive immune responses are highly specific responses dependent upon the recognition of specific antigen by B cell receptors and T cell receptors expressed on lymphocyte cell membranes. In the most general sense, an antigen is any substance that, when introduced into the body, elicits an immune cell response. In practice, T cell receptors can recognize peptide antigen only, whereas B cell receptors can recognize and bind to a much broader diversity of antigen, including proteins, carbohydrates, and lipids. Upon antigen recognition by a B cell receptor, B cells may proliferate and differentiate into antibody-producing plasma cells. Several analytical methodologies of importance to forensic toxicologists rely upon the unique properties of antibody–antigen binding.

C.2 ANTIBODIES

Antibodies, also called immunoglobulins, are the secreted form of the B cell receptor, and the antigen specificity of an antibody is therefore identical to the specificity of the B cell receptor responsible for the initial antigen recognition. The immune system must produce antibodies capable of binding to a wide variety of antigenic substances, while at the same time maintaining the ability to interact with a more limited number of effector cells and molecules; the physical structure of antibodies is vital to this function. The overall protein structure of antibodies is often described as a "Y" shape, comprises three equally sized sections connected by a flexible polypeptide chain called the hinge region. The two arms of an antibody can move freely and independently on the hinge region, and at the tip of each arm is a highly variable sequence of amino acids called the variable region (Figure C.1). The unique antigen-binding surface area formed by the sequence of amino acids in the variable region of an antibody determines the antigen specificity of a given antibody. The sequence of amino acids found in the variable regions of antibodies is in turn dictated by a specialized process of gene rearrangement that occurs during B lymphocyte development; this process, called V(D)J recombination, is responsible for the generation of a highly diverse repertoire of B cell receptors and antibodies, each capable of binding to a specific antigen. The stem of the antibody is called the constant region, as and is reflected in the name, consists of an amino acid sequence that is much less variable among antibodies. There are, however, five classes of immunoglobulins, IgG, IgM, IgD, IgA, and IgE, which are distinguished by the amino acid composition of their constant regions. Whereas the function of the variable region of an antibody is to recognize and bind to antigen, the function of the constant region is to interact with various effector cells and/or molecules to elicit an appropriate immune response to the detected threat.

In general, antibodies bind to antigens that have surfaces that are complementary to the antigen-binding site in the variable regions of the antibody arms. Antigens can be small or large, and may bind in pockets, grooves, or extended regions of the antigen-binding sites. However, antibodies typically recognize and bind to only a small region on the surface of any antigen, this region is called the antigenic determinant or epitope. Antibody—antigen binding is noncovalent and reversible and can be disrupted by high salt concentrations, pH changes, detergents, and high concentrations of epitope. The four most significant forces responsible for facilitating

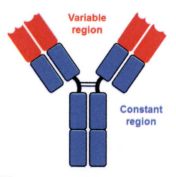

FIGURE C.1 Antibody Structure

Antibodies, or immunoglobulins, are the secreted form of the B cell receptor. Antibodies are comprised of three equally sized sections connected by a flexible hinge region. At the tip of each arm is a highly variable sequence of amino acids called the variable region; the variable region facilitates antigen binding. The five classes of immunoglobulins (IgG, IgM, IgD, IgA, and IgE) are distinguished based upon the amino acid composition of their constant regions, which interact with various effector cells and/or molecules.

antibody—antigen binding are electrostatic forces, hydrogen bonds, van der Waals forces, and hydrophobic interactions.

C.3 ANTIBODY PRODUCTION

The specificity with which antibodies bind to antigen can be exploited for use in drug detection assays. Immunoassays, which are typically utilized as presumptive or screening tests, are analytical techniques that rely upon the interactions between antibodies and antigens; the "antigens" in toxicological immunoassays, rather than being invading pathogens, are generally drugs or drug metabolites. The application of immunoassays to toxicological analyses therefore depends upon the generation of specific antidrug antibodies. There are two main types of antibodies that may be generated for use in immunoassays: polyclonal and monoclonal antibodies. Polyclonal antibodies are antibodies that recognize the same antigen, but because they are produced by B cells of differing lineages, recognize different epitopes. Conversely, monoclonal antibodies are produced by B cells of a single lineage, and therefore recognize a single, identical, epitope on a given antigen.

Polyclonal antibodies are straightforward to produce. The immunization of a sensitized laboratory animal with a compound of interest will stimulate the production of polyclonal antibodies that can be collected from blood serum and purified. Although the generation of compound-specific antibody by such an in vivo method of stimulation is theoretically straightforward, it is important to note that the resulting antibodies will bind with varying affinities to varying antigenic epitopes. Furthermore, the repertoire of antibodies generated will often vary within and between animals, making it difficult to obtain a predictable and well-characterized population of compound-specific antibodies. The inherent variability of polyclonal antibodies, and the resultant unpredictability of their binding interactions with a drug analyte of interest, makes them less than optimal for use in toxicological immunoassays. It is preferable, therefore, to utilize monoclonal antibodies, which bind in a uniform manner to a single antigenic epitope.

The generation of compound-specific monoclonal antibody is initiated similarly to the generation of polyclonal antibody: a sensitized animal is immunized with the compound of interest. During the production of polyclonal antibody, significant volumes of blood must be collected from the immunized animals in order to purify meaningful amounts of antibody. Therefore, larger animals such as sheep, goats, or rabbits are generally employed. During the generation of monoclonal antibody, however, mice are typically utilized because antibody is not collected from blood serum, but rather antibody-producing plasma cells are purified from the peripheral lymphoid organs and fused with myeloma cells to form long-lived antibody-producing hybridomas. Each hybridoma line produces a unique, monoclonal, antibody population, and the binding affinity, and antigenic specificity of each antibody can be characterized. The hybridoma(s) determined to produce the most optimal monoclonal antibody for a specific drug analyte of interest generally is(are) cloned and propagated in culture to produce large amounts of the desired antibody.

C.4 IMMUNOASSAYS

Most immunological techniques utilized by forensic toxicologists are competition binding assays based upon the principle that drug analytes in biological samples of interest will compete with reagent drugs in a reaction mixture for binding to a specific antidrug antibody. To monitor the binding kinetics of the antibody—antigen reactions, most immunoassays rely upon the labeling of either the antibody or the antigen with a radioisotope, fluorophore, or enzymatic tag.

There are two main types of competitive binding assays—homogeneous and heterogeneous reactions. In heterogeneous reactions, after the completion of the binding reaction, any unbound labeled component must be removed from the reaction mixture before the quantification of binding is performed. This separation step is not required in homogeneous reactions, however, because the quantification of antibody—antigen binding relies not merely upon the quantity of the labeled component present (as in heterogeneous reactions), but upon the modulation of some property of the label by antibody—antigen binding. Although heterogeneous reactions have the advantage of a greater signal to noise ratio and lower limits of detection, homogeneous reactions are more easily automated; both heterogeneous and homogeneous reactions are utilized in forensic toxicology laboratories. The four major types of immunoassays of importance to forensic toxicologists are the radioimmunoassay (RIA), enzyme-multiplied immunoassay technique (EMIT), enzyme-linked immunosorbent assay (ELISA), and fluorescence polarization immunoassay (FPI or FPIA).

C.4.1 RADIOIMMUNOASSAY

The technique of RIA was first described by Yalow and Berson in 1959. RIA is a competitive binding assay based upon the principle that radioactively labeled drug will compete with unlabeled drug in a biological sample for binding to a specific antidrug antibody. In practice, a known amount of drug, which has been labeled with a radioisotope (generally ^{125}I), is added to a biological sample of interest, after which antidrug antibody is added to the sample. After an established period of time, unbound drug is removed from the reaction tube and the amount of radioactivity remaining is measured. Because the binding of labeled drug to antidrug antibody is inhibited by unlabeled free drug in the sample, the amount of radioactivity present in the antibody—drug complexes is inversely proportional to the concentration of drug in the biological sample (Figure C.2). Reactions utilizing reference standards, that is, known concentrations of unlabeled drug, must also be performed to generate a standard curve of counts per minute versus drug concentration; the drug concentration in the biological sample of interest can then be determined by interpolation

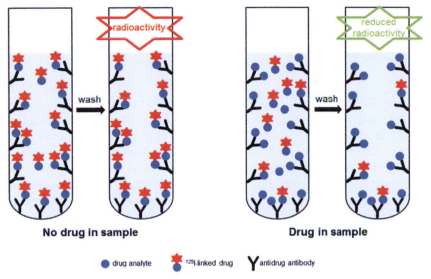

No drug in sample   **Drug in sample**

● drug analyte   ✶ ^{125}I-linked drug   Y antidrug antibody

FIGURE C.2 Radioimmunoassay (RIA)

The technique of RIA is a heterogeneous competitive binding assay in which radioactively labeled drug competes with unlabeled drug in a biological sample for binding to a specific antidrug antibody. Because the binding of labeled drug to antidrug antibody is inhibited by unlabeled free drug in the sample, the amount of radioactivity present in the antibody—drug complexes is inversely proportional to the concentration of drug in the biological sample.

wherein the counts per minute in the experimental reaction are compared to the standard curve.

The quantification of radioactivity in an RIA reaction mixture must only be performed after any unbound drug is removed from the sample; thus, RIA is a heterogeneous assay. There are two widely used methods for the separation of free drug from antibody bound drug: the use of antibody-coated reaction tubes and the use of secondary antibody. In the coated tube technique, the primary, antidrug antibody is adhered to the reaction tube before the addition of the biological sample and the radioactively labeled drug. Any drug that binds to the adhered antibodies will therefore also be adhered to the reaction tube, and upon the completion of the biding assay, the unbound drug can be easily removed by the removal of the supernatant. An alternative method for the separation of unbound drug from bound drug is the use of a secondary antibody with specificity for the primary antidrug antibody. Upon the completion of the binding assay, the secondary antibody is added directly to the reaction mixture. The binding of the secondary antibody to the primary antibody triggers a precipitation reaction in which the cross-linked antibodies (and any bound drug) precipitate out of solution. The precipitated components of the reaction mixture can be centrifuged, the supernatant (containing unbound drug) discarded, and the radioactivity in the precipitated pellet measured. RIA has been successfully utilized for the detection of numerous drugs in various biological matrices, including urine, saliva, plasma, hair, oral fluid, and tears. RIA has high sensitivity and relatively low background. However, it can be difficult to automate and requires the use of radioactivity.

C.4.2 ENZYME-MULTIPLIED IMMUNOASSAY TECHNIQUE

The EMIT is based upon the principle that, for specific enzymes, if the enzyme is linked to an antigen, the binding of an antibody to the antigen can modulate the activity of the enzyme. EMIT assays are competition binding assays in which free drug in a biological sample competes with enzyme-bound reagent drug in the reaction mixture for binding to the drug-specific antibody. The EMIT assay is performed by adding enzyme-labeled drug and antidrug antibody to the biological sample of interest. If the antidrug antibody binds to the enzyme-linked drug, the enzymatic activity will decrease. If however, the antibody binds to free, unlabeled drug in the biological sample, the enzymatic activity will not be affected. Therefore, there is a direct relationship between drug concentration in the sample and enzymatic activity; higher concentrations of unlabeled drug in the sample will result in more competition for antibody binding and subsequently less binding of the antibody to the enzyme-linked drug (Figure C.3).

Several different enzymes have successfully been utilized in EMIT assays, but the enzyme most commonly used is glucose-6-phosphate dehydrogenase. Glucose-6-phosphate dehydrogenase uses NAD as a cofactor to catalyze the oxidation of glucose-6-phoshate to glucuronolactone-6-phosphate; as a by-product of the oxidation reaction, NAD is reduced to NADH, which has a characteristic absorbance at 340 nm. The quantity of NADH produced during the course of the binding reaction can therefore be quantified by measuring absorbance at 340 nm. Because enzyme activity is suppressed by antibody binding to the enzyme-linked drug complex, and enzymatic activity is correlated with the amount of NADH produced (and therefore absorbance at 340), it follows that because the free drug in the sample competes with the enzyme-linked drug complex for antibody binding, the concentration of free drug is directly proportional to the absorbance at 340 nm. When performing EMIT assays, the absorbance at 340 nm is measured over a period of time, and a decrease in enzymatic activity is manifested as a decrease in absorbance over the time period of observation. The drug concentration in a sample can be interpolated by comparing the absorbance of an experimental reaction to the absorbance of several standards.

The EMIT is a homogeneous assay that does not require the separation of unbound drug from bound drug; for this reason the technique is relatively efficient. EMIT assays have been utilized to detect the presence of various drugs in many biological matrices, including blood, plasma, saliva, with the added advantage of no radioactivity being required. EMIT assays cannot, however, be utilized if the biological matrix of interest contains components that absorb at 340 nm, as this would interfere with the quantification of enzymatic activity.

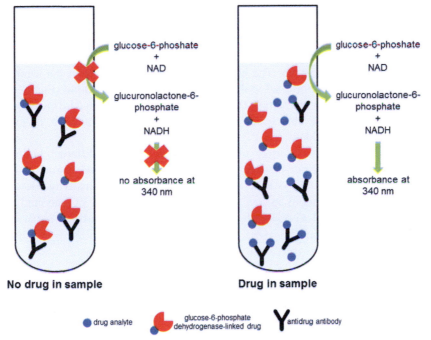

No drug in sample   **Drug in sample**

● drug analyte   glucose-6-phosphate dehydrogenase-linked drug   Y antidrug antibody

FIGURE C.3 Enzyme-Multiplied Immunoassay Technique (EMIT)

The EMIT is a homogeneous assay based upon the principle that, for specific enzymes, if the enzyme is linked to an antigen, the binding of an antibody to the antigen can modulate the activity of the enzyme. Therefore, there is a direct relationship between drug concentration in the sample and enzymatic activity; higher concentrations of unlabeled drug in the sample will result in more competition for antibody binding and subsequently less binding of the antibody to the enzyme-linked drug.

C.4.3 ENZYME-LINKED IMMUNOSORBENT ASSAY

ELISAs are arguably the most widely used immunoassays in forensic toxicology. Similar to EMIT assays, ELISAs are competition binding assays in which enzyme-linked drug competes with unlabeled drug for binding to antidrug antibody. ELISAs are typically performed in microplates that have been coated with primary, drug-specific antibody. A biological sample of interest and enzyme-linked drug are added to the wells of the microplate; as in EMIT assays, the unlabeled drug will compete with the enzyme-linked drug for antibody binding. After an appropriate incubation period, the wells of the microplate are washed to remove any unbound drug or unbound enzyme-linked drug, and enzymatic activity is measured. Because the unlabeled drug in the sample competes with the enzyme-linked drug for antibody binding, the amount of enzyme activity remaining in the microplate after the removal of unbound drug is inversely proportional to the concentration of free drug in the sample. The most common enzyme utilized in ELISA assays is horseradish peroxidase, which, in the presence of peroxide, oxidizes tetramethylbenzidine to tetramethylbenzidine diimine, which has a characteristic blue color. The catalytic reaction can be stopped by the addition of a dilute solution of sulfuric acid, which will convert the blue color to a yellow color, which can be measured at an absorbance of 450 nm. The concentration of drug present in the sample is therefore inversely proportional to the absorbance reading at 450 nm (Figure C.4). The drug concentration in a sample can be interpolated from a standard curve generated by measuring the absorbance of wells to which drug standards of known concentrations were added.

ELISAs can detect a variety of drug analytes in many different biological matrices, including urine, plasma, oral fluid, sweat, bile, and tissue extracts. Compared to EMIT, ELISAs have increased specificity and sensitivity. However, ELISAs are heterogeneous assays that require the separation of unbound drug from bound drug, and thus are slightly less time efficient and somewhat more

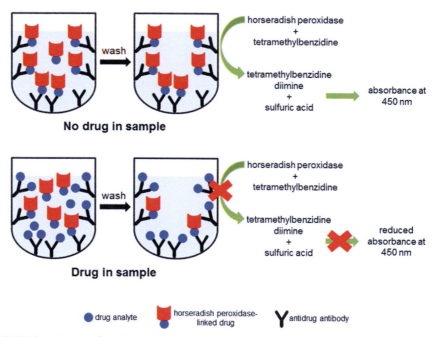

FIGURE C.4 Enzyme-Linked Immunosorbent Assay (ELISA)

ELISAs are heterogeneous competition binding assays in which enzyme-linked drug competes with unlabeled drug for binding to antidrug antibody that has been adhered to the walls of microplate wells. Because the unlabeled drug in the sample competes with the enzyme-linked drug for antibody binding, the amount of enzyme activity remaining in the microplate after the removal of unbound drug is inversely proportional to the concentration of free drug in the sample.

difficult to automate than EMIT. Nonetheless, due to the versatility of the assay ELISAs often utilized as the presumptive test of choice in forensic toxicology laboratories.

C.4.4 FLUORESCENCE POLARIZATION IMMUNOASSAY

FPI or FPIA was first applied to the detection of drugs in the 1960s, although the principles of the method were established in the 1920s. FPI is based upon the principle that when fluorescent molecules (fluorophores) are excited with a specific wavelength of light, some of the light is rapidly reemitted at a longer emission wavelength. If the fluorophore is stationary, the emitted light will be in the same polarization plane as the excitation light. For instance, if vertically polarized light is used to excite a stationary fluorophore, the emitted light will also be in the vertical plane. If, however, a fluorophore rotates during the brief period between excitation and emission, the emitted light will not be polarized. For instance, if a rotating fluorophore is excited with light in the vertical plane, the emitted light will be in both the vertical and horizontal planes; the degree to which the emission light intensity moves from the vertical to the horizontal plane is proportional to the mobility of the fluorophore. FPI exploits the fact that small molecules rotate more quickly than large molecules; thus, free drug molecules rotate more quickly than antibody–drug complexes. Therefore, if a fluorophore is linked to a free drug molecule and the complex is excited, the emission light will be nonpolarized relative to the excitation plane, due to the rotation of the small complex. However, if a specific antidrug antibody is bound to the fluorophore-linked drug and the complex is excited, the large antibody will inhibit the fluorophore rotation and the emission light will be polarized.

FPI is a competition binding assay in which fluorophore-linked drug, antidrug antibody, and a biological sample of interest are added to a reaction tube; the unlabeled free drug in the sample and the fluorophore-linked drug compete for antibody binding. The greater the concentration of free drug in the sample, the more competition there is for antibody binding. Drug concentration in the sample is therefore directly correlated with the amount of unbound fluorophore-linked drug in the reaction, and inversely correlated with the resulting degree of polarization, with increasing free drug concentration resulting in reduced emission polarization (due to the greater rotational potential of the unbound fluorophore-linked drug) (Figure C.5). Standard curves illustrating the relationship between free drug concentration and the resultant emission polarization (generally represented in millipolarization units) can be generated and utilized to interpolate the drug concentration in a biological sample of interest. FPI can be used to detect a wide diversity of drugs of abuse in a variety of biological matrices, including blood, bile, hair, and tissue extracts. Notably, FPI may not be useful for the analysis of drug concentration in urine as certain components of the matrix may interfere with the assay. A homogeneous assay, FPA does not require the separation of unbound from bound drug and it does not require the use of radioactivity, but it is less sensitive than RIA or the EMIT.

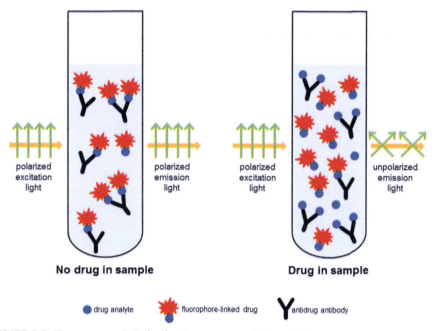

No drug in sample   **Drug in sample**

● drug analyte   ✹ fluorophore-linked drug   Y antidrug antibody

FIGURE C.5 Fluorescence Polarization Immunoassay (FPI or FPIA)

FPI assays are homogeneous assays based upon the principle that when fluorophores are excited, some of the light is rapidly reemitted. If the fluorophore is stationary, the emitted light will be in the same polarization plane as the excitation light, but if the fluorophore rotates during the brief period between excitation and emission, the emitted light will not be polarized. FPI assays are competition assays in which free drug in a biological sample competes with fluorophore-linked drug for binding to an antidrug antibody. If a fluorophore—drug complex is excited, the emission light will be nonpolarized, but if a specific antidrug antibody is bound to the fluorophore-linked drug and the complex is excited, the large antibody will inhibit the fluorophore rotation and the emission light will be polarized.

SUGGESTED READING

Agius, R., Nadulski, T., Moore, C., 2012. Validation of LUCIO-Direct-ELISA kits for the detection of drugs of abuse in urine: application to the new German driving licence re-granting guidelines. Forensic Sci. Int. 215 (1–3), 38–45.

Allen Jr., L.V., Stiles, M.L., 1981. Specificity of the EMIT drug abuse urine assay methods. Clin. Toxicol. 18 (9), 1043–1065.

Appel, T.A., Wade, N.A., 1989. Screening of blood and urine for drugs of abuse utilizing diagnostic products corporation's Coat-A-Count radioimmunoassay kits. J. Anal. Toxicol. 13 (5), 274–276.

Armbruster, D.A., Schwarzhoff, R.H., Hubster, E.C., Liserio, M.K., 1993. Enzyme immunoassay, kinetic microparticle immunoassay, radioimmunoassay, and fluorescence polarization immunoassay compared for drugs-of-abuse screening. Clin. Chem. 39 (10), 2137–2146.

Armbruster, D.A., Schwarzhoff, R.H., Pierce, B.L., Hubster, E.C., 1994. Method comparison of EMIT 700 and EMIT II with RIA for drug screening. J. Anal. Toxicol. 18 (2), 110−117.

Asselin, W.M., Leslie, J.M., 1992. Modification of Emit assay reagents for improved sensitivity and cost effectiveness in the analysis of hemolyzed whole blood. J. Anal. Toxicol. 16 (6), 381−388.

Asselin, W.M., Leslie, J.M., McKinley, B., 1988. Direct detection of drugs of abuse in whole hemolyzed blood using the EMIT d.a.u. urine assays. J. Anal. Toxicol. 12 (4), 207−215.

Barnes, A.J., Spinelli, E., Young, S., Martin, T.M., Kleete, K.L., Huestis, M.A., 2015. Validation of an ELISA synthetic cannabinoids urine assay. Ther. Drug Monitor. http://dx.doi.org/10.1097/FTD.0000000000000201.

Basilicata, P., Pieri, M., Settembre, V., Galdiero, A., Della, C.E., Acampora, A., Miraglia, N., 2011. Screening of several drugs of abuse in Italian workplace drug testing: performance comparisons of on-site screening tests and a fluorescence polarization immunoassay-based device. Anal. Chem. 83 (22), 8566−8574.

Beck, O., Lin, Z., Brodin, K., Borg, S., Hjemdahl, P., 1997. The online screening technique for urinary benzodiazepines: comparison with EMIT, FPIA, and GC-MS. J. Anal. Toxicol. 21 (7), 554−557.

Beck, O., Rausberg, L., Al-Saffar, Y., Villen, T., Karlsson, L., Hansson, T., Helander, A., 2014. Detectability of new psychoactive substances, "legal highs," in CEDIA, EMIT, and KIMS immunochemical screening assays for drugs of abuse. Drug Test. Anal. 6 (5), 492−499.

Bogusz, M., Aderjan, R., Schmitt, G., Nadler, E., Neureither, B., 1990. The determination of drugs of abuse in whole blood by means of FPIA and EMIT-dau immunoassays—a comparative study. Forensic Sci. Int. 48 (1), 27−37.

Borggaard, B., Joergensen, I., 1994. Urinary screening for benzodiazepines with radioreceptor assay: comparison with EMIT d.a.u. benzodiazepine assay and high-performance liquid chromatography. J. Anal. Toxicol. 18 (5), 243−246.

Bress, W.C., Bidanset, J.H., Lukash, L., 1982. Analysis of post mortem brain tissue using EMIT. J. Anal. Toxicol. 6 (5), 264−265.

Castro, A., Mittleman, R., 1978. Determination of drugs of abuse in body fluids by radioimmunoassay. Clin. Biochem. 11 (3), 103−105.

Cheong, J.C., Suh, S., Ko, B.J., Lee, J.I., Kim, J.Y., Suh, Y.J., In, M.K., 2013. Screening method for the detection of methamphetamine in hair using fluorescence polarization immunoassay. J. Anal. Toxicol. 37 (4), 217−221.

Choi, J., Kim, C., Choi, M.J., 1998. Comparison of capillary electrophoresis-based immunoassay with fluorescence polarization immunoassay for the immunodetermination of methamphetamine using various methamphetamine antibodies. Electrophoresis 19 (16−17), 2950−2955.

Cirimele, V., Etienne, S., Villain, M., Ludes, B., Kintz, P., 2004. Evaluation of the One-Step ELISA kit for the detection of buprenorphine in urine, blood, and hair specimens. Forensic Sci. Int. 143 (2−3), 153−156.

Cleeland, R., Christenson, J., Usategui-Gomez, M., Heveran, J., Davis, R., Grunberg, E., 1976. Detection of drugs of abuse by radioimmunoassay: a summary of published data and some new information. Clin. Chem. 22 (6), 712−725.

Coccini, T., Crevani, A., Acerbi, D., Roda, E., Castoldi, A.F., Crespi, V., Manzo, L., 2008. Comparative HPLC and ELISA studies for CDT isoform characterization in subjects with alcohol related problems. Prospective application in workplace risk-prevention policy. G. Ital. Med. Lav. Ergon. 30 (2), 119−127.

Cone, E.J., 1989. Validity testing of commercial urine cocaine metabolite assays: III. Evaluation of an enzyme-linked immunosorbent assay (ELISA) for detection of cocaine and cocaine metabolite. J. Forensic Sci. 34 (4), 991−995.

Datta, P., 2009. Immunoassay design for drugs of abuse testing. In: Dasgupta, A. (Ed.), Critical Issues in Alcohol and Drugs of Abuse Testing. AACC Press, Washington, DC, pp. 105−115.

Debrabandere, L., Van, B.M., Daenens, P., 1993. Development of a radioimmunoassay for the determination of buprenorphine in biological samples. Analyst 118 (2), 137−143.

Diosi, D.T., Harvey, D.C., 1993. Analysis of whole blood for drugs of abuse using EMIT d.a.u. reagents and a Monarch 1000 Chemistry Analyzer. J. Anal. Toxicol. 17 (3), 133−137.

Fraser, A.D., Worth, D., 2002. Monitoring urinary excretion of cannabinoids by fluorescence-polarization immunoassay: a cannabinoid-to-creatinine ratio study. Ther. Drug Monitor. 24 (6), 746−750.

Gross, S.J., Worthy, T.E., Nerder, L., Zimmermann, E.G., Soares, J.R., Lomax, P., 1985. Detection of recent cannabis use by saliva delta 9-THC radioimmunoassay. J. Anal. Toxicol. 9 (1), 1−5.

Han, E., Miller, E., Lee, J., Park, Y., Lim, M., Chung, H., Wylie, F.M., Oliver, J.S., 2006. Validation of the immunalysis microplate ELISA for the detection of methamphetamine in hair. J. Anal. Toxicol. 30 (6), 380−385.

Harwood, C.T., 1974. Radioimmunoassay: its application to drugs of abuse. Pharmacology 11 (1), 52−57.

Hindin, R., McCusker, J., Vickers-Lahti, M., Bigelow, C., Garfield, F., Lewis, B., 1994. Radioimmunoassay of hair for determination of cocaine, heroin, and marijuana exposure: comparison with self-report. Int. J. Addict. 29 (6), 771−789.

Juhascik, M., Habbel, S., Barron, W., Behonick, G., 2006. Validation of an ELISA method for screening methadone in postmortem blood. J. Anal. Toxicol. 30 (8), 617−620.

Kaul, B., Davidow, B., 1980. Application of a radioimmunoassay screening test for detection and management of phencyclidine intoxication. J. Clin. Pharmacol. 20 (8−9), 500−505.

Keller, T., Schneider, A., Dirnhofer, R., Jungo, R., Meyer, W., 2000. Fluorescence polarization immunoassay for the detection of drugs of abuse in human whole blood. Med. Sci. Law 40 (3), 258−262.

Kemp, P., Sneed, G., Kupiec, T., Spiehler, V., 2002. Validation of a microtiter plate ELISA for screening of postmortem blood for opiates and benzodiazepines. J. Anal. Toxicol. 26 (7), 504−512.

Kirschbaum, K.M., Musshoff, F., Wilbert, A., Rohrich, J., Madea, B., 2011. Direct ELISA kits as a sensitive and selective screening method for abstinence control in urine. Forensic Sci. Int. 207 (1−3), 66−69.

Klinger, R.A., Blum, L.M., Rieders, F., 1990. Direct automated EMIT d.a.u. analysis of N,N-dimethylformamide-modified serum, plasma, and postmortem blood for amphetamines, barbiturates, methadone, methaqualone, phencyclidine, and propoxyphene. J. Anal. Toxicol. 14 (5), 288−291.

Knittel, J.L., Clay, D.J., Bailey, K.M., Gebhardt, M.A., Kraner, J.C., 2009. Comparison of oxycodone in vitreous humor and blood using EMIT screening and gas chromatographic-mass spectrometric quantitation. J. Anal. Toxicol. 33 (8), 433−438.

Laloup, M., Tilman, G., Maes, V., De, B.G., Wallemacq, P., Ramaekers, J., Samyn, N., 2005. Validation of an ELISA-based screening assay for the detection of amphetamine, MDMA and MDA in blood and oral fluid. Forensic Sci. Int. 153 (1), 29−37.

Lewis, M.G., Lewis, J.G., Elder, P.A., Moore, G.A., 2003. An enzyme-linked immunosorbent assay (ELISA) for methylphenidate (Ritalin) in urine. J. Anal. Toxicol. 27 (6), 342−345.

Lu, N.T., Taylor, B.G., 2006. Drug screening and confirmation by GC-MS: comparison of EMIT II and online KIMS against 10 drugs between US and England laboratories. Forensic Sci. Int. 157 (2−3), 106−116.

Maier, R.D., Erkens, M., Hoenen, H., Bogusz, M., 1992. The screening for common drugs of abuse in whole blood by means of EMIT-ETS and FPIA-ADx urine immunoassays. Int. J. Legal Med. 105 (2), 115−119.

Marin, S.J., Keith, L., Merrell, M., McMillin, G.A., 2009. Comparison of drugs of abuse detection in meconium by EMIT II and ELISA. J. Anal. Toxicol. 33 (3), 148−154.

Miki, A., Katagi, M., Tsuchihashi, H., 2002. Application of EMIT d.a.u. for the semiquantitative screening of methamphetamine incorporated in hair. J. Anal. Toxicol. 26 (5), 274−279.

Miller, E.I., Torrance, H.J., Oliver, J.S., 2006a. Validation of the Immunalysis microplate ELISA for the detection of buprenorphine and its metabolite norbuprenorphine in urine. J. Anal. Toxicol. 30 (2), 115−119.

Miller, E.I., Wylie, F.M., Oliver, J.S., 2006b. Detection of benzodiazepines in hair using ELISA and LC-ESI-MS-MS. J. Anal. Toxicol. 30 (7), 441−448.

Miyaguchi, H., Takahashi, H., Ohashi, T., Mawatari, K., Iwata, Y.T., Inoue, H., Kitamori, T., 2009. Rapid analysis of methamphetamine in hair by micropulverized extraction and microchip-based competitive ELISA. Forensic Sci. Int. 184 (1−3), 1−5.

Mule, S.J., Whitlock, E., Jukofsky, D., 1975. Radioimmunoassay of drugs subject to abuse: critical evaluation of urinary morphine-barbiturate, morphine, barbiturate, and amphetamine assays. Clin. Chem. 21 (1), 81−86.

Narongchai, P., Sribanditmonkol, P., Thampithug, S., Narongchai, S., Chitivuthikarn, C., 2002. The duration time of urine morphine detection in heroin addicts by radioimmunoassay. J. Med. Assoc. Thai. 85 (1), 82−86.

Noe, E.R., Lathrop, G.D., Ainsworth III, C.A., Merritt, J.H., 1976. Radioimmunoassay technology in mass drug screening: an evaluation of an absorbent paper disk transport system. J. Forensic Sci. 21 (2), 390−397.

Oellerich, M., Kulpmann, W.R., Haeckel, R., 1977. Drug screening by enzyme immunoassay (EMIT) and thin-layer chromatography (Drug Skreen). J. Clin. Chem. Clin. Biochem. 15 (5), 275−283.

Perez-Bendito, D., Gomez-Hens, A., Gaikwad, A., 1994. Direct stopped-flow fluorescence polarization immunoassay of abused drugs and their metabolites in urine. Clin. Chem. 40 (8), 1489−1493.

Pujol, M.L., Cirimele, V., Tritsch, P.J., Villain, M., Kintz, P., 2007. Evaluation of the IDS One-Step ELISA kits for the detection of illicit drugs in hair. Forensic Sci. Int. 170 (2−3), 189−192.

Rodrigues, W.C., Catbagan, P., Rana, S., Wang, G., Moore, C., 2013. Detection of synthetic cannabinoids in oral fluid using ELISA and LC-MS-MS. J. Anal. Toxicol. 37 (8), 526−533.

Sarris, G., Borg, D., Liao, S., Stripp, R., 2014. Validation of an EMIT(R) screening method to detect 6-acetylmorphine in oral fluid. J. Anal. Toxicol. 38 (8), 605−609.

Schutz, H.W., 1989. THC-carbonic acid determination in serum with fluorescence polarization immunoassay (FPIA, TDX) and GCMS. Beitr. Gerichtl. Med. 47, 95−96.

Sloop, G., Hall, M., Simmons, G.T., Robinson, C.A., 1995. False-positive postmortem EMIT drugs-of-abuse assay due to lactate dehydrogenase and lactate in urine. J. Anal. Toxicol. 19 (7), 554–556.

Smith, F.P., 2005. Handbook of Forensic Drug Analysis. Elsevier Academic Press, San Diego.

Smith-Kielland, A., Olsen, K.M., Christophersen, A.S., 1995. False-positive results with Emit II amphetamine/methamphetamine assay in users of common psychotropic drugs. Clin. Chem. 41 (6 Pt 1), 951–952.

Spiehler, V., 1975. Drugs of abuse radioimmunoassay directory. Clin. Toxicol. 8 (2), 257–265.

Spiehler, V.R., Sedgwick, P., 1985. Radioimmunoassay screening and GC/MS confirmation of whole blood samples for drugs of abuse. J. Anal. Toxicol. 9 (2), 63–66.

Standefer, J.C., Backer, R.C., 1991. Drug screening with EMIT reagents: a quantitative approach to quality control. Clin. Chem. 37 (5), 733–738.

Sulkowski, T.S., Lathrop, G.D., Merritt, J.H., Landez, J.H., Noe, E.R., 1975. A semiautomated radioimmunoassay for mass screening of drugs of abuse. J. Forensic Sci. 20 (3), 524–536.

Taylor, J., 1989. Presence of inhibitors to the EMIT test in postmortem urine samples. J. Forensic Sci. 34 (5), 1055–1056.

Venkatratnam, A., Lents, N.H., 2011. Zinc reduces the detection of cocaine, methamphetamine, and THC by ELISA urine testing. J. Anal. Toxicol. 35 (6), 333–340.

Wang, S., Wei, Y., Chen, G., Liu, X., Jin, H., Yan, Z., Wu, Q., Du, H., 2009. Generation and utilization of anti-drug monoclonal antibodies for screening of 36 drug users by dot-ELISA. Hybridoma (Larchmt.) 28 (2), 145–148.

Ward, C., McNally, A.J., Rusyniak, D., Salamone, S.J., 1994. 125I radioimmunoassay for the dual detection of amphetamine and methamphetamine. J. Forensic Sci. 39 (6), 1486–1496.

Toxicogenomics

Toxicogenomics, broadly defined, is the study of genetic variation on individual differences in adverse drug responses. Every individual possesses a unique genotype, differentiated from the genotypes of every other individual by the specific nucleotide sequence contained within each chromosome. The genetic polymorphisms, or differences in nucleotide sequence, present within the human population account for the distinct phenotype (or, observable characteristics) of each individual. Although the majority of human chromosomal DNA is noncoding, small portions of the human genome, called genes, contain the information necessary to direct the synthesis of proteins. Polymorphisms within protein-encoding genes may result in altered protein structure and/or function, leading to distinct phenotypes within a population. A variety of polymorphisms have been identified within the human genome, but the most common type of polymorphism is a single nucleotide polymorphism, or SNP, which is a difference in nucleotide sequence of a single base. Toxicogenomic studies generally focus on the impact of genetic variation on the pharmacokinetic and pharmacodynamic profiles of drugs, but they may also be used to investigate individual differences in susceptibility to the development of drug dependency and/or addiction. In practice, the subdiscipline of toxicogenomics of most interest to forensic toxicologists is the study of the effects of genetic polymorphism on drug disposition: absorption, distribution, metabolism, and secretion. It is known that sequence variation within the genes encoding for a variety of proteins involved in drug disposition results in individual differences in response to many common drugs of abuse. Although inherited variation in the genes encoding for any of the proteins involved in drug disposition could potentially modulate the effects elicited by drug administration, drug disposition appears to be affected most commonly by polymorphisms in genes encoding for transport proteins and metabolic enzymes.

D.1 TRANSPORT PROTEINS

Although drug transport proteins are responsible for a minority of the movement of drugs into and out of cells, they play a vital role in the distribution of several drugs of interest to forensic toxicologists. Genetic polymorphisms in the genes encoding several drug transport proteins have been characterized, with the variant alleles identified influencing protein expression, activity, and/or ligand binding.

D.1.1 MULTIDRUG-RESISTANT PROTEIN

The multidrug-resistant protein (MDR1), which is encoded by the ABCB1 gene, is an ATP-binding cassette transmembrane transporter. An efflux transporter, MDR1 is a p-glycoprotein that is expressed on the luminal surfaces of many barrier tissues such as the intestinal epithelium and capillary endothelium of the blood—brain barrier. The broad expression of the MDR1 transporter, coupled with its ability to transport structurally diverse compounds from intracellular to extracellular spaces, underscores the importance of the transporter in protecting tissues from the accumulation of potentially toxic drugs and metabolites via their excretion into the bile, urine, and intestinal lumen. At the choroid plexus of the blood—brain barrier, in particular, MDR1 expressed in the capillary endothelium plays an important role in preventing the entry into and/or limiting the accumulation of drugs in the central nervous system. Among the substrates for MDR1 are digoxin, morphine, methadone, fentanyl, vinblastine, cyclosporine, and dexamethasone and tramadol. Several genetic polymorphisms in the ABCB1 gene have been identified and found to contribute to individual differences in the disposition of drugs. The most common SNPs in the ABCB1 gene are a C1236T variant, a G2677T base substitution, and a C3435T polymorphism. The C3435T SNP in exon 26 does not alter the amino acid sequence of the MDR1 protein, but it is associated with variable expression of MDR1 in the duodenum, with individuals who are homozygous for the C3435T substitution expressing half the level of MDR1 as individuals homozygous for the wild-type allele; individuals who are homozygous for the C3435T allele experience greater bioavailability of digoxin as compared to individuals homozygous for the wild-type allele. The G2677T base substitution in exon 21 results in an amino acid substitution of alanine to serine at position 893 in the MDR1 protein, which is associated with an increased transporter activity that has been correlated with decreased plasma fexofenadine concentrations after drug administration. The C1236T variant also encodes for an MDR1 protein that demonstrates increased activity as compared to the wild-type allele, and individuals who are homozygous for the G2677T and/or C1236T allele are significantly more likely to require elevated doses of methadone to achieve the desired effects. Polymorphisms in the ABCB1 gene have also been demonstrated to play a role in tramadol bioavailability as well as physiological response to some protease inhibitors, morphine, and fentanyl.

D.1.2 THE DOPAMINE TRANSPORTER

The dopamine transporter gene (DAT1) encodes for the dopamine transporter which has two major functions: to facilitate the release of dopamine into the synapse and to facilitate the reuptake of dopamine from the synapse into the presynaptic neuron. The release of dopamine by the dopamine transporter is known to be stimulated by amphetamines, and the reuptake of dopamine is inhibited by cocaine. Several polymorphisms have been identified in the DAT1 gene, with the most common variants caused by a variable number of tandem repeats (VNTR) of a 40 nucleotide sequence located in the 3′ untranslated region of exon 15. The most common genotype at this region is a 10 repeat VNTR of the 40 nucleotide sequence. However, a variant containing 9 repeats of the sequence has been identified, and individuals possessing at least one 9 repeat allele are at increased risk of experiencing cocaine-induced paranoia. Although the mechanism by which the VNTR effects dopamine transporter activity is not entirely clear, it has been suggested that the 9 repeat allele has altered transcriptional expression, potentially affecting transporter expression levels. Two additional polymorphisms, a T265C base substitution (which results in the substitution of alanine for valine at amino acid position 33) and a T1246C variant (which results in the substitution of alanine for valine at amino acid position 382), have been suggested to alter the reuptake of dopamine by the dopamine transporter and influence the affinity of cocaine binding to the transporter. Several polymorphisms in the DAT1 gene have also been shown to affect the susceptibility of individuals to addiction and to influence individual responses to stimulants.

The function of the serotonin transporter is analogous to that of the dopamine transporter in that it regulates the levels of the neurotransmitter serotonin in the synapse (whereas the dopamine transporter regulates the levels of dopamine in the synapse). The serotonin transporter is encoded for by the SLC6A4 gene, which can exist in several variant forms. The most common polymorphisms in the SLC6A4 gene are caused by the presence or absence of a 44 nucleotide sequence in the promoter region, which results in a long or short allele, respectively. The short variant, which lacks the specific 44 nucleotide promoter sequence, results in reduced levels of protein expression as compared to the long allele, and has been correlated with a predisposition to addiction to various drugs of abuse including cocaine. A second common polymorphism in the serotonin transporter gene is a VNTR in intron 2; three alleles have been identified, consisting of 9, 10, or 12 repeats of a 16−17 nucleotide sequence. A correlation between the presence of the 10 repeat VNTR allele and heroin addiction has been shown, and specific combinations of the VNTR variants and the short or long variant alleles have been suggested to modulate individual responses to amphetamine. The norepinephrine transporter, encoded by the SLC6A2 gene, is involved in the facilitation of norepinephrine and dopamine reuptake. Several polymorphisms of the SLC6A2 gene have been identified, including SNPs within the promoter regions and intron variants. A common variant results in a proline substitution at amino acid position 457 and results in an altered response to cocaine, potentially playing a role in addiction.

D.2 METABOLIC ENZYMES

Metabolism can be defined as the biochemical modification of drugs by enzymatic systems.[1] The end products of a metabolic reaction, the metabolites, may elicit

---

[1]Nonenzymatic metabolism can also occur, such as the conversion of cocaine to benzoylecgonine under acidic conditions, but the metabolism discussed in this chapter will be confined to enzymatic metabolism.

greater physiological effects than the parent drug, lesser effects, or different effects, depending upon the specific drug. The physiological effects elicited by a drug may therefore be influenced by the rate and extent of drug metabolism, which in turn are influenced by the expression level and/or catalytic activity of the metabolic enzyme(s) responsible for metabolism. The expression and activity of both phase I and phase II metabolic enzymes involved in the metabolism of drugs of abuse are known to be affected by various genetic polymorphisms within the genes encoding for these enzymes.

D.3 PHASE I METABOLIC ENZYMES

The cytochrome p450 (CYP) enzymes are responsible for the metabolism of a wide variety of drugs and are therefore arguably the most important class of phase I metabolic enzymes. Genetic polymorphisms in the genes encoding for the CYP enzymes have been well established and are responsible for the considerable individual differences in the expression levels and activity of the enzymes observed within populations. For a given CYP gene, there are often several common alleles and many more less common alleles, which may be present in characteristic frequencies within populations of differing ethnicities. Many types of genetic polymorphisms have been identified in the CYP genes, including SNPs, deletions, duplications, and insertions. Variant forms of the CYP alleles may result in enzymes with reduced catalytic activity, enhanced catalytic activity, normal catalytic activity, or no catalytic activity/no enzyme expression. Additionally, individuals may possess more than two alleles for a CYP gene. Based upon their genotype for a given CYP gene, individuals can therefore be categorized as ultrarapid metabolizers, extensive metabolizers, intermediate metabolizers, or poor metabolizers. Ultrarapid metabolizers generally express more than two active genes encoding for a specific CYP enzyme and/or express alleles that encode for an enzyme with increased enzymatic activity; ultrarapid metabolizers are therefore able to metabolize certain drugs with increased efficiency. The increased metabolic activity of ultrametabolizers results in blood concentrations of drug that are lower than anticipated for a given dose, resulting in decreased physiological responses; in the case of prodrugs,[2] the increased metabolism of the prodrug to the active form of the drug results in greater physiological responses. Extensive metabolizers express two functional alleles of a given CYP gene that encode for an enzyme with normal activity; extensive metabolizers may be considered to be the "wild-type" genotype. Intermediate metabolizers possess one or more alleles that encode for CYP enzyme with reduced enzymatic activity, and poor metabolizers possess fewer than two functional alleles for a specific CYP enzyme and/or possess alleles that encode for an enzyme that is nonfunctional or exhibits severely reduced catalytic activity. The decreased metabolic

---

[2]Drugs that are inactive, but are metabolized to active metabolites.

activity of poor metabolizers (and to a lesser extent, intermediate metabolizers) results in blood concentrations of drug that are higher than anticipated for a given dose, resulting in increased physiological responses and an increased risk of adverse effects or accidental overdose; in the case of drugs that produce active metabolites, the decreased metabolism of the drug to the active metabolite of the drug results in decreased physiological responses.

D.3.1 CYP2D6

CYP2D6 is the most polymorphic of the CYP enzymes, with more than 90 variant alleles identified, including variants that encode for nonfunctional enzymes, enzymes with reduced activity, enzymes with normal activity, and enzymes with increased activity. Of the multiple alleles identified, there are 3—5 common alleles that are found in approximately 95% of the population, with 75—85% of the population considered extensive metabolizers, 10—15% intermediate metabolizers, 5—10% poor metabolizers, and 1—10% ultrarapid metabolizers; the specific alleles' frequencies found within populations vary with ethnicity. CYP2D6 metabolizes 25—30% of all drugs, including a number of opioids such as codeine, tramadol, dihydrocodeine, oxycodone, hydrocodone, ethylmorphine, and methadone. Genetic polymorphisms at the CYP2D6 gene significantly affect the conversion of codeine to morphine and the metabolism of oxycodone to oxymorphone, a potent opioid. Therefore, CYP2D6 polymorphisms that alter the metabolic activity of the enzyme and its ability to produce active metabolites have been shown to alter the physiological effects of drug administration—either increasing the risk of accidental overdose or adverse effects (in ultrarapid metabolizers) or decreasing the physiological response (poor metabolizers). CYP2D6 is also involved in the metabolism of a variety of other drugs of interest to forensic toxicologists, including tricyclic antidepressants and selective serotonin reuptake inhibitors. The metabolism of several selective serotonin reuptake inhibitors is facilitated by CYP2D6, and plasma concentrations of fluoxetine and paroxetine specifically have been correlated with polymorphisms in the CYP2D6 gene, with elevated blood concentrations found in poor metabolizers as compared to extensive metabolizers, resulting in poor metabolizers being more susceptible to adverse reactions after drug administration. Correlations have also been shown between the number of functional copies of the CYP2D6 gene and the ratio the tricyclic antidepressant amitriptyline to its hydroxylated metabolites. Additionally, the decreased metabolism of 3,4-methylenedioxymethamphetamine (MDMA) by poor metabolizers likely makes these individuals more prone to adverse effects, although to date there have been no published reports definitively linking CYP2D6 polymorphisms to adverse outcomes following MDMA administration.

D.3.2 CYP2C9

CYP2C9 metabolizes warfarin, phenytoin, and a number of nonsteroidal anti-inflammatory drugs, as well as Δ9-tetrahydrocannabinol (Δ9THC). There have been several identified variants of the CYP2C9 gene, including two SNPs resulting in amino acid substitutions in the protein: a C430T substitution in exon 3 resulting in arginine being substituted for cysteine at amino acid position 144 and an A1075C substitution in exon 7 resulting in leucine replacing isoleucine at amino acid position 359. The C430T variant is associated with the impaired 6-hydroxylation and 7-hydroxylation of S-warfarin, resulting in intermediate metabolizers (who express one normal and one C430T allele) requiring a significantly lower maintenance dose of warfarin to maintain anticoagulation than extensive metabolizers. The A1075C variant allele encodes for a CYP2C9 enzyme with significantly reduced catalytic activity for all enzyme substrates. It has been shown that the CYP2C9 encoded by the A1075C allele exhibits a significantly lower maximum catalytic rate and/or lower affinities for S-warfarin, tolbutamide, and phenytoin as compared to the wild-type form of the enzyme. Individuals expressing the A1075C allele are therefore poor metabolizers of CYP2C9 substrates, including S-warfarin phenytoin, glipizide, tolbutamide, losartan, and acenocoumarol. The reduced clearance of anticoagulants such as S-warfarin observed in carriers of the C430T and/or A1075C CYP2C9 variants result in increased susceptibilities to adverse effects including bleeding, and a high incidence of these polymorphisms have been found in individuals who have experienced severe gastric bleeding after nonsteroidal anti-inflammatory drug use.

D.3.3 CYP2C19

CYP2C19 catalyzes the metabolism of several drugs, including diazepam, some barbiturates, tricyclic antidepressants, proguanil, and omeprazole. Although the majority of all ethnicities can be classified as extensive metabolizers, at least nine variant alleles have been identified, some of which affect the catalytic activity of the enzyme causing individuals to be poor metabolizers of CYP2C19 substrates. The two most common variant alleles encode for nonfunctional enzyme: a G681A SNP in exon 5 results in an altered splice site causing a change in the reading frame of the mRNA and a truncated nonfunctional protein; a G636A SNP in exon 4 produces a premature stop codon, resulting in a truncated nonfunctional protein. The presence of a G681A allele and/or a G636A allele accounts for the vast majority of poor metabolizers of CYP2C19 substrates, however, correlations have also been shown between the number of functional copies of the CYP2C19 gene and the ratio the tricyclic antidepressant amitriptyline to its demethylated metabolites, with fewer copies correlated with an increased ratio.

D.3.4 CYP3A4

Approximately 20–40% of the total hepatic CYP activity is composed of CYP3A4, which metabolizes the greatest number of drugs, including fentanyl, buprenorphine, methadone, and benzodiazepines. Although more than 28 SNPs have been identified in the CYP3A4 gene, no inactivating polymorphisms have been identified, and surprisingly few reports of definitively altered drug metabolism resulting in adverse effects have been published. However, a hypoactive variant CYP3A4 allele has been correlated with the inhibited N-dealkylation of fentanyl to its inactive metabolite norfentanyl, and variant alleles have been correlated with the differing metabolism of the calcineurin inhibitors, cyclosporine and tacrolimus. Additionally, the significant individual variability in CYP3A4 expression levels (varying by up to 20-fold) may account for the wide range of individual variability in the disposition of drugs metabolized by the enzyme. CYP3A4 also metabolizes Δ9THC, but none of the variant alleles identified to date have been correlated with an altered Δ9THC metabolism. Interestingly, up to 90% of the Caucasian population has been shown to carry a null allele of a second member of the CYP3A family, CYP3A5. A decrease or lack of CYP3A5 expression has been shown to amplify the fentanyl metabolism deficiencies observed in individuals carrying a variant CYP3A4 allele.

D.4 PHASE II METABOLIC ENZYMES

Phase II metabolic reactions include glucuronidation, glycine conjugation, acetylation, and mercapturic acid synthesis reactions, with glucuronidations being the most common phase II reaction. The metabolites produced by phase II reactions are typically larger, more water soluble, and less lipid soluble than their parent drugs. Toxicogenomic studies have heretofore focused predominantly on genetic variations in the phase I cytochrome p450 family of enzymes, but genetic polymorphisms may also affect the activity of any of the metabolic enzymes involved in phase II reactions.

The most well-established examples of genetic polymorphisms in phase II metabolic enzymes are found in the genes encoding glucuronyl transferase, N-acetyltransferase, and S-methyltransferase. Glucuronyl transferase, which is responsible for the glucuronidation of a variety of drugs including opioids, is encoded for by the UGT2B7 gene. Two common variants of the UGT2B7 gene have been identified: a C802T variant allele that is associated with an elevated efficiency of morphine glucuronidation and a resulting decreased incidence of adverse effects of codeine and/or morphine administration, and an A840G allele that is associated with decreased glururonidation of morphine. N-acetyltransferase is encoded for by two genes: the NAT1 gene and NAT2 gene. Interestingly, there seems to be significant ethnic variation in the prevalence of variant NAT1 and NAT2 variant alleles, with most individuals of East Asian descent being ultrarapid metabolizers of N-acetyltransferase substrates. S-methyltransferase (or thiopurine S-methyltransferase) catalyzes the metabolism of the thiopurine drugs, mercaptopurine and azathioprine. Several genetic variants of the S-methyltransferase gene have been identified, with the two most common genetic polymorphisms resulting in amino acid alterations in the enzyme (Ala154Thr and Tyr240Cys), which result in significantly reduced levels of enzyme expression, likely due to the rapid degradation of the mutated proteins. Approximately 0.3% of the Caucasian population exhibits little or no S-methyltransferase activity (due mostly to the presence of the Ala154Thr and/or Tyr240Cys mutation), 10%

demonstrates intermediate activity, and approximately 90% of the population possesses high enzymatic activity. Low levels of S-methyltransferase expression and/or activity result in a greatly increased risk of drug-induced myelosuppression and other adverse drug effects, whereas elevated enzymatic activity results in decreased drug responsiveness.

D.5 CONCLUSION

With the advance of modern molecular biology techniques and the increased accessibility of genetic sequencing facilities, the identification of genetic polymorphisms within gene encoding for proteins involved in drug disposition has become more feasible. As the field of toxicogenomics expands, it is likely that there will be accumulating evidence linking variant alleles to individual drug responses and predisposition to adverse drug effects. It is therefore important that forensic toxicologists are familiar with the literature of toxicogenomics in order to properly assess and potentially correlate drug concentrations collected in body fluids to the anticipated drug dosage and physiological effects of drug administration, as these parameters may be influenced by individual differences in drug disposition resulting from genetic polymorphisms.

SUGGESTED READING

Afshari, C.A., Hamadeh, H.K., Bushel, P.R., 2011. The evolution of bioinformatics in toxicology: advancing toxicogenomics. Toxicol. Sci. 120 (Suppl. 1), S225—S237.

Agrawal, Y.P., Rennert, H., 2012. Pharmacogenomics and the future of toxicology testing. Clin. Lab Med. 32 (3), 509—523.

Cropp, C.D., Yee, S.W., Giacomini, K.M., 2008. Genetic variation in drug transporters in ethnic populations. Clin. Pharmacol. Ther. 84 (3), 412—416.

Daly, A.K., Fairbrother, K.S., Smart, J., 1998. Recent advances in understanding the molecular basis of polymorphisms in genes encoding cytochrome P450 enzymes. Toxicol. Lett. 102—103, 143—147.

Daly, A.K., 1995. Molecular basis of polymorphic drug metabolism. J. Mol. Med. (Berl) 73 (11), 539—553.

Dasgupta, A., Langman, L.J., 2012. Pharmacogenomics of Alcohol and Drugs of Abuse. Taylor and Francis Group, Boca Raton, FL.

Evans, W.E., McLeod, H.L., 2003. Pharmacogenomics—drug disposition, drug targets, and side effects. N. Engl. J. Med. 348 (6), 538—549.

Fuke, S., Suo, S., Takahashi, N., Koike, H., Sasagawa, N., Ishiura, S., 2001. The VNTR polymorphism of the human dopamine transporter (DAT1) gene affects gene expression. Pharmacogenomics. J. 1 (2), 152—156.

Glatz, K., Mossner, R., Heils, A., Lesch, K.P., 2003. Glucocorticoid-regulated human serotonin transporter (5-HTT) expression is modulated by the 5-HTT gene-promotor-linked polymorphic region. J. Neurochem. 86 (5), 1072—1078.

Gomes, A.M., Winter, S., Klein, K., Turpeinen, M., Schaeffeler, E., Schwab, M., Zanger, U.M., 2009. Pharmacogenomics of human liver cytochrome P450 oxidoreductase: multifactorial analysis and impact on microsomal drug oxidation. Pharmacogenomics 10 (4), 579−599.

Ingelman-Sundberg, M., Oscarson, M., McLellan, R.A., 1999. Polymorphic human cytochrome P450 enzymes: an opportunity for individualized drug treatment. Trends Pharmacol. Sci. 20 (8), 342−349.

Jacobsen, L.K., Staley, J.K., Zoghbi, S.S., Seibyl, J.P., Kosten, T.R., Innis, R.B., Gelernter, J., 2000. Prediction of dopamine transporter binding availability by genotype: a preliminary report. Am. J. Psychiatry 157 (10), 1700−1703.

Jannetto, P.J., Wong, S.H., Gock, S.B., Laleli-Sahin, E., Schur, B.C., Jentzen, J.M., 2002. Pharmacogenomics as molecular autopsy for postmortem forensic toxicology: genotyping cytochrome P450 2D6 for oxycodone cases. J. Anal. Toxicol. 26 (7), 438−447.

Jin, M., Gock, S.B., Jannetto, P.J., Jentzen, J.M., Wong, S.H., 2005. Pharmacogenomics as molecular autopsy for forensic toxicology: genotyping cytochrome P450 3A4*1B and 3A5*3 for 25 fentanyl cases. J. Anal. Toxicol. 29 (7), 590−598.

Khan, S.R., Baghdasarian, A., Fahlman, R.P., Michail, K., Siraki, A.G., 2014. Current status and future prospects of toxicogenomics in drug discovery. Drug Discov. Today 19 (5), 562−578.

Klein, K., Winter, S., Turpeinen, M., Schwab, M., Zanger, U.M., 2010. Pathway-targeted pharmacogenomics of CYP1A2 in human liver. Front Pharmacol. 1, 129.

Kupiec, T.C., Raj, V., Vu, N., 2006. Pharmacogenomics for the forensic toxicologist. J. Anal. Toxicol. 30 (2), 65−72.

Lee, M., Liu, Z., Kelly, R., Tong, W., 2014. Of text and gene−using text mining methods to uncover hidden knowledge in toxicogenomics. BMC Syst. Biol. 8, 93.

Leeder, J.S., 2001. Pharmacogenetics and pharmacogenomics. Pediatr. Clin. North Am. 48 (3), 765−781.

Low, Y., Uehara, T., Minowa, Y., Yamada, H., Ohno, Y., Urushidani, T., Sedykh, A., Muratov, E., Kuz'min, V., Fourches, D., Zhu, H., Rusyn, I., Tropsha, A., 2011. Predicting drug-induced hepatotoxicity using QSAR and toxicogenomics approaches. Chem. Res. Toxicol. 24 (8), 1251−1262.

Meyer, U.A., 2000. Pharmacogenetics and adverse drug reactions. Lancet 356 (9242), 1667−1671.

Musshoff, F., Stamer, U.M., Madea, B., 2010. Pharmacogenetics and forensic toxicology. Forensic Sci. Int. 203 (1−3), 53−62.

Rioux, P.P., 2000. Clinical trials in pharmacogenetics and pharmacogenomics: methods and applications. Am. J. Health Syst. Pharm. 57 (9), 887−898.

Rushmore, T.H., Kong, A.N., 2002. Pharmacogenomics, regulation and signaling pathways of phase I and II drug metabolizing enzymes. Curr. Drug Metab. 3 (5), 481−490.

Sistare, F.D., Degeorge, J.J., 2008. Applications of toxicogenomics to nonclinical drug development: regulatory science considerations. Methods Mol. Biol. 460, 239−261.

Sistonen, J., Fuselli, S., Palo, J.U., Chauhan, N., Padh, H., Sajantila, A., 2009. Pharmacogenetic variation at CYP2C9, CYP2C19, and CYP2D6 at global and microgeographic scales. Pharmacogenet. Genomics 19 (2), 170−179.

Snozek, C.L.H., Langman, L.J., 2009. Pharmacogenomics of drugs of abuse. In: Dasgupta, A. (Ed.), Critical Issues in Alcohol and Drugs of Abuse Testing. AACC Press, Washington, D. C., pp. 83−103.

Vandenbergh, D.J., Rodriguez, L.A., Hivert, E., Schiller, J.H., Villareal, G., Pugh, E.W., Lachman, H., Uhl, G.R., 2000. Long forms of the dopamine receptor (DRD4) gene VNTR are more prevalent in substance abusers: no interaction with functional alleles of the catechol-o-methyltransferase (COMT) gene. Am. J. Med. Genet. 96 (5), 678–683.

Wang, T., Papoutsi, M., Wiesmann, M., DeCristofaro, M., Keselica, M.C., Skuba, E., Spaet, R., Markovits, J., Wolf, A., Moulin, P., Pognan, F., Vancutsem, P., Petryk, L., Sutton, J., Chibout, S.D., Kluwe, W., 2011. Investigation of correlation among safety biomarkers in serum, histopathological examination, and toxicogenomics. Int. J. Toxicol. 30 (3), 300–312.

Weinshilboum, R., 2003. Inheritance and drug response. N. Engl. J. Med. 348 (6), 529–537.

White, Sr., R.M., Wong, S.H., 2005. Pharmacogenomics and its applications. Med. Lab Obs. 37 (3), 20–27.

Wong, S.H., Wagner, M.A., Jentzen, J.M., Schur, C., Bjerke, J., Gock, S.B., Chang, C.C., 2003. Pharmacogenomics as an aspect of molecular autopsy for forensic pathology/toxicology: does genotyping CYP 2D6 serve as an adjunct for certifying methadone toxicity? J. Forensic Sci. 48 (6), 1406–1415.

Wood, A.J., Zhou, H.H., 1991. Ethnic differences in drug disposition and responsiveness. Clin. Pharmacokinet. 20 (5), 350–373.

Wu, A.H., Kearney, T., 2013. Lack of impairment due to confirmed codeine use prior to a motor vehicle accident: role of pharmacogenomics. J. Forensic Leg. Med. 20 (8), 1024–1027.

Xie, H.G., Kim, R.B., Wood, A.J., Stein, C.M., 2001. Molecular basis of ethnic differences in drug disposition and response. Annu. Rev. Pharmacol. Toxicol. 41, 815–850.

Yang, X., Zhang, B., Zhu, J., 2012. Functional genomics- and network-driven systems biology approaches for pharmacogenomics and toxicogenomics. Curr. Drug Metab. 13 (7), 952–967.

Zhang, M., Chen, M., Tong, W., 2012. Is toxicogenomics a more reliable and sensitive biomarker than conventional indicators from rats to predict drug-induced liver injury in humans? Chem. Res. Toxicol. 25 (1), 122–129.

Famous Cases in Forensic Toxicology

A familiarity with significant cases in the history of forensic toxicology is useful for the modern forensic toxicologist. Many of the questions, problems, and issues encountered by forensic toxicologists of today may have also been encountered by those of the past. Therefore, an awareness of the strategies, both successful and unsuccessful, employed by forensic toxicologists over the years in response to challenges of analysis, interpretation, and reporting may prove useful to current forensic toxicologists.

E.1 THE CASE OF WILLIAM PALMER

The case of William Palmer exemplifies the importance of transparent, accessible, and objective reporting of toxicological evidence by forensic toxicologists.

Dr William Palmer was born in Rugeley, Staffordshire, England and trained as a physician in London. After spending time at St Bartholomew's Hospital in London and passing the Royal College of Surgeon's membership examination, Palmer returned to Rugeley to establish a medical practice. Using funds from his father's estate and his mother's generosity, Palmer established his medical practice in 1846, and a year later married Ann Thorton, the daughter of wealthy parents who had established an annual income for their daughter. Ann gave birth to five children between 1851 and 1854, but only one survived beyond infancy. Although the Palmers lived a seemingly idyllic life in Rugeley, William quickly became ensnared in a life of gambling and racehorses. Shortly after his return to Rugeley, William had purchased a stable and several racehorses, upon which he frequently bet. William soon found himself deep in debt—due both to his heavy gambling losses and the loans he had procured to fund his stable and horses.

On January 19, 1849, Ann Mary Thorton, William's mother-in-law, died while visiting the Palmer home. William's wife inherited her mother's fortune, but due to a stipulation in the estate, any remaining money would return to the Thorton family after her death. William, reportedly fearing the loss of income should his wife die, took out several life insurance policies on Ann's life naming himself as the beneficiary; the insurance purchased totaled £13,000. The insurance policies took effect in early 1854, and shortly thereafter, Ann became ill with symptoms that were described by William as being consistent with cholera, which was rampart in the area at the time. William cared for his wife until her death on September 29, 1854, at which time the local physician, in accordance with William's suggestion, reported that the cause of death was cholera. William subsequently collected the £13,000 from Ann's insurance policies, a sum that fell short of covering his accumulated debt. At the time of Ann's death, William was having an affair with the family's housemaid Eliza Tharme, who gave birth to his child in June 1855. Reportedly in debt to various creditors in the amount of £15,000, in January 1855, William insured the life of his brother Walter, who was known to be in relatively poor health, for £13,000. On August 16, 1855, after his health had progressively deteriorated while being cared for by a personal physician and his brother William, Walter died. William attempted to collect the insurance money, but due to the somewhat suspicious timing of the claim, the insurance company did not immediately pay the premium, but rather enlisted a private detective to investigate the death. At this time, Palmer was also being blackmailed by one of his former mistresses, the daughter of a Staffordshire police officer.

Shortly after the death of his brother, on November 13—15, 1855, William and Jon Parsons Cook attended the Shrewsbury Handicap Stakes horse race. Cook and Palmer had been long-standing gambling partners and were coowners of several racehorses. On November 13, at the Shrewsbury races, Cook won a large sum of money, whereas Palmer's wagering was fruitless. Cook collected a portion of his winnings immediately, but in accordance with the racing regulations, the remainder would be collected the following week in London with the presentation of the betting book. After the races on November 13, Palmer and Cook went to the local pub to celebrate, after which Cook complained of feeling ill. On November 15, Palmer and Cook returned to Rugeley and Cook, whose health had recovered, stayed at the Talbot Arms Inn, which was next to Palmer's home. Cook's residence at the Inn proved to be short-lived; on November 16, after having lunch with Palmer, Cook became violently ill and began having convulsions as well as other distressing physical symptoms. Palmer took control of Cook's medical treatment until Cook's death on November 20. Interestingly, on November 18, a chambermaid tasted the broth prepared for Cook by Palmer and she too became ill. After Cook's death, his stepfather, William Stevens, arrived in Rugeley to represent the family. The circumstances surrounding his son's death, including Cook's then missing betting book, quickly raised Steven's suspicions of foul play and he requested that a postmortem examination be performed of Cook's body.

An inquest was initiated on November 26, and an autopsy was performed by a team of local physicians, with Palmer in attendance. During the course of the autopsy, Palmer reportedly tampered with evidence by bumping into one of the physicians as he lifted Cook's stomach out of the body, causing the contents of the stomach to spill out. The remaining stomach contents were placed in a sealed jar for analysis, and Palmer was accused of tampering with the seal on the jar. The local coroner enlisted the help of Dr Alfred Swaine Taylor, a distinguished physician/scientist at the forefront of the burgeoning discipline of toxicology, to analyze Cook's stomach contents and viscera. Taylor, a lecturer in medical jurisprudence at Guy's Hospital in London, was the author of the well-known text, *A Treatise on Poisons in Relation to Medical Jurisprudence, Physiology, and the Practice of Physic*. It had been discovered that Palmer had purchased a quantity of strychnine shortly before Cook's death. Taylor's laboratory therefore analyzed the stomach contents for this, as well as other poisons: Taylor reported that the only notable finding in the stomach contents was a small amount of antimony, the active ingredient of tarter emetic, a commonly used medicine. It was also noted, however, that nothing in the internal organs was identified as being indicative of death by natural causes.

The Cook inquest was held from December 12−15, 1855, and based upon the results of his toxicological analyses Taylor initially testified that he could not make a determination as to Cook's cause of death, but could only state that Cook took antimony at some point before his death. Immediately following Taylor's testimony, however, Elizabeth Mills, a chamber maid at Talbot Arms who had helped to care for Cook during his brief illness, testified to the physical symptoms exhibited by Cook during his final days. Mills recounted Cook's convulsions, a general wild look about his eyes, and the stiffening of his limbs following the convulsive episodes. Taylor, upon learning that no external lacerations were evident upon Cook's body, immediately declared that he could now give a definitive opinion as to Cook's cause of death: strychnine poisoning. Taylor explained that the symptoms described by Mills indicated that Cook must have died from tetanus, and that in the absence of any natural cause of tetanus, it must have resulted from the administration of a pharmacological agent: strychnine was the only known compound capable of eliciting the symptoms described, and Taylor proclaimed that he had "not the slightest hesitation" in identifying it as the cause of death. As the coroner reminded the jury in his subsequent testimony, no strychnine had been found in Cook's body, and Taylor's conclusions were based solely on the eye witness testimony of a chambermaid. Taylor, however, asserted that because strychnine is an organic compound, it would likely be absorbed very rapidly by the body and no analytical methods of the time could be expected to detect it. The jury ruled that Cook had "died by poison willfully administered by William Palmer," and Palmer was promptly charged with murder. With speculation running rampant in Rugeley, the deaths of Ann and Walter Palmer were reexamined, and within a week of the Cook inquest, the bodies of Ann and Walter Palmer were exhumed and inquests regarding their causes of death were initiated. It was ultimately determined, however, that there was insufficient evidence to implicate William in their deaths.

The trial of William Palmer for the murder of Jon Cook was held in May of 1856. In the interval between the end of the Cook inquest and the beginning of the Palmer trial, several newspapers published articles sensationalizing both the case and the discipline of toxicology. As a result of newspaper editorials, which alternately professed staunch support of and significant wariness of toxicology, the discipline of toxicology itself was seemingly on trial along with Dr Palmer. A public discourse regarding the applicability and appropriateness of applying toxicology to legal proceedings were centered on opinions such as the following, which were presented by various newspapers:

- "We do not remember any case exemplifying so remarkably the great advance made in our time by science, not only as our helper in everyday life, but as a power bearing witness against crime" (The *Examiner*).
- "How precarious is the evidence, if such it may be called, of learned professors as to the alleged existence of symptoms indicative of a vegetable poison of which it is on all hands admitted that we have no available tests in the present state of chemical knowledge!" (The *Saturday Review*).
- "Every day new names, sometimes conventional, sometimes expressing a new, often false theory, are applied to common things only to be altered upon the day that follows... It this becomes absolutely impossible for the ordinary administrators of the law to test a skilled medical witness, who becomes, in fact, himself, a jury sole..." (The *Dublin University Magazine*).
- "We are afraid, in short, that this trial may be made so much an opportunity for Dr. A. to fight Dr. B. that, between both, the jury may get puzzled and the prisoner off... We can only hope that it will be remembered that it is not science only, but the application of science to a particular question, which is required" (The *Illustrated Times*).

Owing to the charged atmosphere in the area, it was believed that Palmer would not receive a fair trial in Staffordshire, and an Act of Parliament was issued to allow the trial to be held at The Old Bailey in London. The prosecution team was composed of Alexander Cockburn and John Walter, and the defense was led by William Shee. Although evidence detailing Palmer's financial difficulties, his suspicious behavior at Cook's autopsy, his purchase of strychnine, and other circumstantial evidence was presented, the crux of the prosecution's case was the testimony of Dr Taylor, which was focused on the following key points:

1. Although no strychnine was found in Cook's body, this did not mean that strychnine had not been administered.
2. The poor quantity and quality of postmortem tissue samples provided to Taylor for analysis may have interfered with the detection of the poison.
3. Due to the rapid absorption of strychnine, if small amounts had been administered to Cook, its detection in the tissue samples would be difficult to accomplish with the available analytical methodologies.
4. The physical symptoms exhibited by Cook and described by eyewitnesses were characteristic of strychnine poisoning, and were distinguishable from the "tetanic" symptoms resulting from a natural cause.

Due to the lack of concrete scientific evidence, the prosecution's case relied heavily on the expert opinion of Dr Taylor as to the cause of Cook's death, and thus the overriding strategy of the defense was to discredit the scientific expertise of Taylor. As the defense mounted its case, Shee first introduced multiple expert witnesses who testified that a skilled analyst would easily be able to detect strychnine in body tissues regardless of the dose that had been administered or the quality or quantity of the tissue samples. Shee then more directly attacked the expertise of Taylor with the following arguments:

1. Shee questioned Taylor about the extent of his personal experience with strychnine in either the clinical or laboratory setting. Taylor remarked that he had never observed a human case of strychnine poisoning but that he had performed an experiment in which he had injected 10 rabbits with the poison. Shee asserted that this lack of experience resulted in Taylor overlooking a key piece of information when formulating his opinion as to the cause of Cook's death: victims of strychnine poisoning generally have engorged hearts, whereas Cook's heart was virtually devoid of blood.
2. Taylor, Shee argued, was not appropriately qualified to offer an expert opinion as to Cook's cause of death, as his knowledge of strychnine was no greater than the layperson.
3. Taylor's interpretation of the available evidence was biased because he was aware of the suspicions of Cook's stepfather, who believed that Palmer was involved in his son's death.
4. Taylor was not an unbiased witness: his participation, and behavior, in the initial inquest indicated that he was in support of the prosecution and believed Palmer to be a murderer. Furthermore, following the inquest Taylor had invited the press to his laboratory and encouraged a newspaper columnist to report that strychnine was often undetectable in human tissues. These actions, Shee argued, indicated that Taylor was far from a dispassionate participant, but rather was an individual who had staked his reputation on a questionable scientific interpretation and was now determined to convince the jury and the public of the accuracy of his claims.

Although Shee attempted to persuade the jury to reject the testimony of Taylor simply because, he nonetheless lamented that, as was evident at the inquest, the jurors were likely to believe that "…whatever Dr Alfred Swaine Taylor says, must be true: if he says is it poison, poison it is." At the conclusion of the 12-day trial, Shee's prediction proved to be accurate: the jury found William Palmer guilty of murder and he was hanged on June 14, 1856. More than 30,000 people attended the execution, at which Palmer's last words reportedly were "I am innocent of poisoning Cook by strychnine." In the years following the trial, Dr Taylor was often criticized for his actions during the course of the case. To some, he served as an example of the dangers of a partisan expert witness willing to exploit his position of scientific authority, and in doing so diminish the discipline of toxicology, for personal or professional interests. Taylor, however, defended his actions in the Palmer trial in subsequent editions of "*On Poisons.*"

E.2 THE CASE OF MARIE BESNARD

The case of Marie Besnard demonstrates the necessity of proper sample handling, the importance of utilizing validated analytical methodologies, and the benefits of being well versed in the current scientific literature.

Marie Besnard, a 53-year-old citizen of Loudun, France was arrested on July 21, 1949 and charged with 11 counts of murder. Born in 1896, Marie married her cousin, Auguste Antigy in 1919. Together, Marie and Auguste worked as caretakers at the Chateau des Martins until Auguste's death in 1927. In 1929, two short years after Auguste's death, Marie married Leon Besnard, the owner of a rope-making business. Marie and Leon were married until 1947 when, after a short illness, Leon died of what was consecutively ruled to be a liver attack, angina pectoris, and finally uremic poisoning. Marie's troubles began when the local postmistress, Madame Pintou, told her friend Auguste Massip that shortly before his death Leon had confided in her that he believed he was being poisoned by his wife Marie. Massip relayed this information to the police who alerted the Examining Magistrate Pierre Roger. Upon examination by Inspector Nocquet and Inspector Chaumier, who had been assigned to investigate the case, Madame Pintou recanted her story and asserted that Leon had not, in fact, expressed any such fears to her. Rumors circulated among the townspeople of Loudun, however, that Marie had been having an affair with a German prisoner of war named Dietz who had moved in with the Besnards in 1947 to work on their farm. It was determined that in fact, not only did Marie go on several trips with Dietz after her husband's death, but also she remained in touch with him after he returned to Germany in 1948, and in 1949 she persuaded him to return to Loudun. The reported affair between Marie and Dietz raised the suspicions of Inspector Nocquet, who came to believe that Marie may have killed her husband Leon in order to continue her relationship with Dietz unimpeded.

The suspicions of Nocquet were only amplified when, in 1949, Marie's 87-year-old mother Marie-Louise Davaillaud died after a short illness. Although there was a flu epidemic in the Loudun area at the time, and the attending physician ruled the virus to be the cause of death, it was believed that Marie-Louise had been staunchly opposed to Marie inviting Dietz back into the home that they shared. The Loudun townspeople and Inspector Nocquet were suspicious of the timing of Marie-Louise's death and wondered if Marie had killed her own mother, as they suspected she had killed her husband, in order to facilitate the continuation of her affair with Dietz. Because of his mounting suspicion of Marie, Nocquet revisited Madame Pintou and once again implored her to recount what Leon had told her shortly before his death. At this point, Pintou admitted that from his sick bed, Leon had claimed that he observed an unknown liquid on his dinner plate, upon which Marie placed soup. Shortly after consuming the soup Leon stated that he felt ill. Leon had suspected that either Marie or Dietz had poisoned him. Additionally incriminating was Nocquet's discovery that Marie had hired a private detective to intimidate Madame Pintou in order to prevent her from telling her story.

On May 9, 1949 Nocquet obtained a court order for the exhumation of Leon Besnard's body from the Loudun cemetery. The exhumation was performed by Jean Morin, Dr Seta, and Dr Guillon. Tissues and organs from the body were placed in glass jars and sent for toxicological examination by Dr Georges Beroud, a renowned scientist and the Director of the police laboratory in Marseilles. Utilizing the Marsh apparatus for analysis, Beroud reported arsenic levels as high as 39 mg/kg in the body tissues—a concentration that Beroud concluded was consistent with lethality. Following the identification of arsenic in Leon's body, the exhumation of Marie-Louise was ordered. Body tissues were once again collected in glass jars and sent to Dr Beroud for analysis. In this case, arsenic levels reaching 58 mg/kg were detected in various organs collected from the corpse. With this evidence in hand, Inspectors Nocquet and Normand arrested Marie Besnard and Dietz on July 21, 1949 and took them to Magistrate Roger for interrogation. During his examination, Dietz staunchly denied having a romantic relationship with Marie and claimed to be innocent of poisoning either Leon or Marie-Louise; Dietz was released and immediately returned to Germany. Marie also denied poisoning her husband and mother, but these pleas notwithstanding, she was imprisoned.

Due to their strong conviction that Marie was guilty of murder, and in the hopes of strengthening the case against her at trial, Magistrate Roger and the inspectors reviewed Marie's history in the hopes of finding additional evidence that would prove her guilt beyond a reasonable doubt. During the course of the next several years, Roger and the inspectors, with the assistance of Dr Beroud, identified several other suspicious deaths that they came ultimately to believe were the result of Marie's murderous utilization of arsenic:

1. The body of Marie's first husband, Auguste Antigy, was exhumed in 1949—22 years after his death. Although it was presumed that Auguste had died of tuberculosis, various organs were sent to Beroud for analysis, and concentrations of arsenic as great as 60 mg/kg were found in the exhumed body tissues.

2. Leon Besnard's great aunt, Louise, with whom Leon had a strained relationship, but with whom Marie maintained a close relationship was known to have died shortly after drafting a will that bequeathed half of her property to Marie and the other half to Leon's sister. Marie was said to have sent wine to Louise and visited her shortly before her death. The exhumation of Louise's body and the subsequent toxicological analysis by Dr Beroud revealed 35 mg/kg of arsenic in the body organs.

3. Marie was known to have visited Leon's grandmother shortly before her death in 1940. The exhumation of her body showed trace amounts of arsenic.

4. Marie visited her father-in-law, Marcellin Besnard, frequently. When Marcellin fell ill in 1940 Marie was a constant presence at his sick bed. Marcellin's death in 1940 was initially ruled to be the result of a stroke, but an arsenic concentration of 38 mg/kg was detected by Beroud in Marcellin's exhumed body. It was noted by the inspectors that Marcellin had come into a large sum of money shortly before his death.

5. Less than a year after her husband's death, Leon's mother, Marie-Louise Besnard died after a nine-day illness: Marie was reported to have been at her bedside during her illness, which was initially diagnosed as pneumonia. Following Marie-Louise's death, the money inherited from Marcellin by Marie-Louise was divided equally between Marie and Leon and Leon's sister. Marie-Louise's body was exhumed 8 years after her death and 60 mg/kg of arsenic was found.

6. In 1941, shortly after the death of her parents, the body of Leon's sister Lucie was found hanging in her parent's home. Ruled a suicide, Lucie's body was nevertheless ordered to be exhumed by Magistrate Roger. The tissues from Lucie's body were analyzed by Beroud who determined an arsenic concentration of 30 mg/kg in various organs.

In addition to Marie's six close family members whose deaths Roger and the inspectors found to be extremely suspicious, several other family members and friends were found to have died under suspicious conditions. In all, during the 31 months of investigation, Roger ordered the exhumations of 13 Besnard relatives and friends who had died since 1927. Among the bodies exhumed were Marie's mother, father, two husbands, father-in-law, mother-in-law, sister-in-law, grandmother-in-law, two cousins, great aunt, and two close friends. Marie was known to have benefited financially from many of these deaths, and upon exhumation, at least trace amounts of arsenic were found in each body. Ultimately, Marie was charged with the murder by arsenic of 11 individuals. It is notable, however, that there was only circumstantial evidence linking Marie to any of the deaths—there were no records or eyewitnesses that Marie had ever purchased arsenic or tampered with the food of any of the deceased. Due to the lack of direct incriminating evidence, Roger hoped to coerce a confession out of Marie and placed informants in her prison cell. Marie, however, never wavered from her proclamation of innocence.

The first trial of Marie Besnard began on February 20, 1952. Marie was represented by several well-known attorneys, including Rene Hayot and Albert Gautrat. The prosecution, as expected, called Dr Beroud to the stand to present his toxicological findings. Beroud described the manner in which the organs, or portions of organs, from the exhumed bodies were placed in glass jars and sent to his laboratory, upon which he and his laboratory technicians analyzed the tissues for arsenic content using the Marsh test. The results from the toxicological analyses were presented by Beroud, with the concentrations of arsenic measured in the organs from each exhumed body described in some detail. The testimony of Dr Beroud, and the accompanying laboratory data from his analyses, formed the framework of the prosecution's case, and it was therefore important that Gautrat identified a strategy by which to discredit this testimony. In his cross-examination of Beroud, Gautrat did indeed attack several key aspects of Beroud's toxicological analyses, as well as his credibility as a scientist and expert witness:

1. Gautrat presented an inventory of glass jars, and their tissue contents, that was prepared by Dr Seta at the Loudun cemetery. He then presented a similar inventory of the glass jars that were received and analyzed at Beroud's laboratory

in Marseilles. To Beroud's surprise and embarrassment, there were significantly more jars listed on his laboratory inventory than were reported to have been mailed from Dr Seta, who had participated in the exhumation of Leon Besnard, in Loudun. Additionally, several of the tissues that Beroud reported having analyzed were not included in the inventory of organs exhumed and collected from the various corpses. Gautrat asked Beroud, since it could be reasonably concluded that the jars did not spontaneously multiply during their trip from Loudun, could it not be concluded that some of the organs that were analyzed as part of the Besnard case were in fact tissues that had been collected from unrelated corpses?

2. Gautrat asked Beroud if his laboratory routinely washed and sterilized the glass collection jars before sending them back to Loudun for additional organ samples. Beroud asserted that, yes, this was standard practice. However, upon questioning by Gautrat, Dr Seta admitted that the jars that were returned to the cemetery, and which were subsequently used for the collection of exhumed tissue, were often very obviously dirty.

3. Gautrat produced a set of letters written by Beroud to Magistrate Roger. In one such letter, Beroud had written "If the report of my analysis is not satisfactory to you, kindly let me know so that I can make the necessary changes." Although it is most likely that Beroud was not suggesting that he would make alterations to his scientific data or expert opinions, but rather was simply asking if the writing style and format would be palatable to a layman, Gautrat nonetheless implied the Beroud was willing to modify his toxicological results in order to strengthen the prosecution's case.

4. Gautrat presented a letter written to Roger in which Beroud had asserted that he was capable of distinguishing, with his naked eye, arsenic mirrors from mirrors formed by other metals in the Marsh apparatus. Gautrat challenged this assertion by producing six sealed glass jars containing, he claimed, either arsenic or antimony mirrors. Beroud was asked to identify which of the jars contained arsenic. After some deliberation, Beroud selected three containers that he believed to contain arsenic mirrors, upon which Gautrat proclaimed that in fact, none of the jars contained arsenic, they all contained antimony mirrors. Although this exercise was irrelevant to the toxicological analyses performed in Beroud's laboratory (determinations of arsenic content were not made by with the naked eye!), it nonetheless served to diminish Beroud's credibility.

Gautrat's cross-examination of Dr Beroud introduced sufficient doubt regarding the accuracy of Dr Beroud's toxicological analyses that Magistrate Roger adjourned the trial, returned Marie to prison and appointed a new panel of scientific experts to perform additional toxicological testing of the corpses. Among the experts appointed to the case were Rene Fabre, E. Kohn-Abrest, Henri Griffon, and Rene Piedelievre. To facilitate the additional analyses, the 11 bodies were exhumed for a second time, and tissues were collected. Unfortunately, because no great care had been taken when the organs and tissues from the bodies were returned to the

Loudun cemetery following Dr Beroud's initial analyses, in many cases the bodies had decomposed to such an extent that the only portion of the corpses remaining for analysis was the hair. Fortunately, it had been demonstrated previously that hair was in fact a very good sample in which to detect the presence of arsenic. Piedelievre supervised the collection of the organ and hair samples, and also directed the collection of soil samples from the regions surrounding the buried bodies. The organ samples and some of the soil samples were analyzed in the laboratory of Dr Kohn-Abrest, who utilized both the Marsh apparatus and spectroanalytic methods to determine arsenic content. Consistent with Beroud's findings, Kohn-Abrest found as much as 20 mg/kg of arsenic in many of the samples, even after the bodies had been buried for many years, exhumed twice, and decomposed significantly. The hair samples and some soil samples were analyzed by Dr Griffon, who utilized atomic physics in his analysis of the samples. Arsenic is not naturally radioactive, but when placed in a nuclear reactor and barraged with neutrons, arsenic will capture the neutrons and be converted into radioactive isotopes that will emit radiation that can be detected. Griffon utilized this relatively new method of analysis that had not been thoroughly validated by the scientific community to test for arsenic in the hair and soil samples collected from the cemetery. In order to quantify the levels of arsenic in the test samples, a known quantity of arsenic was placed in the nuclear reactor at the same time as the test sample, and the amount of radioactivity emitted by the two samples was compared. Utilizing this method, Griffon identified significantly elevated levels of arsenic in the hair and soil samples collected from the cemetery.

The toxicological findings of Dr Kohn-Abrest and Dr Griffon were relatively consistent with the previous findings of Dr Beroud: both scientists found significantly elevated levels of arsenic in the bodies of the alleged victims of Marie Besnard, whereas relatively low levels of arsenic were found in the cemetery soil. To mount an effective defense of Marie, Gautrat therefore sought a way to refute this second set of analyses. Gautrat, upon learning of the experimental methods utilized by Dr Griffon and reviewing the available relevant scientific literature, developed two main arguments that he believed would discredit the scientists and their data:

1. Gautrat discovered that Griffon had made a key mistake in his experimental protocol. It had recently been determined that the half-life of radioactive arsenic decay, 26.5 h, was also the optimal length of time required to activate the arsenic in the nuclear reactor. However, Gautrat found that Griffon had placed the test samples in the reactor for only 15 h. This was a significant mistake because arsenic is not the only element that will become radioactive when placed in a nuclear reactor—in fact several other elements commonly found in human hair, including carbon, hydrogen, potassium, magnesium, and sodium will also absorb the neutrons and become radioactive. Many of these elements possess half-lives of radioactive decay that differ significantly from that of arsenic; therefore, the optimal length of time for these elements to be placed in

the reactor is therefore significantly different than the optimal time required to make arsenic radioactive, and the radioactivity emitted from these elements can be easily distinguished from the emission produced by arsenic. However, the half-life of radioactive decay of sodium is 18 h, and therefore, the 15-h time period that Griffon selected to use in his nuclear reactor protocol would be expected to convert sodium to a radioactive state, and Gautrat speculated that the radioactivity measured by Griffon could therefore be the result of the presence of either arsenic or sodium in the test samples.

2. Gautrat suspected that his best defense tactic would be to argue that the arsenic found in the exhumed bodies had originated within the cemetery soil.[1] A significant weakness in this argument was the widely held belief within the scientific community that arsenic, even if found in high concentrations in soil, is relatively insoluble and would therefore not enter into the tissues of bodies buried in the soil. In fact, a study performed previously by Rene Truhaud had demonstrated that the arsenic content of hair, when buried in arsenic rich soil for more than a year, was not significantly altered. During the course of his research, however, Gautrat came upon the work of Ollivier and Lepeintre who demonstrated that the presence of certain anaerobic bacterial species in soil samples causes a significant increase in the solubility of soil arsenic. Further-more, Gautrat learned that the anaerobic bacteria in cemetery soil had been shown to facilitate the influx of arsenic into hair; in fact, it had been observed that as a result of the respiration of anaerobic bacterial species, the arsenic contents of hair or tissue within a body could exceed that of the concentration in the soil surrounding the body. Ollivier and Lepeintre did acknowledge, how-ever, that the effect of anaerobic bacterial species on arsenic solubility was somewhat unpredictable. These principles, although novel and not widely accepted within the scientific community, nonetheless provided Gautrat with the basis of an argument in defense of Marie.

The second trial of Marie Besnard began in 1954. In an effort to strengthen their case, the prosecution eliminated 5 of the original 11 victims due to a lack of solid toxicological evidence—presumably due to the deterioration of the bodies resulting in only trace amounts of arsenic being found in the corpses during the second set of analyses. Marie was therefore charged with six counts of murder by poisoning. The panel of scientists appointed by the court presented the results of the toxicological analyses, which indicated that there were significantly elevated levels of arsenic in the remains of the six bodies in question, with markedly lower concentrations of arsenic found in the cemetery soil. As anticipated by Gautrat, the experts asserted that the lethal levels of arsenic found in the exhumed corpses could not have entered the bodies from the surrounding soil due to the low solubility of soil arsenic.

---

[1]A similar defense had been raised in the trial of another Marie, Marie LaFarge, more than 100 years previously (Chapter 1).

However, upon cross-examination, Gautrat attacked the method employed by Griffon, as well as the assumption of low arsenic solubility. By successfully introducing reasonable doubt as to the accuracy of the toxicological findings, Gautrat once again succeeded in undermining the scientific data presented by the prosecution's witnesses, to the extent that even Dr Kohn-Abrest admitted that he could not definitely say that the solubility of the soil arsenic had not be affected by the presence of bacteria. Once again, the trial was adjourned and the court ruled that a new panel of experts must be appointed to investigate the claims of Ollivier and Lepeintre regarding the effect of anaerobic bacteria on the arsenic solubility. Marie was released on bail.

For the next 7 years, various scientists investigated the toxicological data collected in the Besnard case and performed a series of experiments aimed at determining, once and for all, if the arsenic found in the exhumed bodies of Marie's supposed victims could have originated in the cemetery soil. Upon review of the scientific evidence several determinations were made:

1. Although Griffon was determined to have made errors in his experimental protocol utilizing the nuclear reactor, it was concluded that his findings were relatively accurate; subsequent studies confirmed the presence of lethal doses of arsenic in the hair samples collected from the bodies.
2. It was acknowledged that the soil in the Loudun cemetery did indeed contain low concentrations of arsenic, but the arsenic concentrations in the soil were markedly lower than the arsenic concentrations in the bodies of Marie's alleged victims. Furthermore, bodies unrelated to the Besnard case, which had been buried in close proximity to the Besnard "victims" were found to contain no traces of arsenic. However, upon repeated investigation, the scientists could come to no clear consensus as to whether the solubility of the soil arsenic could have been influenced by soil bacteria, or other factors, to such an extent that could enter the bodies. Nonetheless, the prosecution experts, after weighing all of the available evidence, concluded that in their expert opinions, the arsenic found in the tissue samples had not originated in the cemetery soil.

The third trial of Marie Besnard commenced in 1961, and once again, the prosecution and defense presented opposing views of the validity of the available scientific data. The prosecution asserted that the lethal levels of arsenic in the exhumed bodies were most likely to have originated from some source other than the soil, whereas the defense repeated its claims that, due to the unpredictable nature of soil arsenic solubility, it was impossible to determine if the arsenic in the bodies entered from the soil. Ultimately, due to the continued lack of clarity regarding the source of the arsenic in the exhumed bodies, the court concluded that the toxicological methodologies of the time could not determine definitively if the six deceased had been victims of arsenic poisoning. After an astounding 12 years, Marie was acquitted of murder on December 12, 1961 due to lack of evidence.

E.3 THE CASE OF DR MARIO JASCALEVICH

The case of Dr Mario Jascalevich underscores the importance of utilizing a proper analytical strategy and scientifically validated methodologies.

Dr Mario Jascalevich was a surgeon at Riverdell Hospital in Oradell, New Jersey. After noticing an increase in patient mortality at the hospital, several of Dr Jascalevich's colleagues became suspicious. Dr Stanley Harris, a surgeon, and Dr Allan Las, an osteopathic physician, suspected Jascalevich of murdering their patients with curare, which contains D-tubocurarine, a noncompetitive antagonist of nicotinic cholinergic receptors found at the neuromuscular junction. The result of this antagonistic mechanism is paralysis of voluntary skeletal muscles, such as the diaphragm, resulting potentially in respiratory arrest. Although neither Harris nor Las had witnessed Jascalevich administering curare to any patients at Riverdell, they nonetheless broke into his surgical locker in the hopes of finding some evidence of wrongdoing. In the locker, Harris and Las found 18 vials of curare, as well as several syringes. In November of 1966, Harris and Las reported their suspicions to the Bergen County Prosecutor's office and an investigation was initiated. Upon questioning, Dr Jascalevich denied administering curare to any patients at Riverdell and told investigators that he had utilized the curare in animal experiments that he had performed at Seton Hall College, a claim that was supported by documentation he provided to the investigators.

The curare samples and syringes found in Dr Jascalevich's locker by his colleagues at Riverdell were analyzed by Dr Milton Helpern, Chief of the New York City Medical Examiner's office, and, consistent with Dr Jascalevich's claims, dog hair and animal blood were found on the vials of curare and the syringes. During the course of the initial investigation, Dr Jascalevich reviewed the medical records of the recently deceased patients of Riverdell Hospital and he reported to the investigators that he believed that the patients had died, not from curare poisoning, but rather from misdiagnosis and medical malpractice. Due to the lack of any evidence indicating that Dr Jascalevich had murdered any patients at Riverdell, the Prosecutor's office closed the investigation of Dr Jascalevich.

Ten years later, however, interest in the case was reignited when in 1976 the New York Times published a series of articles describing the investigation of a physician who was suspected of murdering patients at Riverdell Hospital. The newspaper did not reveal Dr Jascalevich's name, but rather called him "Dr X." Concomitantly to the New York Times articles, Dr Michael Baden, the Deputy New York Medical Examiner, submitted a report stating that 20 patients who died at Riverdell Hospital in 1966 had died from causes other than those listed on their death certificates. Furthermore, Dr Baden stated that it was his professional opinion that the patients' deaths were consistent with respiratory depression, such as that which could be caused by curare overdose. Dr Baden asserted that curare is a stable compound that could persist in body tissues for years, and thus argued that the bodies of the alleged victims of Dr X should be exhumed. Dr Baden emphasized that, in his opinion, modern methods of toxicological analyses, which were unavailable in 1966, could be used to detect even small amounts of curare in the tissues from the exhumed bodies, even though the bodies had been buried for 10 years. In accordance with Dr Baden's recommendation, a Superior Court judge issued a court order for the exhumation of the bodies of five Riverdell patients whose deaths were considered to be suspicious; included were the bodies of Nancy Savino, Emma Arzt, Frank Biggs, Margaret Henderson, and Carl Rohrbeck. All five of these individuals had visited Riverdell Hospital during the years of 1965 and 1966 for routine surgical procedures, and all five were reported to have had uneventful surgeries and normal recoveries before dying unexpectedly several days after surgery.

The first body to be exhumed was the body of 4-year-old Nancy Savino. Dr Baden performed an autopsy of the body, and toxicological analyses were performed by Dr Leo Dal Cortivo, Chief Toxicologist for Suffolk County New York, and Dr Richard Coumbis, Chief Toxicologist for the New Jersey Medical Examiner's office. Although Dr Baden subsequently reported to a Grand Jury that the experts could not be certain if there was curare present in the body, on May 18, 1976, Jascalevich was indicted on five counts of murder. In 1977, prosecution and defense experts began thorough forensic analyses of tissues from the five exhumed bodies. Dr Cortivo and Dr Coumbis served as exerts for the prosecution, and Dr Frederick Rieders and Dr Bo Holmstedt were retained as experts for the defense. The state's forensic scientists utilized radioimmunoassay (RIA) and high-performance liquid chromatography (HPLC), as well as ultraviolet (UV) spectrophotometry and thin-layer chromatography (TLC), to analyze the exhumed tissue samples. Tissue samples and samples of the embalming fluid from the exhumed bodies were also provided to the defense.

The trial of Dr Jascalevich began on February 28, 1978, and the defense immediately requested a hearing to determine if RIA and/or HPLC were valid methods to utilize for the detection of curare in human tissue. Defense experts contended that RIA had only been shown to detect drugs in blood and other bodily fluids, but had never been validated for use in the identification of drugs in human tissues. The presiding Superior Court Judge, William J. Arnold, denied the request of the defense for a hearing, but ruled that the request could be resubmitted later in the trial when the analytical techniques and toxicological data were to be presented. Thus, the trial began with the prosecution introducing various medical personnel from Riverdell Hospital who generally asserted that each of the alleged victims of Dr Jascalevich had been recovering well after surgery, but then suddenly died. Upon cross-examination, however, several of the physicians admitted that some of the patients had been misdiagnosed and several had received less than optimal postoperative care.

After the completion of the testimony by the medical personnel, the defense once again requested a hearing on the admissibility of the analytical data collected by the state's experts via RIA, HPLC, UV spectrophotometry, and TLC. The prosecution was opposed to the hearing on the grounds that the four techniques were not new techniques, but rather were considered to be standard toxicological methods of analysis. Therefore, it was asserted by the prosecution, it was not necessary for the court to rule on the reliability of the methods as analytical tools. Judge Arnold, however, ruled in the favor of the defense and a hearing, outside the presence of the jury, was granted.

The prosecution presented arguments that relied heavily upon legal precedence that had been established by decisions in prior cases. Among the key arguments presented by the prosecution in support of the admissibility of the evidence collected via RIA, HPLC, UV spectrophotometry, and TLC were legal rulings that had established that:

- The scientific community need not be unanimous regarding the validity of an analytical method, nor must the method be infallible, in order for it to be deemed admissible in court.
- Courts should allow for the admissibility of evidence that has been collected by qualified scientists. Such evidence may be applied to the demonstration of fact, but the significance of the evidence should be left to the discretion of the jury.
- The "newness" of an analytical method should not preclude its admissibility in court.
- Analytical methods developed specifically for a case at hand, and for the purpose of detecting previously undetectable drugs in the human body, should be admissible.
- If scientific analyses are performed utilizing methods that have been proven to have high degrees of reliability, and they are performed by qualified scientists, the evidence is admissible.

The defense, in turn, presented statements and affidavits from experts, which contended that:

- RIA, HPLC, UV spectrophotometry, and TLC, although established analytical methods within the scientific community, had not been demonstrated to be reliable for the specific purses employed in this case: that is, the detection of curare in embalmed human tissues.
- Although RIA, HPLC, UV spectrophotometry, and TLC are extremely sensitive methods (i.e., capable of detecting small quantities of various substances), sensitivity does not necessarily correlate with specificity (i.e., the ability to identify a specific compound). The four methods utilized by the state's experts were known to possess high levels of sensitivity, but they had not been demonstrated to be highly specific in their ability to differentiate curare from other compounds in embalmed human tissue.

After considering the arguments of both the prosecution and the defense, Judge Arnold ruled that the analytical results obtained by means of RIA, HPLC, UV spectrophotometry, and TLC were admissible. Judge Arnold did not comment on the reliability of the evidence, but rather asserted that it should be up to the jury to make the determination of whether or not the evidence was scientifically valuable. The trial therefore resumed, and the prosecution presented the remainder of its case, including testimony from several expert witnesses who testified regarding both the toxicological results, as well as the analytical methods utilized:

1. Dr Coumbis testified that he identified curare in four of the five exhumed bodies, and he found presumptive evidence of curare in the fifth body. Dr Coumbis maintained that the RIA and HPLC methods that he utilized were valid methods of analysis, and that it was his expert opinion that no other substances interfered with the detection of curare (i.e., the test was specific). Dr Coumbis did state that the efficiency of the analytical instruments he utilized in the RIA analyses was subject to varying degrees of error, and that the determinations of what was deemed a positive result for curare and what was deemed a negative result were somewhat arbitrary and established at his own discretion!

2. Dr Cortivo testified that he found curare in three of the five bodies using RIA and HPLC.

3. Dr David Beggs, a scientist from Hewlett—Packard, testified that utilizing Gas chromatography—mass spectrometry (GC/MS) he had found curare in several tissues collected from the Savino body, and in tissues collected from the Biggs and Arzt bodies he had found presumptive positive results for curare. Beggs did admit the GC/MS was likely not an "absolute test" for curare but that his expert opinion was that the test was likely accurate and that the bodies did contain curare.

4. Dr Sidney Spector, a scientist from Roche Institute, testified about his role in the development of the anticurare antibody that was utilized in the RIA test. Dr Spector testified that he had used the antibody in RIA tests for curare in urine and blood, but not in solid tissues. He stated that although the antibody, if used in an RIA test, could possibly detect curare in tissues, he had not demonstrated this. Spector also testified that the RIA and HPLC methods might be able to detect curare in human tissues, but the results should be considered to be presumptive findings only.

After the completion of the prosecution's case, Judge Arnold dismissed the charges against Jascalevich for the murder of Emma Artz and Margaret Henderson due to a lack of evidence. The defense then presented its case, with two experts testifying about the toxicological evidence:

1. Dr Frederick Rieders asserted that, due to a lack of specificity, RIA must be considered a presumptive test only, and although it might indicate that curare "might" be present, it was not conclusive. Dr Rieders testified that in his opinion, GC/MS would be an appropriate methodology to utilize for the detection of curare in human tissues, but a full spectrum analysis, rather than selected ion monitoring, should have been used. Dr Rieders also described a set of experiments he had conducted in which he determined that both embalming fluid and tissue fluids triggered the degradation of curare within a few days, indicating that the detection of curare in the tissues from exhumed bodies that had been buried in embalming fluid for more than 10 years would be very

unlikely unless there were extremely large quantities of the curare present in the tissue initially, which was unlikely. Dr Rieders further testified that he had identified curare in the liver of the Savino body, but not in the muscle tissues, which was, he claimed, a significant inconsistency.

2. Dr Bo Holmstedt testified that due to the effects of bacteria and alterations in temperature, curare would not persist in embalmed bodies for 10 years. Furthermore, he described experiments that had shown that when curare is injected into humans, the concentration of curare in the muscle tissue is equal to or greater than the concentration in the liver, supporting the claims of Dr Rieders that it was very unusual to detect curare in the liver, but not the muscles, of the Savino body.

After deliberating for only 2 h following the conclusion of the trial, on October 24, 1978, the jury returned a verdict of not guilty on all counts and Dr Jascalevich was released.

E.4 THE CASE OF BRIAN EFTENOFF

The case of Brian Eftenoff illustrates the significance of interpretation and highlights the requirement that toxicological interpretations must be based upon a sound foundational knowledge of pharmacokinetics and pharmacodynamics.

On September 24, 1999, Brian Eftenoff arrived home from a night of gambling to find his wife Judi dead on the bathroom floor with cuts and bruises on her body and blood dripping out of her nose. The Eftenoffs had two young children, ages 3 and 5, who were home at the time. The cause of death was not immediately evident, but there were no signs of a break-in. Upon questing by Phoenix Detective Joe Petrosino, Brian stated that he had left home at approximately 10 pm the previous night to go gambling with a friend, and at that time Judi was putting the children to bed and acting normally. Although videotaped footage from the casino confirmed Brian's story of his whereabouts, Judi's family, who had never approved of Brian, immediately suspected that he had played a role in Judi's death. The mystery of Judi's cause of death was clarified to some extent on November 16, 1999 when the Maricopa County Medical Examiner's office announced that Judi had died of a cocaine-induced stroke. Large amounts of cocaine had been found in Judi's stomach and blood, and the Medical Examiner reported that "the cocaine in her blood may have caused severe hypertension that resulted in intracerebral hemorrhage." Large amounts of unmetabolized cocaine were found in Judi's stomach, suggesting that she had swallowed the drug—an uncommon route of administration. The toxicological findings further indicated that Judi may have ingested cocaine up to 72 h prior to her death. A secondary cause of death was listed as blunt force had injury. However, the Medical Examiner was unable to rule if the death was caused by an accidental overdose, or was, in fact, homicide, and the manner of death was therefore listed as undetermined.

Lead Detective Joe Petrosino, quickly became convinced that Judi's death was not accidental.

In conversations with Detective Perosino shortly after Judi's death, Brian disclosed that Judi used cocaine regularly as a weight loss aid, and also routinely took diet pills. Brian also admitted that he and his wife had been involved in physical altercations—a contention that was supported by Rikki Eftenoff, the 5-year-old daughter of Brian and Judi, who told social workers that she had observed her parents fighting on several occasions, including in the period shortly before Judi's death. Several of Judi's friends and family members, including her best friend Tamara Coalwell and her sister Janell Harding, told Detective Perosino that Judi had confided in them that Brian had physically abused her. Although Tamara, and several other friends, admitted that Judi did use cocaine regularly, it was attributed to the pressure put on her by Brian to remain thin. Brian admitted to Detective Perosino that he and Judi had participated in extramarital affairs, but asserted that they "had an understanding" about such behavior. Detective Perosino quickly became aware of Brian's criminal record, which included time spent in prison for robbery and multiple allegations of assault. Additionally, Brian's auto parts business was having financial difficulties, due largely to Brian's neglect of outstanding accounts. The Brian's behavior, coupled with the accounts of a troubled marriage and a largely absent and/or abusive husband, provided by Judi's friends and family members, solidified in Detective Perosino's mind that Judi's death had not been accidental. Brian, however, staunchly maintained that he had done nothing to injure his wife, and was in no way involved in her death.

Detective Perosino's suspicions notwithstanding, sufficient evidence was not present to immediately file charges against Brian Eftenoff for the murder of his wife. In an unexpected turn of events, it was a different charge that first led to the arrest of Brian Eftenoff; Brian allegedly mailed 1.1 g of cocaine, along with several of Judi's personal items, to Judi's parents. Brian denied knowingly mailing cocaine and was released on bail in February 2000. On May 30, 2000, however, Brian was arrested and charged with one count of second degree murder, and on May 25 Deputy County Attorney Kurt Altman presented his case to a grand jury. Altman presented the results of the autopsy, which revealed that Judi had bruises on her face, abrasions around her mouth, lacerations inside her mouth, and hemorrhages on the inside of her throat. Altman stated that the Chief Medical Examiner advised him that the hemorrhages inside Judi's throat were unusual, and could be caused by grabbing the throat tightly or stroking "the side of the esophagus…as if you were trying to get someone to swallow something." The toxicological findings of the large amounts of cocaine in Judi's stomach and blood, the statements made by Ricki about her parents fighting, and Detective Perosino's testimony were also included in the presentation to the grand jury, resulting in the unanimous vote of the grand jury to indict Brian Eftenoff on charges on second degree murder and mailing cocaine to his in-laws.

The trial of Brian Eftenoff proved to be fraught with anecdotal evidence of physical abuse and other malfeasances by Brain Eftenoff that, as was interpreted by some bystanders, served to "poison" the jury against Brian. In addition to presenting such anecdotal evidence, however, the prosecution also called upon its expert witnesses to present the result of Judi's autopsy as well as the results of the toxicological analyses that had been performed on the body. The prosecution made the case that Brian and Judi had been involved in a physical altercation on the night of her death, during which Brian may have knocked Judi unconscious. In an effort to conceal the physical abuse that he had imparted upon her, Brian forced Judi to swallow a large amount of cocaine, which ultimately led to her death. As was reported to the grand jury, the scientific evidence presented by the prosecution's experts included the following results and interpretations.

1. Large amounts of unmetabolized cocaine were found in Judi's stomach.
2. High levels of cocaine were found in Judi's blood.
3. Based upon the amounts of cocaine found in her body, Judi must have taken at least 1 g of cocaine in the hour or two before her death—an amount that was deemed to be too great for her to have taken on her own.
4. Injuries consistent with "forcing" someone to swallow something were found on both the outside and the inside of Judi's throat.
5. Bruises and lacerations were found on Judi's face and neck.

Although the results of the toxicological analyses were not disputed by the defense experts, the interpretations of these results were. In summary, defense experts emphasized the following:

1. It was impossible to determine if Judi swallowed the cocaine that was found in her stomach. Although the large amount of unmetabolized cocaine in her stomach might be consistent with the ingestion of cocaine, cocaine can also enter the stomach from the blood, and thus Judi may have taken cocaine through the more typical intranasal route.
2. It was not possible to determine the amount of cocaine that Judi had taken (either voluntarily or by force). Because cocaine is subject to postmortem redistribution and metabolism, the blood levels of cocaine measured at autopsy are not indicative of blood concentrations before death, and therefore cannot be utilized in a calculation of the amount of cocaine administered.
3. The amount of cocaine found in Judi's stomach and blood were not as impossibly high as purported by the prosecution.
4. Although it was not possible to determine the exact timing of Judi's cocaine use, the levels of cocaine metabolites present in Judi's body were consistent with her being a regular cocaine user who had used the drug in the day or two before her death.

After a 5-week trial and 36 h of deliberation, the jury returned a verdict of guilty, and Brian Eftenoff was sentenced to 50 years in prison. Whether the verdict was returned as a result of convincing scientific evidence presented by the prosecution, or due to anecdotal evidence that portrayed Brian as a husband eminently capable of murder is unclear. In the years since Eftenoff's 2001 conviction, however, various media outlets have taken an interest in the case and have enlisted several forensic experts (including the Chief Toxicologist for Miami-Dade County, the Chief Toxicologist for Suffolk County and the former Chief Medical Examiner of Seattle, among others) to review the forensic evidence presented at trial. The general consensus of the experts has been that the death of Judi Eftenoff was consistent with an acute, accidental, cocaine overdose resulting in cerebral hemorrhage; neither the physical nor toxicological findings were deemed by these, presumably unbiased, experts to be suggestive of foul play.

SUGGESTED READING

Bates, S., 2014. The Poisoner: The Life and Crimes of Victorian England's Most Notorious Doctor. Penguin Group, New York.

Besnard, M., 1963. The Trial of Marie Besnard. Harper Collins, New York.

Burney, I., 2006. Poison, Detection, and the Victorian Imagination. Manchester University Press, New York.

Farber, M., 1982. "Somebody Is Lying": The Story of Dr. X. Doubleday, New York.

Frankiln, C., 1970. World Famous Acquittals. The Hamlyn Publishing Group Limited, Feltham, Middlesex.

Hall, L.H., Hirsch, R.F., 1979. Detection of curare in the Jascalevich murder trial. Anal. Chem. 51 (8), 812A–819A.

Kohn, D., 2002. In: Moriarty, E. (Ed.), Reasonable Doubt. CBS News, New York.

Peschel, B., 2015. The Times Report of the Trial of William Palmer (The Rugeley Poisoner). CreateSpace Independent Publishing Platform, Seattle.

Rubin, P., 2000a. 'Til Death Do Us Part: Part One. Phoenix New Times, LLC, Phoenix.

Rubin, P., 2000b. 'Til Death Do Us Part: Part Two. Phoenix New Times, LLC, Phoenix.

Rubin, P., 2001. The Final Straw. Phoenix New Times, LLC, Phoenix.

Siegel, H., Rieders, F., Holmstedt, B., 1985. The medical and scientific evidence in alleged tubocurarine poisonings. A review of the so-called Dr. X case. Forensic Sci. Int. 29 (1–2), 29–76.

Thorwald, J., 1966. Proof of Poison; Century of the Detective. Thames and Hudson, Ltd.

Glossary

β-Glucuronidase An enzyme that hydrolyzes a glucuronide version of a drug back to the free, nonglucuronide, version of the drug.

Absorption The process by which drugs enter the circulatory system.

Addiction The phenomenon by which symptoms are produced when a person stops taking a drug.

Adenylyl cyclase An enzyme that catalyzes the conversion of adenosine triphosphate (ATP) to $3'$-$5'$-cyclic adenosine monophosphate (cAMP) and pyrophosphate.

Affinity The stability with which a drug binds to a target molecule.

Agonist A drug that binds to a target molecule with high affinity and possesses high intrinsic activity.

Alexander Gettler The first Director of the forensic toxicology laboratory in the New York City Medical Examiner's office.

Anagen phase The period of active growth of a hair shaft.

Analysis The detection, identification, and often quantitation of drugs and chemicals in biological samples.

Analyte A drug or chemical that is the substance of interest in an analysis.

Antagonist A drug that binds to a target molecule with high affinity but possesses no intrinsic activity.

Antemortem Prior to death.

Apparent volume of distribution (V_d) A theoretical measure of the volume of fluid a drug must be distributed into to result in the measured plasma concentration of free drug.

Assistant Chief Toxicologist A supervisory position held by an upper-level scientist whose duties include management of the day-to-day operation of a forensic toxicology laboratory, personnel training, methods review, development and validation of analytical methods, performance of special or nonroutine analyses, and administration of quality control measures including the design of internal proficiency programs and the participation in external proficiency evaluation programs.

Autolysis The process by which cells are degraded by intracellular enzymes.

Blood—brain barrier (BBB) Arguably the most important barrier to entry into the brain, the blood—brain barrier comprised of both physical and metabolic factors that function to limit the entry of substances into the central nervous system.

Blood—cerebral spinal fluid barrier (BCSF) A barrier against entry of substances into the brain; the blood—cerebral spinal fluid barrier is formed by the choroid plexi of the four ventricles of the brain.

Case manager An individual within a laboratory who acts as a bridge between the acquisition of samples, with the associated case information, and the analyst conducting the analyses.

Catagen phase The period during which the hair follicle begins to degenerate.

Chain of custody (COC) The record of the movement of samples from the time of their collection until the time of their disposal.

Chemicals Substances, e.g., volatile organic compounds, pesticides, carbon monoxide, that are not intended either for medical purposes or to affect the structure or any function of the body of man or other animals, but that are intentionally or unintentionally used or misused for the effects that they produce.

Chief toxicologist Also designated as the laboratory director; a chief toxicologist directs the overall operation of all aspects of a forensic toxicology laboratory.

Chromatography Methods that facilitate the separation of drugs and metabolites by introducing them into a mobile phase that passes over and/or through a stationary phase designed to affect their movement based on their partitioning between the two phases.

Color tests Methods of identification based upon the production of a product of specific color when the analyte reacts with specific reagents.

Common strategy A two-phase approach to analysis that is widely recognized as the standard analytical strategy in forensic toxicology laboratories. The common strategy consists of an initial presumptive (screening) test followed by a secondary confirmatory test if needed.

Competitive antagonists Drugs or chemicals that compete for receptor binding sites and bind reversibly to a receptor.

Confirmatory test Analytical tests designed to confirm the presence of an analyte or analytes that have been presumptively identified in a sample with a presumptive/screening test. Confirmatory tests generally possess detection limits that are equal to or less than those of presumptive tests.

Contextual bias A bias that develops as a result of using existing information to reinforce a position.

Cooperativity A phenomenon in which the affinity of a drug for its receptor is influenced by the prior binding of some other receptor ligand.

Creatinine The breakdown product of creatine, which is involved in the production of energy in muscle tissue; creatinine is found in normal urine at a relatively constant concentration.

Cyclic AMP (cAMP) A second messenger that plays an integral role in the regulation of multiple cellular processes including cell metabolism, cell differentiation, ion channel activity, and cell division.

Cytochrome p450 enzymes A family of phase I metabolic enzymes, sometimes called mixed function oxidase systems (MFOs). The basic reaction catalyzed by these enzymatic systems is the reaction of oxygen with a drug in the presence of the cofactor NADPH to form an alcohol, water, and NADP+.

Diffusion A form of passive transport by which substances move across a membrane from a region of high concentration to a region of lower concentration.

Directed search The analytical strategy by which the only analyses conducted are those intended to detect exogenous substances that are reasonably suspected of being present in the sample based upon the information collected from the nonanalytical investigation of the case, including police reports, eyewitness testimony, and medical and autopsy reports.

Distribution The transport of a drug throughout the body to various cells and tissues.

Dose–response curve A plot of the dose of a drug administered versus the effect elicited by the drug.

Drug disposition A term that is used to describe the four major events that occur to a drug in the body—absorption, distribution, metabolism, and excretion.

Drugs Substances that are intended to furnish pharmacological activity or to affect the structure or any function of the body of man or other animals and are used intentionally or unintentionally for appropriate or inappropriate purposes.

Effective dose 50 (ED_{50}) The dose of a drug at which 50% of the population experiences the desired effect (a single drug may have several different ED_{50} values depending upon which desired effect is being measured).

Enterohepatic circulation A state of localized circulation between the gastrointestinal tract and the liver.

Enzyme-linked immunosorbent assays (ELISA) Competition binding assays in which enzyme-linked drug competes with unlabeled drug for binding to antidrug antibody.

Enzyme-linked receptors Receptors that either possess intrinsic enzymatic activity or are associated with an intracellular enzyme.

Enzyme-multiplied immunoassay technique (EMIT) An immunoassay based upon the principle that, for specific enzymes, if the enzyme is linked to an antigen, the binding of an antibody to the antigen can modulate the activity of the enzyme.

Equilibrium dissociation constant (Ka) A quantitative measure of the amount of dissociation of an acid or base in solution.

Excretion The process by which a drug and/or its metabolites are eliminated from the body.

Expert reports Written statements prepared by forensic toxicologists that offer expert opinions on any of a number of matters within the purview of their expertise.

Extraction The process by which analytes are separated from the matrix and a number of nonanalyte substances in a sample.

First-pass metabolism The process by which drugs are metabolized before they enter systemic circulation.

Flavin monooxygenase enzymes A family of five phase I metabolic enzymes that oxidize nucleophilic heteroatoms present in drugs, including nitrogen, sulfur, and phosphorous atoms.

Fluorescence polarization immunoassay (FPI or FPIA) An immunoassay based on the principle that if a fluorophore is stationary when excited, the emitted light will be in the same polarization plane as the excitation light, but if the fluorophore rotates during the brief period between excitation and emission, the emitted light will not be polarized.

Fortified samples Samples that have been spiked with an analyte or analytes.

G protein-coupled receptors (GPCRs) A class of receptors that are comprised of a single polypeptide chain containing seven membrane-spanning a-helices, with an extracellular amino terminus and an intracellular carboxy terminus. GPCRs interact with a class of proteins called G proteins.

General unknown screening (GUS) An analytical strategy that is designed to detect analytes when no prior information is present to suggest the identity or presence of the analytes.

Genetic polymorphisms Differences in nucleotide sequence among individuals.

Gibbs free energy The portion of a system's energy that can perform work when temperature and pressure are uniform throughout the system; the free energy represents the total usable energy in a system.

Glomerular filtration rate The amount of blood filtered by the glomerulus per minute.

Glucuronyl transferase A phase II metabolic enzyme that catalyzes glucuronidation reactions in which glucuronic acid is transferred to a drug substrate to form a drug-glucuronide.

Glutathione-S-transferases (GST) A family of phase II metabolic enzymes that catalyze mercapturic acid synthesis reactions, which are a major pathway for the detoxification of electrophiles.

Headspace The vapor phase above the sample in a closed container.

Henderson–Hasselbalch equation A method for the determination of the degree of ionization of acids and bases at various pH values.

Heterogeneous reactions Competition binding assays in which, after the completion of the binding reaction, any unbound labeled component must be removed from the reaction mixture before the quantification of binding is performed.

Homogeneous reactions Competition binding assays in which it is not necessary to separate the unbound labeled component from the reaction mixture before the quantification of binding is performed.

Homogenization The process by which a sample is made by blending.

Hormesis The phenomenon in which relatively low doses of a drug elicit beneficial effects that are not achieved by higher doses of the drug.

Immunoassays Analytical tests that are typically utilized as presumptive/screening tests and which rely upon the interactions between antibodies and antigens; the antigens in toxicological immunoassays are generally drugs or drug metabolites.

Interpretation Providing opinions as to the meaning of the presence of detected substances, e.g., the effects that the drugs and/or chemicals may have produced on a subject.

Intrinsic activity The ability of a drug to initiate signal transduction.

Ion channels Transmembrane receptors that can exist in open or closed conformations. When open, ion channels facilitate the passage of specific ions across the plasma membrane and into the interior of a cell, and when closed, ion passage is prevented.

K_D A constant that is equal to the concentration of drug resulting in 50% receptor occupancy at equilibrium.

Law of mass action A rule that states that the rate of a homogeneous chemical reaction at a constant temperature is proportional to the product of the concentrations of the reactants.

Lethal dose 50 (LD_{50}) The dose at which a drug is lethal to 50% of a population.

Levey–Jennings chart A graphical representation of control data attained for the purpose of determining whether a method of analysis produces the results it is designed to produce.

Limit of detection (LOD) A measure of the lowest analyte concentration that can be detected reliably.

Limit of quantitation (LOQ) The lowest analyte concentration that can be quantitated reliably; it is greater than the LOD.

Lineweaver–Burke plot A method by which to convert a hyperbolic saturation curve into a linear plot from which the value of K_D can more easily be extrapolated.

Liquid–liquid extraction (LLE) An extraction process based on the principle that nonvolatile analytes can be transferred from the aqueous milieu of biological samples into organic solvents in which they have a high partition coefficient and thus a greater solubility than in water. Following this initial extraction of the analyte into an organic solvent, the analyte may be transferred or "back-extracted" into an aqueous solution of appropriate pH in which they form water-soluble salts.

Litigation packet A packet of materials produced by a laboratory, which contains essential information pertaining to the analyses conducted as well as the chain of custody of a sample.

Margin of safety A measure of drug toxicity, calculated as LD1/ED99, where LD1 is the dose that elicits lethality in 1% of the population, and ED99 is the dose that elicits the therapeutic effect in 99% of the population.

Marsh test A method for the detection of arsenic in biological samples.

Mees lines Transverse white lines sometimes present in nails.

Metabolism The biochemical modification of drugs by enzymatic systems.

Metabolites The end products of a metabolic reaction.

Michaelis—Menton constant A constant that is equal to the substrate concentration at which the velocity of the reaction is one-half of the maximum velocity.

Minimum reports Forensic toxicology laboratory reports that contain a bare minimum of information regarding the case, the sample, and the qualitative or quantitative results.

Monoclonal antibodies Antibodies that bind in a uniform manner to a single antigenic epitope.

Negative cooperativity A phenomenon in which the prior binding of a ligand decreases the affinity of a drug for its receptor.

Noncompetitive antagonists Drugs and chemicals that compete for receptor binding and bind irreversibly to the receptor.

Occupancy theory A receptor theory based on several key assumptions, some of which are not valid in all situations.

Oral fluid A fluid that contains several types of secretions including saliva, crevicular fluid, and secretions from the pharynx and nasal cavity.

Paracelsus Philippus Theophrastus Aureolus Bombastus von Hohenheim; an alchemist, theologian, physician, and "protoscientist" who formulated the famous maxim: "In all things there is a poison, and there is nothing without a poison. It depends only upon the dose whether a poison is poison or not."

Partial agonist A drug that binds to a target molecule with high affinity and possesses moderate intrinsic activity.

Partition coefficient The solubility of a drug in an organic solvent divided by the solubility of the drug in water.

Pharmacodynamics The study of the effects a drug has on the body; included in this study is the examination of the various factors that influence drug effects.

Pharmacokinetics The study of the rates at which dispositional events occur after the administration of a drug. The major events of pharmacokinetics include drug absorption, distribution, metabolism, and excretion.

Phase I metabolic reactions Nonsynthetic metabolic reactions, including oxidation, reduction, and hydrolysis reactions.

Phase II metabolic reactions Synthetic, or conjugation, reactions, including glucuronidation, glycine conjugation, acetylation, and mercapturic acid synthesis reactions.

Phospholipase C (PLC) An enzyme that catalyzes the breakdown of the membrane lipid phosphatidylinositol 3,4-bisphosphate (PIP2) into two products: the membrane lipid diacylglycerol (DAG) and the soluble second messenger inositol 1,4,5-triphosphate (IP3).

Photodecomposition The degradation of chemicals by radiant energy.

Postmortem After death.

Postmortem redistribution The postmortem movement of drugs and chemicals from one site in the body to another.

Precision The measure of the closeness of agreement between a series of measurements obtained from multiple samplings of the same homogenous sample.

Presumptive test (see also screening test) Generally, nonanalyte specific analytical methods used to determine the possible presence of drugs or chemical in biological samples; results must be confirmed by a more specific method. Presumptive tests generally possess low detection limits, are easy to perform, inexpensive, and are compatible with rapid, batch analysis.

Proficiency program A program designed to evaluate the performance of laboratory personnel and instrument function.

Protein kinases Enzymes that trigger the covalent attachment of a phosphate group to a protein through a process called protein phosphorylation.

Putrefaction The process by which the soft tissues of the body are converted into gasses, liquids, and small molecules by microorganisms.

Qualitative analysis An analysis performed with the intent of determining whether exogenous substances and/or their metabolites are present in a sample.

Quality assurance (QA) The procedures and policies that have been established by the laboratory management to ensure, to the greatest degree possible, that the analytical results are accurate and reliable.

Quality control (QC) The policies and procedures employed by the laboratory to ensure that the QA procedures are being implemented appropriately and effectively.

Quantitative analysis An analysis performed with the intent of correlating the analyte concentrations in a sample with the effects produced by the analytes.

Radioimmunoassay (RIA) An immunoassay based on the principle that radioactively labeled drug will compete with unlabeled drug in a biological sample for binding to a specific antidrug antibody.

Rate theory A receptor theory designed as an alternative to the occupancy theory. The rate theory proposes that the intrinsic activity of a drug, its ability to cause an effect, is a function of the rate of association and dissociation of the drug–receptor complex.

Receptor desensitization A phenomenon caused by a decreasing ability of an agonist to stimulate signal transduction (decreasing intrinsic activity).

Receptor theory A theory of drug action based on the principle that structurally specific drugs interact with a small number of target molecules, called receptors, which are distributed with characteristic and varying density among the cells and tissues of the body. The molecular structure of a specific drug determines which receptor(s) the drug will interact with.

Reliability The combination of the sensitivity, specificity, reproducibility, etc. that can be achieved by the use of a specific method.

Renal clearance The volume of blood plasma cleared of a drug in 1 min.

Renal elimination rate The half-life of drug elimination by the kidneys.

Receptor A target molecule with which a drug must interact in order to elicit a physiological effect. Drug receptors have four defining characteristics: specificity, saturability, high-affinity binding, and reversibility.

Reporting The presentation, either in written or oral form, of the analytical results and interpretation derived from them.

Salting out The process by which substances are precipitated from solution by the addition of salt.

Side effects All of the effects that are produced by a therapeutic dose of a drug and that are not the desired therapeutic effects.

Signal transduction The process by which an extracellular signal (i.e., the binding of a drug to its receptor) is transmitted across the plasma membrane, into the cell, and along intracellular signaling pathways, to ultimately cause a biochemical change within the cell.

Single nucleotide polymorphism (SNP) A difference in nucleotide sequence of a single base.

Solid-phase extraction (SPE) An extraction process similar to liquid–liquid extraction with the exception that the organic solvent used in LLE has been replaced by a solid phase to which analytes will bond.

Solid-phase microextraction (SPME) An adaptation of solid-phase extraction in which the solid-phase column has been replaced by a fused silica fiber coated with a suitable stationary phase polymer.

Spare receptors Systems in which there are more receptors present than are needed to produce the maximum effect are described as having spare receptors.

Specificity A measure of the degree to which the analyte is differentiated from other compounds that are present in the sample.

Standard operating procedure (SOP) manual An up-to-date record of the validated analytical methods employed for the detection, identification, and quantitation of analytes.

Storage period I The period between the time of an event and the time of sample collection.

Storage period II The period between the collection of a sample and the initial analysis of the sample.

Storage period III The long-term storage of a sample in anticipation of a future need to repeat the initial analysis or conduct additional analyses.

Structurally nonspecific drugs Substances that produce effects due to their physical properties, not their structures.

Structurally specific drugs Substances that exhibit structure–activity relationship, in which the structure of the drug determines its effects.

Systematic toxicological analysis (STA) A comprehensive and systematic analysis of samples for the presence of chemicals of toxicological importance. The STA strategy includes methods for sampling, sample preparation, differentiation, detection, as well as identification of analytes.

Target molecule A molecule with which a drug must interact in order to elicit a physiological effect.

Technician A support position within a forensic toxicology laboratory with duties, including the preparation of solutions and reagents, maintenance of reagent and chemical inventories, and care of noninstrumental materials. Technicians do not handle samples or conduct analyses.

Telogen phase The period during which hair growth comes to a halt.

Therapeutic effects The specific, desired effects of drug administration.

Therapeutic index A measure of drug toxicity, calculated as LD_{50}/ED_{50}.

Threshold dose The dose at which the desired effect of the drug is first observed.

Tolerance A state in which, after repeated administration of a drug, a greater than initial dose of the drug is required to produce the desired effect.

Toxic effects The effects produced by a drug when the drug is administered at a greater than therapeutic dose.

Toxicogenomics The study of the influence of genetic variation on individual differences in adverse responses to drugs.

Toxicologist I An entry-level position within a forensic toxicology laboratory that generally requires a bachelor's or master's degree. Duties of a toxicologist I include performing routine analyses such as presumptive (screening) tests, maintaining instruments, and record keeping.

Toxicologist II A position within a forensic toxicology laboratory that generally requires a bachelor's or master's degree as well as relevant laboratory experience. Duties of a toxicologist II include performing confirmatory tests and participation in the development and validation of new analytical methods.

Toxicology The study of the adverse effects of chemical, physical, and/or biological agents on living organisms.

Two-state theory A receptor theory that proposes that receptors exist in two conformations: an active state called the relaxed, or R, state and an inactive state called the tense, or T, state. The relaxed state of a receptor produces a biological effect and the tense state produces no effect.

Ultrafiltration The process by which membranes restrict the passage of substances based on their molecular weights.

Validation The process by which an analytical method is determined to be reliable for its intended purposes.

Vitreous humor The fluid-like gel located in the posterior chambers of the eyes.

V_{max} The maximum reaction velocity.

Voir dire The procedure by which attorneys elicit information concerning the qualifications of experts in order to demonstrate their qualifications and competence to testify as expert witnesses and thus provide opinion testimony in the area of their expertise.

Volatilization The process by which substances are transferred from a liquid phase into a vapor phase.

Water loading The process by which large amounts of water are ingested prior to the submission of urine samples in an attempt to dilute the urine, thereby decreasing the concentrations of analyte drugs and metabolites to levels below their detection limits.

Westgard rules Rules that provide criteria for the identification of out-of-control methods.

Index

Note: Page numbers followed by "b," "f" and "t" indicate boxes, figures and tables respectively.

CPI Antony Rowe
Eastbourne, UK
August 13, 2020